D1336449

The Geopolitics of Hunger, 2000–2001

THE GEOPOLITICS OF HUNGER, 2000–2001

Hunger and Power

ACTION AGAINST HUNGER

LYNNE
RIENNER
PUBLISHERS

BOULDER
LONDON

Published in the United States of America in 2001 by
Lynne Rienner Publishers, Inc.
1800 30th Street, Boulder, Colorado 80301
www.rienner.com

and in the United Kingdom by   169439X
Lynne Rienner Publishers, Inc.
3 Henrietta Street, Covent Garden, London WC2E 8LU

A previous version of this work was published in French in 1999 as
Géopolitique de la faim, 2000.
© 1999 by Presses Universitaires de France,
108, boulevard Saint-Germain, 75006 Paris, France.

Library of Congress Cataloging-in-Publication Data
The geopolitics of hunger, 2000–2001: Hunger and power   /
   by Action Against Hunger.
      p.   cm.
   Includes bibliographical references and index.
   ISBN 1-55587-925-X (alk. paper)—ISBN 1-55587-901-2 (pbk. : alk. paper)
   1. Food relief—Political aspects.   2. Hunger—Political aspects.
   3. Humanitarian assistance—Political aspects.   I. Action Against Hunger.
HV696.F6G388   2000
363.8'8—dc21

                                                                  00-042552

British Cataloguing in Publication Data
A Cataloguing in Publication record for this book
is available from the British Library.

Printed and bound in the United States of America

∞   The paper used in this publication meets the requirements
     of the American National Standard for Permanence of
     Paper for Printed Library Materials Z39.48-1984.

   5   4   3   2   1

Contents

Part 2
Confronting Unjust Food Distribution:
Which Strategies for Humanitarian Intervention?

Part 3
Food Policies to Eradicate Hunger

Foreword: Hunger and the New Humanitarianism

Barnett R. Rubin

On 24 June 1859, Jean-Henri Dunant, a Genevan traveling in northern Italy, watched as the armies of Napoleon III of France and Emperor Franz Josef of Austria butchered six thousand of each other's soldiers. When the Austrians abandoned the field, both armies left the wounded to die and the dead to rot, while peasants plundered the corpses. Dunant organized the women of the neighboring village of Castiglione to help tend the wounded. His powerful account of his experience, published three years later, led to the founding of the International Committee of the Red Cross (ICRC).[1]

The new humanitarianism was born in the ICRC hospitals of Biafra. In September 1968, the French Red Cross Society lent the ICRC a team of five French doctors to care for the victims of the war in Biafra, the name given by leaders of the Ibo ethnic group of Nigeria to the new state they wished to found through secession from Nigeria. The French doctors' team, soon joined by doctors from other countries, set up two hospitals. In one, in the tradition of Dunant, they treated the war wounded, though they were shocked to find that most of the wounded seemed to be civilians, and notably a large number of children. At the other hospital they treated a new kind of war victim: malnourished children, starving not from a natural disaster but from hunger intentionally inflicted on innocents as an act of war against a whole people. Despite the ICRC's code of silence, considered necessary to assure unimpeded access to all victims, one of the doctors, Bernard Kouchner, asked himself: "What use were doctors if they did not warn the world about the murderous use of a food blockade as a weapon of war? If we remained silent, we would be accomplices to the systematic massacre of a population."2

Just as classic humanitarianism was founded to ensure that soldiers wounded in battles between states were cared for as human beings, the new humanitarianism was founded to challenge the use of violence against noncombatants in civil wars. Under the slogan *soigner et témoigner* (provide care and bear witness), Doctors Without Borders was created in 1972. Other organizations followed suit. This volume, with its extensive testimony drawn from the experience of its aid workers in thirty-six countries around the world, shows that Action Against Hunger, founded in 1979 to fight hunger worldwide, has upheld and expanded this new movement.

In the world in which the ICRC was founded, wars pitted uniformed soldiers of recognized states against each other. The business of killing and maiming was pursued without quarter, and cruelty was accepted as the task of warriors, but the carnage was confined to those under arms. The warrior profession was inspired by a common code of honor, and despite their political antipathies, men were bound by the profession of arms in a kind of solidarity that transcended borders. The ICRC counted on that code and solidarity and on the recognition of a common interest in humanitarian standards to make its confidential interventions effective. We should not romanticize those days: No code of honor saved the victims of colonial wars and extermination campaigns in Africa, Asia, or the Americas. The Nazi regime abjured the very idea of a common humanity and showed the results of systematic antihumanitarianism. In response, the postwar Geneva Conventions (1948) codified basic humanitarian obligations in wartime and made adherence to its conventions a mark of sovereignty.

In the massive violence of postcolonial and post–Cold War civil conflict, however, the worst traditions of total war have returned. Biafra, the first postcolonial war of secession, was only a taste of what was to come. In the immediate postcolonial euphoria, international efforts and postcolonial states focused on "development" as the means to abolish poverty and hunger, considered as remnants of colonial exploitation. Famine resulted, it seemed, from a combination of natural disasters and mass poverty.

Biafra taught otherwise: Hunger was a weapon of war. In total wars where the aim is to subordinate, expel, or eliminate a whole population, control of food, as the reports in this book amply demonstrate, becomes the means of choice to impose submission, flight, or death. As a result, even peacetime economic decisions about food production can no longer be considered, alas, solely in the light of economic rationality. An economically rational division of labor that leaves populations dependent on purchased food while they concentrate on cash crops may leave them vulnerable to later assault by those who control roads, ports, or a few marketplaces. Control of food is an aspect of security. Many warriors in today's conflicts recognize no code. Rulers employ private militias to insulate themselves from responsibility. Both they and the rebels may be answerable to no one but the criminal syndicates that market the commodities that fund their war, whether these are looted diamonds or illegal drugs. Humanitarian assistance itself is seen only as another weapon of war: supplies to be stolen for their troops or manipulated to starve the "enemy."

Self-interest may lead such leaders to allow humanitarian access, but the rising toll among humanitarian workers and journalists bearing witness shows the intentional violation of standards by the new warlords. To expose and oppose such crimes, including those masquerading as natural disasters or poverty, those present in the field have a duty to alert the wider public and call for international action beyond the humanitarian response. As the reports in this book show, these deeply committed workers are better placed than anyone to elucidate the complex ways in which the basic human need for food can be manipulated to diminish and destroy humanity. In this book, the humanitarians of Action Against Hunger present us, the international community, with overwhelming evidence of how hunger is used as a weapon of war. It is for us now to assume the responsibilities these testimonies have given us.

Notes

Barnett R. Rubin was director, Center for Preventive Action, Council on Foreign Relations. He now works at the Center for International Cooperation of New York University.

1. Michael Ignatieff, *The Warrior's Honor: Ethnic War and the Modern Conscience* (New York: Henry Holt, 1997), pp. 109–124.

2. "A quoi servaient les médecins s'ils n'alertaient pas le monde sur l'usage assassin du blocus alimentaire comme arme de guerre? Silencieux, nous étions complices du massacre systématique d'une population." Bernard Kouchner, *Le malheur des autres* (Paris: Armand Colin, 1993), pp. 57–69.

Preface

Sir Ronald Grierson
Chairman,
Action Against Hunger–UK

Burton K. Haimes
Chairman,
Action Against Hunger–USA

Founded in France some twenty years ago with the aim of combating hunger and advocating the legal right to food (as stated in the United Nations Charter of 1945), Action Against Hunger is now firmly established in Paris, Spain (Madrid), the United Kingdom (London), and the United States (New York). As the twenty-first century begins, hunger is still a reality in many parts of the world.

It is indeed a sad state of affairs that we are entering a new century of technology and globalization, a century of the Internet and information, while such deleterious human conditions persist.

The end of the Cold War took us all by surprise. In the last ten years we have failed to see the realization of the hopes raised at the beginning of the 1990s. Absent the balance of power or balance of terror, local and regional conflicts have multiplied, and the number of civilian victims is growing. Nevertheless, progress has been made.

We are no longer impotent witnesses to remote natural disasters in India, Bangladesh, or China. Droughts, hurricanes, El Niño, and earthquakes continue to claim their share of lives, but not as a result of hunger. "Green Revolutions" and disaster response mechanisms have proven their effectiveness. The speed of information sharing and increased global agricultural yields, coupled with the experience and skills of relief organizations, enable us to defeat hunger when a natural disaster occurs. In theory, death by starvation due to natural disasters should not occur. Hunger can no longer be seen merely as the result of natural occurrences.

And yet, Action Against Hunger continues to see widespread hunger even as the world produces more than enough food for all.

This paradox is analyzed in this book, our second report on global issues of hunger. The book gathers together the analyses and testimonies of Action Against Hunger field-workers with contributions from experts and academics, but it is neither a directory of world hunger nor a country-by-country description of the different forms of malnutrition afflicting each. Rather, in this book we explore the use of hunger as a weapon in food crises from Sierra Leone to North Korea; we study the different humanitarian strategies being used to confront unjust food distribution and to avoid manipulation in increasingly complicated contexts where neutrality and impartiality should be the permanent criteria of humanitarian action.

The Kosovo crisis of 1999 showed us that, even when public generosity is combined with the professionalism of humanitarian organizations, we are not free of manipulation. From the legitimization of war to cynical strategies that use discrimination in the distribution of food to displace populations, the Kosovo crisis has highlighted the need for independent humanitarian organizations concerned only with the fate of civilian victims not to be hindered by any political, military, or strategic agenda.

The Geopolitics of Hunger, 2000–2001 is divided into three parts. Part 1 deals with current crises, from the Congo to Somalia and from Nicaragua to Afghanistan and Sierra Leone. It shows that whoever controls food controls power. In Part 2, we seek an answer to a daily concern: how to react when confronted by criminal regimes. What are the principles to be respected and the code of conduct to be followed? What is the role of humanitarian organizations in the present world of international relations? Part 3 analyzes policies that could be implemented to secure the right to food.

Without international recognition of such a right and the establishment of policies, laws, and mechanisms to ensure its application, we are condemned to witness people dying of hunger in a world of plenty, a world in which food supplies are more than sufficient but distribution remains scandalously discriminatory.

PART ONE

FOOD CRISES:
HUNGER AS A WEAPON

He who controls the food supply wields the power. Hunger remains a weapon throughout the world, and certain populations are the victims of deliberate discriminatory practices that are intended to bring about their subjugation, their departure, or the arrival of the international community. In this sense, great famines are always the consequence of human action, even when the point of departure is a natural catastrophe.

1

Sierra Leone: Food at the Heart of the Conflict

Pascal Lefort

In Sierra Leone, civilian populations have been the main victims of the civil war that the Revolutionary United Front (RUF) has been waging since 1991.[1] Food, which has always been used as a political weapon in the country, has gradually become a key factor in the conflict. Used to legitimize the actions of both the government and the rebellion, food also represents a vital resource in the war economy. For its part, the RUF has frequently used hunger and terror as weapons with which to subjugate populations or force political dialogue.

Food and Terror

After being driven out of Freetown by ECOMOG (the Economic Community of West Africa States [ECOWAS] Monitoring Group) forces in February 1998, RUF fighters and the rebel soldiers of the Armed Forces Ruling Council (AFRC) took less than two months to reorganize.[2] Still lacking the military means for a direct confrontation with ECOMOG, the rebels fell back on the two weapons of terror and food that they had previously used to subjugate the civilian population and paralyze agricultural production.

Starting in April 1998, the rebels, who had retreated to their strongholds in the northeast, launched a campaign of terror in the north of the country to brutally refute the government's communiqués announcing victory. ECOMOG had concentrated its efforts on recapturing the towns and controlling the main roadways, thus mak-

3

Chronology

27 April 1961	Sierra Leone achieves independence.
1968	Siaka Stevens gains power.
1985	Siaka Stevens hands power over to his chief of staff, General Joseph Momoh.
23 March 1991	First Revolutionary United Front (RUF) offensive in the Kailahun district, Eastern province.
29 April 1992	Military coup d'état. Captain Valentine Strasser takes power at the head of the National People Revolutionary Council.
16 January 1996	Valentine Strasser is "gently" overthrown by General Julius Maada Bio, who promises to set the path for a transition to democracy.
15 March 1996	Ahmad Tehan Kabbah is democratically elected president of Sierra Leone.
26 March 1996	Cease-fire agreement between the RUF and the armed forces of Sierra Leone.
25 May 1997	Military coup d'état. President Kabbah flees to Guinea. Establishment of a military junta, the Armed Forces Ruling Council, led by Major Johnny Paul Koroma.
28–29 August 1997	Economic Community of West African States summit in Abuja. Embargo imposed on Sierra Leone.
23 October 1997	Conakry Accords (Guinea) provide for the return to power of President Kabbah on 22 April 1998.
6 February 1998	Launch of the Economic Community of West African States Monitoring Group's offensive on Freetown. Flight of junta.
10 March 1998	Return of President Kabbah to Freetown.
6 January 1999	Revolutionary United Front attacks Freetown.
18 May 1999	Cease-fire agreement between the RUF and the Government of Sierra Leone.
7 July 1999	Signing at Lomé of peace agreement between the RUF and the government of Sierra Leone.
May 2000	The peace agreement is de facto broken and the RUF holds several hundred UN peacekeepers hostage.

ing the rural areas an ideal target. Organized in small commando units, the combatants attacked isolated villages, following a well-practiced routine: looting, atrocities, and the burning of houses, all carried out in such a way as to ensure maximum effect. They inflicted mutilations, for example, that left permanent scars on victims and their families. For the farming population, a person's loss of one or sometimes two hands meant that the victim would no longer be able to provide for the needs of his or her family. To maximize the impact, victims were chosen at random, and there was no hesitation to amputate the limbs of very young children or to draw lots to decide which victims would have their limbs amputated.

This zone, which includes much of the Northern province, is the country's rice granary. The consequences of the atrocities committed were immediate: farming ceased, large numbers of people were displaced (150,000 people sought refuge in Guinea to escape the savagery and hunger), and the sale of cereals in the villages was restricted in preparation for the scarce times ahead. Within a few weeks the region was paralyzed, and the country's stocks of cereal declined precipitously. Because of the insecurity and the violence that they had suffered in the past, humanitarian organizations confined their activities to the towns and to areas along the main roadways that were protected by ECOMOG. During 1998, access to the population diminished as the security situation worsened, even as humanitarian needs increased.

When the RUF recaptured the mining town of Koidu in December 1998 and launched an offensive that took it to Freetown in a few weeks, Action Against Hunger teams were forced to abandon Makeni, capital of the Northern province. At the time, 700 severely malnourished children were being treated in our therapeutic nutrition centers.

Since January 1999, one and a half million people have been deprived of humanitarian assistance in the rebel-controlled northern half of the country. The first evaluation missions led by Action Against Hunger in June 1999 and reports from people who had recently returned from Makeni confirmed the acute shortages of food and medicine.[3] Because of the shortage of paddy (rice), very little has been planted. Only the populations living near the border with Guinea have access to food supplies on a more regular basis.

Right up to the start of peace negotiations in May 1999, the fate of these populations was of little concern to either the government or the RUF, who were less interested in managing the territory under their control than in exploiting the wealth that fed their war economy.

Food in the Service of the War Economy

The diamond industry and the importation of food are closely linked in Sierra Leone. Through a subtle compensation mechanism, these

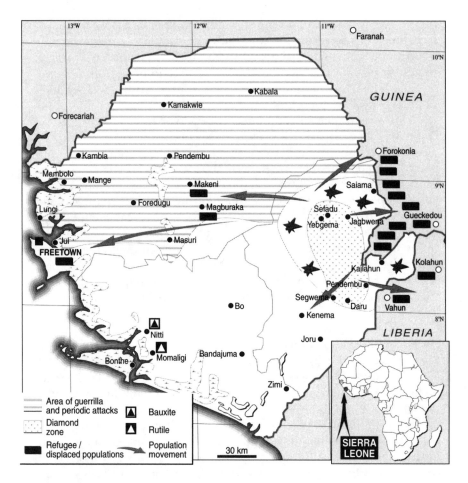

Sierra Leone

two activities complement each other, particularly since the development of mining activities has greatly reduced the level of agricultural activity in the prospecting zones. Miners need food, which is provided to them on credit by a merchant who in return is given first preference for the purchase of the stones. The income derived from the export of diamonds is used to pay the food suppliers in foreign currency, while the money earned from sales of rice inside the country provides the cash needed to purchase the stones. The prospectors' profits are modest, whereas at the other end of the chain the annual income from the diamond industry is estimated to be nearly 200 million dollars.[4] Since 1997, the rebels have controlled most areas that bring in annual revenues of approximately 100 million dollars.

When fighting or unsafe roads make it impossible to transport food from Freetown to the interior of the country or when local production is insufficient, food aid stocks assume critical importance. This food has the double advantage of being available close to the diamond-mining zones and of being less expensive than imported food. The food is diverted to the diamond mines in a variety of ways: repurchase of food distributed to families who are in urgent need of money to cover their basic needs; looting of the warehouses of humanitarian organizations; and requisition of food from civilian populations. Thus, when Makeni was captured by the RUF in December 1998, the fact that humanitarian organizations had left the town was used as a pretext for seizing their food supplies. Soon afterward, the RUF organized the distribution of one sack of bulgur (precooked cracked wheat) per family as a way of reassuring the population that remained in the town and to encourage others to return. This was the only time food was distributed. The bulk of the supplies was transported to the diamond-mining area of Kono. Of course, this source of supply alone could not suffice for the needs of the miners. Mechanisms have been put into place to barter uncut diamonds for food and other basic products or for material needed in the mines. This activity took place mainly between Makeni and Guinea and on the Liberian border.

Food as a Political Weapon

On 6 January 1999, the RUF combatants joined forces with the former AFRC coup plotters and attacked Freetown, occupying the presidential residence and burning and looting the city.[5] President Ahmad Tejan Kabbah's government wavered for the second time. Fleeing the advancing rebel troops, nearly 150,000 people took refuge in the western districts of the city. Citing as justification the withdrawal to Guinea of the expatriate humanitarian personnel in charge of food aid, the Sierra Leonean government organized a food distribution program. The objective was twofold: first, to regroup the displaced population at a few locations; second, above all to reassure people and forestall a revolt by a population that felt betrayed by the government's inability to defend the city. A campaign to register displaced persons was hastily organized, and accessible food supplies were requisitioned for distribution to residents who had fled the eastern suburbs to seek refuge in the western parts of the city, which remained under ECOMOG control.[6] Under the program, 200,000 rations were distributed within a few days. It mattered little that 80 percent of the beneficiaries were from the western suburbs and that, upon verification, only 17,000 displaced people were actually accommodated in the hastily built makeshift camps. The main purpose was to show that the government was taking care of the population.

The same scenario was repeated a few weeks later in the town of Kenema, where the authorities announced the arrival of displaced persons and, in the absence of international staff, organized within a few days the distribution of food aid for 60,000 people. As the level of the available food supplies dwindled, the official number of displaced persons also declined. Having become useless, the displaced population was then relocated outside the town, sometimes by force.

Although aid agencies demanded and managed to regain control of food distribution, the results of the assistance provided over the first six months of 1999 speak for themselves: not a single sack of food went to rebel-held areas. Quite apart from legitimate safety concerns, no attempt was made to deliver food aid to the northern part of the country, which has been the most severely affected by the lack of food. It was not until May 1999, the start of peace negotiations between the government and the RUF leader, Foday Sankoh, that this question was addressed.

President Kabbah's government does not of course have a monopoly over the manipulation of food for political ends. We have seen how, during the capture of Makeni in December 1998, the RUF was also keen to appear generous by arranging for the distribution of food taken from the supplies of humanitarian organizations. William Reno and Paul Richards have shown how each regime in Sierra Leone, and in particular that of Siaka Stevens, has used food as a means of retaining political support.[7] What is so shocking in the recent history of Sierra Leone is not that a democratically elected president—supported by Great Britain, the Commonwealth, ECO-WAS, and the United Nations Department of Political Affairs—has taken advantage of humanitarian aid in order to improve his political image and to support the population in the south of the country, which constitutes his electoral base. Rather it is that, faced with a rebellion that will stop at nothing to achieve its ends, priority has been given to a military action that was doomed from the start, given the lack of interest on the part of the international community, which has left ECOWAS to deal with the conflict. In doing so, the government and its allies have deliberately remained silent about the tragic humanitarian situation of more than a million people living in RUF-controlled zones and have discouraged any humanitarian assistance on the grounds that it would be used to support the rebellion. Fearing for the safety of its personnel, no humanitarian organization has agreed to take the risk of involvement in such a confused situation, and it is the civilian population, already suffering terribly from this conflict, that has paid the price.

Notes

Pascal Lefort is a desk officer at Action Against Hunger.

1. The RUF began an armed rebellion in 1991 in Liberia, where it gained the support of Charles Taylor's National Patriotic Front of Liberia (NPFL). Charles Taylor is today president of Liberia. Foday Sankoh, leader of the RUF, who had been imprisoned in Freetown, was condemned to death in late 1998 for treason. He was released under the peace agreement signed between the Sierra Leone government and the RUF on 7 July 1999 at Lomé.

2. ECOMOG was a peacekeeping force established in 1990 by the member countries of the ECOWAS. In February 1998, ECOMOG drove the military junta allied with the RUF from power and reinstated President Ahmad Tejan Kabbah. The ARFC was a military junta led by Major Johnny Paul Koroma; it seized power in the coup of 25 May 1997 that overthrew Ahmad Tejan Kabbah, the democratically elected president.

3. In June 1999, taking advantage of the negotiations that began in Lomé between the RUF and the Sierra Leonean government, Action Against Hunger approached the RUF for authorization to operate in RUF-controlled areas.

4. This valuation is according to Mbendi, *Mining Industry Profile, Sierra Leone*, March 1998 and statistics published by the Diamond High Council at Antwerp. On the diamond economy, see also François Misser and Olivier Vallée, *Les gemmocraties, l'économie politique du diamant africain* (Paris: Desclée de Brouwer, 1997).

5. For more on the brutality to which civilians were subjected during this offensive, see the report of Human Rights Watch, *Sierra Leone, Getting Away with Murder, Mutilation, and Rape* (New York: Human Rights Watch, 1999).

6. Officially, the requisitioned food supplies were recorded as borrowed by the World Food Program (WFP) from the nongovernmental organizations (NGOs) concerned and made available by the WFP to the local NGOs that organized the distribution under government supervision.

7. Siaka Stevens was president of Sierra Leone from 1968 to 1985. See William Reno, *Corruption and State Politics in Sierra Leone* (Cambridge: Cambridge University Press, 1995); Paul Richards, *Fighting for the Rain Forest: War, Youth, and Resources in Sierra Leone* (Oxford: James Currey/Heinemann, 1996); and Action Against Hunger, *Geopolitics of Hunger, 1998–1999* (Paris: PUF, 1998), pp. 7–21.

Bibliography

Human Rights Watch. *Sierra Leone: Getting Away with Murder, Mutilation, and Rape.* New York: Human Rights Watch, 1999.

Misser, François, and Olivier Vallée. *Les gemmocraties, l'économie politique du diamant africain.* Paris: Desclée de Brouwer, 1997.

Reno, William. *Corruption and State Politics in Sierra Leone.* Cambridge: Cambridge University Press, 1995.

Richards, Paul. *Fighting for the Rain Forest: War, Youth, and Resources in Sierra Leone.* Oxford: James Currey/Heinemann, 1996.

2

Congo-Brazzaville: A Civilian Population Held Hostage to Militias

Pascal Lefort

Congo-Brazzaville[1] has been plunged into a spiral of violence caused by the radicalization of political action that accompanied the rise of armed militias controlled by the main political leaders. The civilian population is held hostage to the violence. In a country where petroleum revenues have encouraged a heavy dependence on imported foodstuffs, the growing incidents of atrocities, looting, and destruction of crops have left the displaced populations without access to food and care and in a life-threatening situation.

A Heavy Dependence on Imported Food

Despite its fertile soils, food production in Congo-Brazzaville covers only two-thirds of the country's needs. While farming allows rural populations a measure of self-sufficiency, it does not meet the needs of a growing urban population that demands a wider selection of food than the traditional *saka-saka* made from manioc and ground leaves. Faced with the effects of twenty years of a centralized agricultural policy and prices fixed at levels that discourage small farmers, the government has turned to the importation of goods from European countries: cereals (especially wheat flour), beef, poultry, eggs, and dairy products. It has deliberately reduced customs duties on these goods in order to keep prices low and forestall public discontent. This policy has the effect of making foreign goods more competitive than local products and profoundly changing the eating habits of the urban population.[2] The easy money earned from the oil

Chronology

15 August 1960	Congo-Brazzaville achieves independence.
1968–1991	Marxist-Leninist regime of Denis Sassou N'Guesso in power from 1979 on.
February–June 1991	Meeting of the Sovereign National Conference mandates a peaceful change of regime.
31 August 1992	Pascal Lissouba elected president by universal suffrage with the support of D. Sassou N'Guesso. The following month, Sassou N'Guesso joins the opposition.
1993–1994	Rise of ethnic militias. Violent clashes in Brazzaville between supporters of P. Lissouba and opposition militants. Some 2,000 people killed and 50,000 displaced.
January 1994	Reconciliation between P. Lissouba and Bernard Kolelas, who is elected mayor of Brazzaville.
June 1997	Two months before the presidential elections, civil war erupts in Brazzaville. The Congolese Armed Forces (FAC) for the most part close ranks with D. Sassou N'Guesso, who is supported by the Angolan Armed Forces. B. Kolelas, who had remained on the sidelines, takes the side of P. Lissouba. Between 5,000 and 10,000 persons killed and nearly 800,000 displaced.
25 October 1997	Victory of D. Sassou N'Guesso, who proclaims himself president. The Ninja militias retreat with their weapons to the Pool forests and the Cocoyes to the forests of Bouenza, Niari, and Lekoumou. B. Kolelas and P. Lissouba go into exile.
1997–1998	Failure to disarm the militias leaves them ready to mobilize at a moment's notice. Beginning in August 1998, the Ninjas mount a number of attacks in the Pool forests. The railway lines between Pointe Noire and Brazzaville (the country's economic hub) are cut in September.
18 December 1998	Faced with the Cobra-led repression in the

(continues)

Chronology Continued

18 December 1998 (cont.)	Pool forests, the Ninjas infiltrate the southern districts of Brazzaville. Violent reprisals by progovernment forces ensue: Ninjas hunt down and force evacuation of the residents of the southern districts of Brazzaville (Makélékélé, Kinsoundi, and Bacongo). Some 200,000 people escape to the Pool forests, and nearly 50,000 flee to the northern suburbs of Brazzaville. Progovernment forces loot the southern suburbs, which remain off-limits to the civilian population.
December–January 1999	The Cocoyes militia infiltrates Nkayi (21 December) and Dolisie (January). Progovernment forces counterattack. The towns are evacuated, then sacked and looted by progovernment forces.
May 1999	50,000 people return to the southern suburbs of Brazzaville.

boom has convulsed the system by causing hefty price increases. And when the state, weakened by the economic crisis of the 1980s and by poor management of its petroleum resources, found it increasingly difficult to pay its employees, the situation became intolerable for middle-class citizens. As the country struggled from one crisis to the other, many city dwellers could afford to eat only one full meal a day.

In addition to this heavy dependence on imported foods, Brazzaville, the country's capital city, relies on the surrounding regions and on the Congo-Ocean railway. Manioc and other staples are supplied mainly by the northern regions of the country. The Pool Prefecture supplies the capital with fresh produce and poultry. Most imported goods arrive at Pointe Noire before being freighted by train to Brazzaville. When the railway line is cut, Brazzaville is strangled. In 1997, fighting in the northern suburbs of the city interrupted the supply of basic goods. Since the end of 1998 and the resumption of military activity in the southern suburbs of Brazzaville and in the Pool Prefecture, fresh produce has been in short supply. Each crisis is thus a further step into poverty for the urban population, which finds it increasingly difficult to secure a daily meal. These difficulties have led to a higher incidence of malnutrition.

The growing vulnerability of the poorest sectors of the popula-

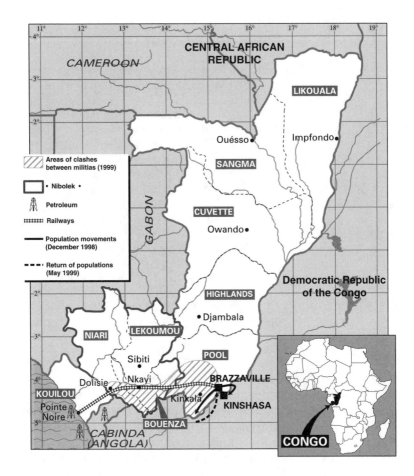

Congo-Brazzaville

tion, whose temptation to respond with violence increases with each new crisis, is also heightened by the specific urban characteristics of Brazzaville itself, whose neighborhoods have long had populations from the same region of origin. Since early in the century, the Bacongo suburbs in the south and the Poto Poto suburbs in the north of the city have been divided into zones around the European center of town, which was the seat of the colonial administration. Bacongo received populations arriving from the Pool region and Poto Poto, those migrating from the north of the country. The construction and development of the Congo-Ocean railway and the demand for workers by the railway management and by trading companies encouraged migration to the cities. This urban phenomenon has not been

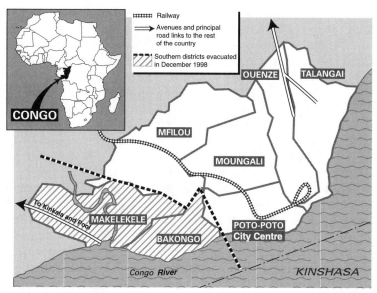

Railway

Avenues and principal
road links to the rest
of the country

Southern districts evacuated
in December 1998

CONGO

OUENZE   TALANGAI

MFILOU

MOUNGALI

To Kinkala and Pool   MAKELEKELE

BAKONGO

POTO-POTO
City Centre

Congo *River*   KINSHASA

The various districts of Brazzaville

restricted to Brazzaville, as the growth of the railway spurred the development of the port of Pointe Noire and of the localities along the 500 kilometers of track.

This accelerating urban spread and the configuration of Brazzaville in the image of a country divided between north and south explain why, up until 1997, most political struggles and dissident activity were concentrated in the capital. During the three successive crises that developed from 1992 to 1997, previously mixed neighborhoods became more polarized. Fighting between the Ninja and Zulu militias in 1993 led to the forced exchange of populations between the Bacongo and Mfilou suburbs.[3] Bacongo residents from Nibolek, who were suspected of supporting Pascal Lissouba's Zulus, were chased out while the Laris, who formed part of the Ninja militia, were in turn driven out of Mfilou.[4]

Progressively cut off from one another with each passing crisis,[5] these districts became fertile grounds for the proliferation of the so-called peoples' militias that were originally established to protect certain political leaders. These militias, however, gradually identified with the area under their protection in which they controlled both legitimate trade and trafficking. By 1997, the militias had become genuine fighting forces and had begun to launch murderous punitive attacks against enemy districts. Unsupervised and operating with impunity, their excesses became a norm.

By the end of 1998, more than 200,000 people had fled the Bacongo and Makelekele suburbs to escape the fighting between the heavily armed Ninja militias from the Pool region and government forces. This fighting marked the culmination of the escalation and spread of political violence that had begun with the failure of the transition to democracy that had started in 1991.

The Sovereign National Conference convened from February to June 1991 in Brazzaville brought a peaceful end to twenty-eight years of Marxist-Leninist–inspired one-party rule. It failed, however, to bring about the emergence of a younger generation representing the desire for change in political practices that had been expressed during the conference. Three members of the older generation—Pascal Lissouba, Denis Sassou N'Guesso, and Bernard Kolelas—dominated the political stage following the presidential elections of 1992. Lissouba, a former prime minister, was elected president in the second round of voting, with the support of the outgoing president, Sassou N'Guesso. Lissouba defeated Kolelas, a longtime opponent of the defunct Marxist regime. Rémy Bazenguissa-Ganga interprets this massive return of the old generation, which was so harshly criticized during the Sovereign National Conference, as a sign that a majority of the people of Congo-Brazzaville were ready to accept the use of political violence.[6]

The instability that quickly followed the shifting alliances fostered this feeling of insecurity and encouraged two actions: The suburbs closed themselves off, and new forces took control by violent means. Left out of the abortive attempts at democracy and shaken by an economic crisis that no longer guaranteed graduates an automatic right to a plush government post, urban youths found an outlet for their frustrations and a place that society had denied them in the militias that were formed around the three leaders.[7] For the "downwardly mobile" (young school dropouts, delinquents, or victims of the crises) who over the years swelled the ranks of the militias, these organizations have often proved to be an unexpected source of income. Identification with a political struggle or with the defense of a group thus served as a justification for factional activities.

From Militarization of Political Action to Open Conflict

The rise of the militia reflected a growing trend toward violence as a means of political action. By reinforcing the isolation of the various suburbs, this violence has also lent legitimacy to the regionalist politics of the principal leaders. Sassou N'Guesso called on the population of the north to rally under his banner for their survival, Lissouba relied on the Nibolek, while Kolelas attempted to unite the Lari population, which was a majority in the southern suburbs of Brazzaville and in the Pool prefecture. The gradual homogenization of the suburbs of Brazzaville and the military clashes that followed the confiscation of oil revenues led to an escalation of violence from the initial clashes in Brazzaville to fighting on a national scale after 1997. The militia groups were now used less for backing political action than for capturing power by force, abandoning any pretext of democracy.

In this strategy of countrywide fighting, the financial support of the oil companies and the countries of the region becomes a valuable asset. Denis Sassou N'Guesso has been the most successful in garnering this support. In 1997, with the aid of the Angolan Armed Forces (FAA) and other combatants, mostly from Chad and Rwanda, he gained a decisive advantage over the Cocoyes and Ninja militias. After five months of fighting that ended in his victory, Sassou declared himself president on 25 October 1997. Lissouba and Kolelas fled the country, and the Cocoyes and Ninjas, left to their own devices and without any real contact with their leaders, retreated to their strongholds in the Nibolek and Pool regions. The fighting resulted in between 8,000 and 10,000 deaths, most of them civilians.

In the spring of 1998, progovernment forces began to face renewed rebel activity in the Pool and Bouenza prefectures. Ninja infiltration into the Bacongo and Makelekele suburbs in December 1998 triggered violent reprisals from progovernment forces. They cut off the two suburbs and began systematic searches that, according to the Congolese Human Rights Monitoring Unit (OCDH), soon degenerated into large-scale massacres of unarmed civilians. The Ninjas, for their part, began arbitrarily executing any person from the Pool region who was suspected of supporting the regime of Denis Sassou N'Guesso. The OCDH estimates the total number of victims at between 5,000 and 6,000.[8]

Eyewitness accounts compiled by Action Against Hunger teams from the population that has been slowly returning from the Pool region since May 1999 confirm the atrocities inflicted on the civilian population. Many families were separated during the exodus in December or during the military offensives in the Pool region. Each account is filled with tales of the inhuman behavior of militia members, young men with no supervision, their minds altered by marijuana, committing the worst atrocities with impunity. Numerous stories of executions carried out by progovernment forces against young people suspected of belonging to the Ninja militia were reported.

Militia were quoted as saying, "If you have 10,000 or 20,000 [francs CFA], we'll let you go. If not, we'll kill you." One mother saw her twenty-year-old son, the father of two children, killed before her eyes. A nineteen-year-old woman, the mother of a month-old baby, related how she has had no news of her husband since he and two friends were detained by the military in Kinkala. She gave birth in Linzozlo before the military took her back to Brazzaville with her child. On the way, they took away two skirts and her sandals.

This war has taken a particularly heavy toll on women. The ethnic-based militias regularly use rape as a weapon of war. There is competition to see who can lay claim to having "truly ravaged the Pool women." Many rapes are committed in the villages and on the road to Brazzaville. To obtain a ride in a truck often requires spending the night at an assembly point. At nightfall, alcohol and drugs push the overexcited men over the edge: "Every woman under the age of forty returning home has been raped," as one old woman reported. "Even us they grope there to see if we are hiding money." One woman, who was eight months pregnant, gave an account of how a group of soldiers tried to rape her, forced her to take off her clothes, but then let her get dressed again after seeing that she was pregnant. She was allowed to return to Brazzaville in their company, but they stole her luggage, including the clothes for the baby she was expecting. Although she had escaped Brazzaville with her husband and their seven children, she returned alone. On 2 April, her husband was killed in a helicopter attack by the army on the village of Mutampa, and in the ensuing panic she was separated from her children, the eldest of whom was eighteen years old. In all cases, the barbarity of the act stems from a desire to humiliate: "Father and mother are forced to watch as their daughter's clothes are removed and she is raped."

The civilian population, in its attempts to escape the fighters, who do not hesitate to use civilians as human shields, has systematically avoided towns and communication hubs that might be considered to be of strategic value, at the risk of dying of hunger or disease.[9] Though less spectacular, this factor is nonetheless crucial. Half of the people returning to Brazzaville suffer from malnutrition edema as a result of poor nutrition. Since the end of the mango season, the displaced populations have survived on wild roots and ground and fermented manioc leaves. The food shortage has been made worse by the fact that all through 1998 farmers in the Pool region did not plant crops because of the upheaval in the region. Children are the first to suffer from this lack of food and medicine. According to a survey of the population returning to Brazzaville in May and June, a quarter of the children under the age of five have perished.[10]

Whether or not intended, the terror inflicted on civilians by the militias has plunged more than 200,000 people into famine with no response from the international community. Repeated calls for action from humanitarian and human rights organizations have most often been met with indifference. The trickle of funds for emergency assistance cannot mask the absence of diplomatic initiatives. The increasing distance between the leaders in exile and their militias, which are in danger of further fragmentation,[11] and the government's refusal to negotiate, faced as it was with its own internal power struggles, do not presage any improvement in the situation in Congo-Brazzaville. The efforts of humanitarian organizations such as Action Against Hunger to help the most vulnerable sectors of the population are inadequate. Barring any new initiatives, the international community's silence and passivity only countenance the militias' continued fighting and their terrorizing of civilians, who are their principal victims.

Notes

Pascal Lefort is desk officer at Action Against Hunger.

1. The Republic of Congo is referred to throughout this book as Congo-Brazzaville to distinguish it from the Democratic Republic of Congo (DRC, or Congo), formerly Zaire.

2. E. Dorier-Apprill, A. Kouvouana, and C. Apprill, *Vivre à Brazzaville* (Paris: Karthala, 1998), p. 258.

3. The Ninja militias in Brazzaville started forming in 1993 in the southern suburbs of Bacongo and Makelekele to support Bernard Kolelas's Congolese Movement for Democracy and Integral Development (MCDDI). Its members are of Lari origin. The Zulus were formed in 1993 by the "movement" supporting President Pascal Lissouba to "secure" the Mfilou district. Not a militia organization like the Cobras and the Ninjas, the Zulus are made up of different armed groups.

4. Nibolek is an acronym designating the prefectures of Niari, Bouenza, and Kekoumouo, which constitute a fictitious regional entity created by Pascal Lissouba to unite around his person the populations in the south of the country.

5. A study carried out in 1997 by the association Agrisud-Agricongo shows how supplies for each sector of the city are provided through a central market and how trade between the northern and southern suburbs is extremely limited.

6. Rémy Bazenguissa-Ganga, "Milices politiques et bandes armées à Brazzaville: enquêtes sur la violence politique et sociale des jeunes déclassés," *Les études* du CERI, no. 13 (Paris: April 1996).

7. The Ninjas formed around Bernard Kolelas, the Cobras around Denis Sassou N'Guesso, and the Aubevillois, Zulus, and later the Cocoyes around Pascal Lissouba.

8. FIDH/OCDH, *Congo-Brazzaville, l'arbitraire de l'État, la terreur des milices* (Paris: FIDH/OCDH, 1999).

9. For security reasons, international humanitarian aid organizations are not authorized to operate in the Pool Prefecture.

10. Study taken from the results of a population survey in the Bacongo and Makelekele suburbs and from the registration of the people returning to Brazzaville.

11. A split has already occurred within the Ninja militia between Kolelas's supporters and the more numerous N'Silulu, a mystical/religious radical group led by Jean N'Toumi

Bibliography

Agir ici/Survie. "Sommet franco-africain au Louvre: la sécurité au sommet, l'insécurité à la base." *Les dossiers noirs de la politique africaine de la France*, no. 12. L'Harmattan, 1998.

Agrisud/Agricongo. *Diagnostic du niveau d'approvisionnement des populations de Brazzaville et identification des circuits de distribution des produits alimentaires.* Paris: Agrisud/Agricongo, 1997.

Bazenguissa-Ganga, Rémy. "Milices politiques et bandes armées à Brazzaville: enquêtes sur la violence politique et sociale des jeunes déclassées." *Les Études* du CERI, no. 13. April 1996.

Bazenguissa-Ganga, Rémy. "La popularisation de la violence au Congo." *Politique Africaine*, no. 73. Karthala, March 1999.

Dorier-Apprill, E., A. Kouvouana, and C. Apprill. *Vivre à Brazzaville*. Paris: Karthala, 1998.

FIDH/OCDH. *Congo-Brazzaville, l'arbitraire de l'État, la terreur des milices*. Paris: FIDH/OCDH, 1999.

Smith, S., and A. Glaser. *Ces Messieurs Afrique 2, Des réseaux aux lobbies*. Paris: Calmann-Lévi, 1997.

3

The Great Lakes:
Avoiding an Ethnic Reading

Jean-François Vidal

Colonial literature abounds with racist clichés that, long after the decolonization of the 1960s, linger on in the consciousness and form the basis for the analysis of crises that are the orphan progeny of the Cold War. The Great Lakes region of Africa is a particularly revealing example in which hunger, power, and politics are all closely intertwined.

A Genocide Rooted in
Colonial History and Struggles for Power

When the first colonial settlers arrived in the Great Lakes area (consisting of Uganda, Rwanda, Burundi, and the eastern part of the Democratic Republic of Congo, known as Kivu), they were surprised to discover societies that had statelike attributes, kingdoms based on systems of well-defined social relationships, with their own laws, justice systems, taxes, and cultures. In short, they discovered other civilizations.

This came as quite a shock, since the nineteenth-century colonization was automatically justified in part by the supposed existence of a single world civilization, namely Western civilization, which had the duty to conquer the rest of the world in order to save the souls of those who, not yet Christian, could only be savages. The pseudoscientific theories of the "superior races" advanced by several authors held center stage at the time and were the compost from which the racist theories of the twentieth century emerged.

Forced then to explain away the existence of these societies in the heart of Africa, the German and later Belgian colonizers discovered a group of people who "could have been white—if they did not have black skin."[1] Who were they? Where did they come from? These were the questions that anthropologists of the period asked themselves.

The "evidence" was quickly unearthed! They (the Tutsi) came from the east, from the mountains of Ethiopia, descendants of the Queen of Sheba and therefore a people of the Bible. And thus was born the myth. Together with their herds, they had brought a civilization of biblical origin to the savage Bantu peoples. Nothing in these societies therefore contradicted the dominant ideology of the nineteenth-century colonizers.

There was no shortage of colonial-era descriptions of the Hutus as "small, thick-lipped, flat-nosed, tillers of the soil" compared with the "tall, slender, majestic, aquiline nosed" lordly Tutsis. This "scientific explanation" led the colonizers to use the "lordly Tutsis" to assure their domination of the "Hutu serfs."[2] Education in colonial Rwanda and Burundi was essentially geared toward the Tutsis, who in the 1960s accounted for approximately 85 percent of the literate class, a proportion that was inverse to their numerical representation in the two countries.

Myths die slowly, and at the time of decolonization a number of European newspapers headlined the "revolt of the serfs" and the "flight of the lords."

The genocide of the Tutsis did not begin in 1994. With independence in 1959, the struggle for power was accompanied by genocidal massacres that forced hundreds of thousands of Rwandan Tutsis out of the country, mostly into neighboring Uganda. The refugees settled in the Ankole area around Fort Portal, Uganda, and twenty-five years later their descendants would form a majority in the Ugandan National Resistance Army (NRA) led by Yoweri Kaguta Museveni in the fight against the second regime of Milton Obote, who had been reinstated following the expulsion of Idi Amin Dada from Uganda by Tanzanian troops. It should be noted that the seizure of power in Uganda by the NRA in 1986 was the first to be achieved by a guerrilla force in Africa in a military victory, without negotiations. Others were to follow.

Flush with their military victory, the descendants of the refugees of 1959, who had been born in Uganda and educated in English, comprised 80 percent of the leadership under Museveni, 50 percent of the senior officer corps, and 35 percent of the soldiers. They also controlled 15 percent of posts in the civil administration. For the first time since the fall of the Kabaka (king of the Buganda) in 1963, northern Ugandans no longer held power.

Despite the massacres committed by Obote's troops from 1983 to 1986 in the Luwero triangle (the triangle of death), fears of NRA retribution did not materialize. President Museveni kept his promises and his pledge. He gradually became one of the so-called darlings of the World Bank. When the International Monetary Fund (IMF) imposed its conditions on Uganda in 1988, most notably a 50 percent reduction within six months in the number of government employees (both civilian and military), it was the Tutsis who bore the brunt of the cuts so that Museveni could reinforce his Ugandan credentials and preempt accusations that he gained power with the help of foreigners and that he himself was a "Rwandan."

Hardened by years of victorious guerrilla warfare, the descendants of the 1959 refugees created the Rwandan Patriotic Front (FPR) and decided to "return home." In one night in 1990, all the Tutsis in Kampala, the capital of Uganda, disappeared. Led by the FPR, they dashed to the frontier and one week later were on the outskirts of Kigali, the capital of Rwanda. Intervention by Belgian, French, and Zairian troops forced them to retreat to northern Rwanda and marked the beginning of a guerilla war between the FPR forces and the Interahamwe militia, which was created, trained, and armed for this purpose and allied with the Rwandan Armed Forces (FAR).

The rest, unfortunately, is all too well known: the planned genocide of the Tutsi by Hutu extremists of 1994; complete failure of the United Nations Blue Helmets; seizure of power by the FPR; Operation Turquoise; flight of the ex-FAR and Interahamwe troops to camps in Goma and Bukavu, Zaire, and Ngara, Tanzania, together with nearly two million Rwandan Hutus; regrouping in camps of the forces that carried out the genocide; and regular incursions into Rwanda and genocidal attacks against Tutsis in Zaire (most notably during the summer of 1995 in the Masisi area).[3] An armed force consisting of officers of the FPR, Zairian Tutsis (Banyamulenge from the southern part of the Zairean province of Kivu and Tutsis from Masisi), and Zairian opponents of Marshal Mobutu Sese Sako was then created, called the Alliance of Forces for Democracy and Freedom (AFDL). The camps were attacked and dismantled in the fall of 1996. There then followed both a massive return of refugees to Rwanda and the flight of hundreds of thousands of people westward, harassed and massacred by the troops of the new AFDL. The AFDL finally drove out Mobutu, and Laurent Désiré Kabila took power in Kinshasa, the capital of Zaire, in May 1997. Zaire became the Democratic Republic of Congo (DRC).

As had happened in Kampala in 1986 and Kigali in 1994, Kinshasa in 1997 fell under the control of troops hardened by nearly fifteen years of victorious guerrilla warfare. Kabila thus found himself in a situation similar to the one in which Museveni had found himself in 1986: accused of having come to power with the help of foreigners. In order to emphasize his Congolese legitimacy, he could no longer rely on the Tutsis of the AFDL, who controlled the army and occupied key posts in the civilian administration.

Rapid Internationalization of the Second War in Kivu

In the spring of 1998, Kinshasa issued instructions for the Banyamulenge soldiers to integrate with units of the new Congolese army and to accept deployment anywhere in the country. The first rebellion erupted in the Uvira area when the Banyamulenge refused to redeploy, since they would no longer be able to protect the highlands.

Unwilling to leave the field open to the Congolese Maï-Maï militia, whether or not these were allied with the ex-FAR, Interahamwe, or the Burundian opposition Hutus of the Palipehutu and the Forces pour la Defense de la Démocratie (the armed branch of the Comité national pour la Defense de la Démocratie [CNDD] in Burundi), the Banyamulenge resisted. Kabila's AFDL dispatched reinforcements to Bukavu, and soon the two camps were facing each other in the Rusisi plain.

It required the intervention of Commander James (James Kabare), Kabila's chief of staff and himself a Tutsi, to avoid a military confrontation. Negotiations were held in Kamanyola, DRC, in the north of the Rusisi plain, near to the Rwandan border. What was negotiated at Kamanyola? Was the second Kivu war promised to the Banyamulenge? There was no official announcement about the results of the negotiations. Whatever occurred, the Banyamulenge agreed to redeploy. One must keep in mind, however, that in the DRC as elsewhere, integrating a segment of the population into a national army has been one way to recognize or acquire nationality.

One of the earliest problems encountered in the Great Lakes region was that of the nationality of the Congolese Tutsis, to whom Zairian citizenship had been granted by Mobutu in 1971 and later revoked in 1981. The Banyamulenge, traumatized by the Rwanda genocide, first and foremost wished to protect the South Kivu highlands that provided shelter for their families and cattle.

The Banyamulenge were not fighting the same battle as the Rwandan authorities, who were more concerned with defending

Rwanda's borders from the repeated incursions of the ex-FAR and Interahamwe guerrillas from North Kivu than with defending their Banyamulenge brothers.

From June 1998 on, the similarities with the Uganda of 1989 grew even more striking: The Kabila government replaced Commander James with a Congolese and in July "foreign soldiers" were asked to return home. On 2 August, a rebellion erupted, Ugandan and Rwandan troops entered Congo, and war resumed in Kivu.

Very soon airplanes were chartered by the forces of the new rebellion, and rebel troops were being flown in from Goma to the lower Congo. The rebels began a march on Kinshasa from Matadi and were finally halted outside the Kinshasa airport by the intervention of troops from Angola, Zimbabwe, and Namibia on the side of Kabila.

For the first time in its history, Africa witnessed a war in which opposing guerrillas and regular troops from several different countries fought within the territory of one of its sovereign states. There is some question as to the actual number of states involved. Officially, the forces of the DRC, allied with troops from Zimbabwe, Angola, Namibia, and Chad, are fighting against the rebel forces, which in turn are allied with troops from Uganda and Rwanda. The involvement of Sudanese contingents fighting on the side of Kabila and troops from Burundi on the side of the rebels has been denied by Khartum and Bujumbura, the Sudanese and Burundian capitals. Libya is thought to be involved, if only in providing financial or even logistical support. It has been confirmed that Kabila's troops have been allowed passage through the Central African Republic to defend Zongo on the Congo River. More than ten African countries are thus involved in the conflict as well as some Israeli and North Korean units, according to witnesses.

To this number must be added the nongovernmental military participants. These consist of ex-FAR and Interahamwe Rwandans; forces opposed to the regime in Bujumbura (CNDD and Palipehutu); Ugandan armed groups based in the Democratic Republic of Congo opposed to President Museveni; National Union for the Total Independence of Angola (UNITA), which is opposed to the regime in Luanda; and the Congolese militia known under the generic name of Maï-Maï in Kivu.

By June 1999, the rebels were in control of half of the DRC but were sharply divided. As further fractures developed within the rebellion, zones of influence emerged that reflected the root causes of the involvement of third parties in the conflict. In the north, units supported by Uganda controlled territory up to Kinsangani; in the center of the rebel country (north Kivu), the Rassemblement Congolais pour la Democratie (RCD), supported by Rwanda, is based in Goma; and in the south of Uvira, conflict developed between troops from Burundi (allied with the Banyamulenge) and the Maï-Maï, who were openly supported by the Kabila regime and allied with rebel forces from Burundi.

By June 1999, the Maï-Maï had gained control of almost the entire Fizi region and threatened to attack the city of Uvira. A new wave of refugees fled the fighting, heading for Tanzania and Burundi or seeking refuge on the slopes of the surrounding hills.

The fault lines within the rebellion deepened with the increase in "bilateral" support from neighboring countries and from the fighting that was taking place within the rebel movement. A split within the RCD created the Congolese Liberation Movement (MLC), openly supported by Uganda, which withdrew its armored cars from Uvira; Burundian troops were ferried by helicopter into Baraka, DRC; fighting broke out between Rwandan and Banyamulenge troops in Uvira; and Uganda and Rwanda fought for control of Kisangani through their proxies, the RCD and the MLC. A second split occurred within the RCD, which thereafter consisted of two separate factions. The Banyamulenge joined the Federalist Republican Forces (FRF). Local, political, strategic, security, and economic interests gradually took precedence over the national rebellion.

These explosions, which were marked by violence and plundering, have reduced even further the level of humanitarian activity, and civilian populations have become increasingly isolated.

Hunger and Malnutrition Used as Weapons

In this chaos of armed groups that lacked any real, unified chain of command, civilian populations found themselves used by all sides. True motives were often concealed, while the professed "democratic" motives proclaimed by all were often a camouflage.

When fighting resumed in South Kivu, the civilian population fled for a second time. During the clashes in 1996, more than 200,000 people had already fled south toward the Shaba province of the DRC (which has since reverted to its old name, Katanga), and nearly 100,000 civilians had crossed Lake Tanganyika into Tanzania, where they hoped to find refuge in Kigoma, a port on Lake Tanganyika in Tanzania. After several months of forced exile, both internal and external, the relative calm of 1997 allowed displaced persons and refugees to return to their homes.

Action Against Hunger developed a comprehensive program of

immediate assistance for their return and began rebuilding the infrastructure that had been destroyed in the fighting. The organization cared for children suffering from malnutrition, repaired water supply systems, protected water sources, distributed seeds and agricultural tools, replaced fishing nets, reopened seventeen health clinics, and curbed a cholera outbreak. The population gradually recovered a measure of autonomy.

The resumption of the fighting on 2 August 1998 interrupted this cycle of recovery. Villagers hastily harvested their last crop and fled again into the forest. Several thousands of them tried in vain to cross Lake Tanganyika but were turned back by rebel guerrillas more concerned with showing the outside world a population that was not in flight than with respecting the right of those populations to seek asylum and refuge in a neighboring country. Their boats were forced to turn around, and today they are still massed on the shores of the lake, without the possibility of planting enough food to feed themselves.

In this example of the use of hunger as a weapon, efforts were made to prevent the movement of populations and to keep them in a situation of internal displacement without any assistance in order to avoid the negative image that always accompanies an outflow of refugees. Famine denied is famine concealed.

No break occurred in the fighting in the Fizi region. Up until the spring of 1999, the coastal road on Lake Tanganyika was controlled by the rebels and the highlands by the Banyamulenge. The Maï-Maï operated between the two, in what is known as the intermediate highlands. Even though the origin of this last-mentioned group of combatants lay in a tradition of ritual initiation, nothing in its recent history can be traced to this tradition. Well-armed and equipped with uniforms, they today constitute a genuine militia that fights against the rebels who are opposed to Kabila and employ a tactic of harassment, which nonetheless includes full control of several dozen villages and even of entire districts. Many eyewitnesses have stated that they are allied with the Burundi rebels, and are said to be directly supported by Kabila's forces.

Rebel commanders usually describe the situation in the following terms: "There are three types of populations: those that are hostages of the Maï-Maï, those that support the Maï-Maï, and those that have fled." In all cases, these populations no longer live in their towns and villages and have instead become a mass of tens of thousands of people hiding in the forest and out of reach of any assistance. What is their condition today? Given the complete lack of access to the areas of conflict, it is very difficult to make an estimate. The few hundred children who manage to reach the Action Against Hunger feeding centers in the coastal plain are proof of a catastrophic food situation. The supplies that villagers carried with them during their flight are now exhausted, and farmers no longer have access to their fields. Cholera is now endemic in the region, and the lack of health care due to the shortage of medicine and trained personnel means that any estimate would be grim indeed.

Fighting also rages in Katanga province in the DRC. Fanning out from Kalemie and Kindu, rebel forces are aiming for Lubumbashi and Mbuji-Mayi, key centers in the south. The air forces of Kabila's allies regularly bombard rebel-held cities, with civilians being the principal victims. Supply roads have been cut, markets are understocked, and prices are skyrocketing.

In September 1998, a particularly poignant event took place: Between ten and twelve thousand Congolese Tutsis living in the Vyura area, some 180 kilometers south of the border with Kivu, sought refuge in Kalemie. The RCD requested international assistance to move this population from Katanga to South Kivu and accused the government in Kinshasa and its allies of continuing the Tutsi genocide in Katanga. Kinshasa in turn denounced the resettlement of these displaced persons in the Rusisi plain as an attempt at "Tutsi colonization" of the land in South Kivu. In any event, the refugees, consisting mainly of women and children, were transported by boat to Uvira and herded into makeshift camps while awaiting their resettlement in the plain.

In Lubumbashi, the capital of Katanga and the center of mining activity in the DRC, Action Against Hunger conducted a nutritional survey that revealed that 34.6 percent of the population suffered from chronic malnutrition and that 20.8 percent of the acute malnutrition among children under five was linked to high levels of malnutrition in their mothers (about one in five). The lack of personnel to care for severely malnourished children in the region led Action Against Hunger to propose the inclusion of treatment for severe malnutrition in the services provided by hospitals.

Also in Katanga, the nutritional situation of the nearly forty thousand Angolan refugees in Kissenge on the Angolan border who had fled the fighting between UNITA and the Luanda government could only be described as disastrous. A nutritional survey conducted in February 1999 revealed catastrophic malnutrition rates (25 percent acute general malnutrition, of which 12.8 percent was severe). These figures were similar to those recorded during the most severe African famines.

Food is in short supply in the capital of Kinshasa. The World Food Program is considering the massive importation of humanitarian aid. Kivu had been the breadbasket of the capital, but the supply system is now dislocated. Moreover, after years of neglect, the basic infrastructure (health, drinking water) is no longer capable of meeting the basic needs of the population. Action Against Hunger has put a system in place to monitor nutritional levels and has improved sanitary conditions in the markets and increased the availability of drinking water in periurban areas.

In Burundi, the government is incapable of controlling its opponents. The civilian population hides in the forest, emerging malnourished and dependent on humanitarian aid. Access to the victims must be continuously negotiated. Action Against Hunger has established its largest nutrition program in Burundi.

In Uganda, the recent fighting between the forces of Kampala and the rebels operating from the DRC has displaced another 100,000 persons at Bundibugyo on the Congolese border. These have now joined the 150,000 refugees (mostly from Sudan) and the approximately 400,000 persons who have been displaced by the ten-year conflict between the Ugandan government and the Ugandan rebel Lord's Resistance Army (LRA) of Joseph Kony, which is now supported by Khartum. Action Against Hunger operates a nutrition program in Uganda and provides clean water for displaced populations (in Gulu and Kitgum). It has also conducted a nutritional survey in the fourteen refugee camps and established a program to settle refugees in the Adjumani district.

In Rwanda, finally, several hundred thousand persons have been displaced in the northwest, victims of the ongoing conflict between government troops and extremist militias, ex-FAR and Interahamwe, based in the DRC.

Redefining International Humanitarian Law: A Dangerous Trend

When fighting resumed in Kivu, all personnel from international humanitarian organizations and United Nations agencies were evacuated. Both Kabila's fleeing troops and troops allied with the RCD commandeered vehicles and communications equipment from humanitarian organizations and systematically looted homes, offices, and warehouses for food and medical supplies. Similar looting had been witnessed in 1996 in both South and North Kivu.

These two incidents of looting have left humanitarian organizations and UN agencies on the defensive. The failure to return the stolen goods and the lack of guarantees for the safety of personnel and property have caused the United Nations agencies to delay their return in order to negotiate the conditions for doing so. It was not until early in March 1999 that the UN reopened an office in Goma, under the responsibility of the United Nations Children's Fund (UNICEF). A second branch office was opened in Bukavu in June 1999.

This prolonged process has involved political discussions between the different actors. The envoy of the United Nations secretary-general to the region, Ambassador Beahanu Dinka, was first met with a refusal and later accepted the position of the Kabila government. Kabila agreed to permit humanitarian aid to be delivered to rebel-controlled areas, but under no circumstances was aid to be allowed to pass through the foreign countries involved in the conflict. Uganda, Burundi, and Rwanda were specifically named. A tentative plan to deliver aid through Tanzania fell through, and supply lines through Zambia were considered.

Many humanitarian organizations, including Action Against Hunger, took umbrage at what they felt amounted to the subordination of humanitarian aid to political considerations. It would require intervention at the highest political level in the United Nations system, in essence a rejection of Ambassador Dinka's position, for the United Nations to consider disregarding Kabila's wishes and basing their logistical support in neighboring countries, which was clearly the most effective solution. The United Nations must be commended for this new position as of January 1999, basing support in Rwanda.

The United Nations, however, has made its return, reinstallation, and thus its humanitarian assistance contingent upon the signing by both the rebel and government authorities of a document enunciating the applicable "principles" that must be respected. These negotiations are over a key issue that concerns the legal framework for humanitarian activities.

Above and beyond the increasing militarization of humanitarian language ("Rules of Engagement" in the DRC or "Strategic Framework" in Afghanistan and elsewhere), there has been a trend toward the redefining of international humanitarian law (Geneva Conventions and the Additional Protocols thereto, Refugee Convention, Conventions on Genocide, Torture, and so on). Why, after all, is it necessary to redefine and negotiate for each conflict principles that already exist and that are enshrined in law, if the purpose is not to rewrite this law?

Under pressure from its member states (including three that are among the five permanent members of the United Nations Security Council) that refuse to sign and thus to recognize the validity of the International Criminal Court, it is feared that the United Nations might be engaged in a de facto process of rewriting a "law" that would end up being no more than an amalgam of "conventions" or "principles" defined in an ad hoc manner for each separate conflict. Ignoring the question of the juridical validity of such a "law," which would no longer be universal, would no longer apply to all parties, and would threaten the very idea of a permanent international court in any form whatsoever, we are witnessing the gradual but formal subordination of the principles of humanitarian action and international law to the political and strategic interests of member states.

The ethnic lenses through which the conflict in the Great Lakes has been viewed since 1994 act as sunglasses, filtering the reality, soothing the view, and reassuring the viewer but falsifying the analysis of the situation.

To view the conflict in the Great Lakes region only as an ethnic rivalry is to fail to understand the situation or to conceive of a permanent solution. The resumption of the war in 1998, the open intervention of neighboring countries, and the recent fighting between Rwandan Tutsi troops and Congolese Tutsis (Banyamulenge) were surprising and unexpected because these events were being viewed, often unconsciously, through the colonial prism as an ethnic conflict between the agricultural Bantu, former serfs, and the pastoral Tutsi, their former masters.

Such an interpretation of events reflects an oversimplification equaled only by the simplifications of the Cold War. The reference points, which the Cold War provided, have been replaced by another simplification. Where the so-called good guys and bad guys were clearly identified during the Cold War, the "good guys" in the Great Lakes region have been, depending on the year and country in question, alternately the Tutsis who were decimated by genocide and the Hutus who were expelled from their farmlands by the Tutsi armies of Burundi or chased into the jungles of what was still Zaire.

Gorbachev had warned Reagan to the effect that the USSR was doing a terrible thing: depriving the United States of an enemy. The hesitations or outright silence of the international community when confronted with the Khmer Rouge in Cambodia or with similar forces in Somalia, Haiti, Chechnya, Kurdistan, and Angola and in the war currently ravaging Ethiopia and Eritrea are perfect illustrations of this.

Balkanization is a term that has been used to describe the Great Lakes region. One could also speak of the Balkans as having been "Great-Laked." In both cases, the conflicts have been inaccurately described as being "ethnic conflicts," "ancient rivalries," "centuries-old conflicts," or even "conflicts that have gone on for millennia," so much so that President Clinton appeared on a CNN television program during the first week of June 1999 to apologize for having justified NATO intervention in Kosovo with such clichés.

On the contrary, the Iraqi conflict and the recent war in Kosovo have placed a spotlight on the political void and the absence of any strategic analysis of these crises. The demons of the Cold War have reemerged. We have found once again (at last!) new and identifiable "bad guys" and thus, by the same token, "good guys." The same fallacious reasoning can therefore be found: The enemy of my enemy is my friend, whoever he might be. We have seen this with Kabila when Mobutu became the number one enemy and with the KLA (Kosovo Liberation Army), which was opposed to Milosevic and therefore our friend. We have also seen it with Joseph Savimbi of Angola, another Mobutu who went from being friend to enemy, and one senses it with Museveni in Uganda, who risks going from international darling to outlaw.

Unlike the situation in Kosovo, the absence of any international response to the conflict in the Great Lakes region and to all African conflicts in general may be attributed to the difficulty in determining who are the "good guys" and the "bad guys" today in the Democratic Republic of the Congo, Congo-Brazzaville, Angola, Sierra Leone, Ethiopia, Eritrea, Somalia, or the Comoros.

Since the Cold War, conflict analysis has found two new buzzwords: *ethnicity* and *humanitarianism*. There are therefore humanitarian crises that require "humanitarian responses." Unfortunately, humanitarian crises do not exist! There are only political crises, which have humanitarian consequences. To seek to provide a humanitarian response to a conflict would therefore be tantamount to seeking to cure a patient suffering from tuberculosis by easing his cough.

Similarly, ethnic conflicts do not exist. There are only political conflicts and power struggles that have ethnic consequences. The response therefore cannot be an ethnic one, and any attempt to use this approach sows the seeds of future instability.

Action Against Hunger has denounced the use of hunger as a weapon of war. We have consistently argued that famines should be considered as political developments and not simply as the mechanical consequences of natural disasters. Because of our commitment to care for civilian populations that are victims of armed conflicts, we must denounce any analysis of these conflicts as being ethnic or humanitarian crises.

To describe a war in ethnic or humanitarian terms is to risk justifying violence and suffering as a means of healing other violence and suffering.

We must at all costs distance ourselves and fight against the growing tendency to claim that there are now "just" humanitarian causes in the same way as there are "just" wars. Such thinking undermines the credibility of humanitarian workers and threatens the survival of international humanitarian law and above all the right of victims to assistance and protection.

Notes

Jean-François Vidal is executive director, Action Against Hunger–USA.

1. Jean-Pierre Chrétien, *Afrique des Grands Lacs* (Paris: Aubier, 1992).

2. Filip Reyntjens, *L'Afrique des Grand Lacs en Crise* (Paris: Karthala, 1995).

3. Action Against Hunger, "The Great Lakes Tragedy," *Geopolitics of Hunger, 1998–1999* (Paris: PUF, 1998).

4

Somalia: A Country Without a State, a Conflict Without End

Michel Anglade

In early 1999, the conflict in Somalia reemerged in its most tragic form: famine. An acute food shortage now threatens over one million people in the south of the country. Drought, poor harvests, but above all war are responsible for this situation. Over the past ten years, the conflict has debilitated the population, brought about the total collapse of the government, and rendered all humanitarian intervention difficult and dangerous.

Conflict Without End

The conflict in Somalia has lasted for over ten years. The January 1991 fall of Siad Barre, who had led the country since 1969, while certainly a contributing factor, merely hastened the decline of the state and intensified a civil war that had begun in the 1980s.

Clashes between opposing Somali militias now rarely gain the attention of the outside world. The failure of the United Nations Operation in Somalia (UNOSOM) between 1992 and 1995 and the country's lack of strategic value offer no incentives for Western countries to reopen the Somali dossier and promote political solutions.

For the time being, no end to the conflict is in sight, and the reconstitution of a Somali state is not in the cards. The "top-down" approach, in which large international conferences bring together heads of factions in a foreign capital, has been a complete failure since 1991. The most recent initiatives, the Cairo Accords of December 1997, which were signed by over thirty factions and which

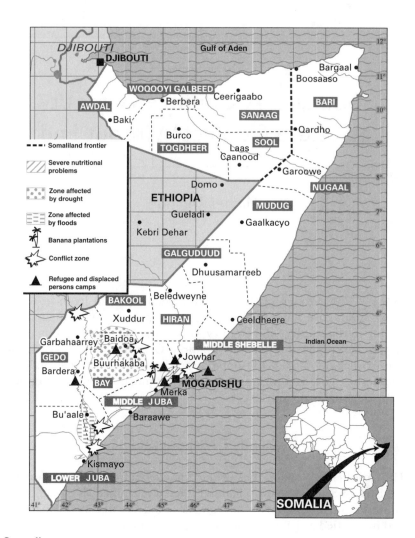

Somalia

provided for national reconciliation, have been completely ignored in Somalia.

Reasons for Failure

Political authority is extremely fragmented, localized, and unstable and is exercised at the village or district level but no further. In a city like Mogadishu, militias control a few blocks while a hundred meters away another militia's territory begins. Borders are marked by a few scraps of metal junk, which close off the street and are guarded by youngsters armed with submachine guns. The borders of these "territories" may change in a matter of hours, as alliances are made and broken in a predatory pattern.

Faction leaders who sign such peace accords simply do not have the means to then implement them. One may well wonder if some of them even have the necessary will to do so, since they depend upon fear and insecurity for their power. War and a state of lawlessness make it easy for them to traffic in arms and drugs. The young militiamen whom they employ know that a return to peace would marginalize them. The extortion in which they engage at checkpoints set up along the roads often constitutes their only source of income. Furthermore, the militia of certain warlords illegally occupy territory that is seized by force and exploited for its meager resources, as in the case of a number of banana plantations in Lower Shebelle. If peace were restored, they would be obliged to return this property to its rightful owners, and this they have no desire to do. Many interests are therefore aligned against peace, and force of arms seems incontestable for the time being.

Most faction leaders conceive of their political power only in terms of control and the appropriation of economic resources. They show little interest in providing minimum health or education services to the population, which they purport to represent. Divisions exist not only between different Somali clans but even within clans. The interests of faction leaders, militia members, religious authorities, and businessmen are in conflict, and each party seeks to assert authority, thereby creating a situation that is often confused and very volatile.

During 1998 and the first half of 1999, Mogadishu was the theater of sporadic clashes between partisans and opponents of a new city administration. Interestingly enough, this division was based not on clan loyalties but solely on the competing interests of individuals fighting for control of the city's resources.

In addition, certain regional powers, including Egypt, Eritrea, Ethiopia, and Libya, are indirectly confronting each other on Somali territory by openly supporting with weapons and money one or the other faction, which can switch sides in accordance with supply and demand. This foreign interference only contributes to the further destabilization of the country, as the Rahaweyne Resistance Army (RRA) militia, which is strongly backed by Ethiopia, demonstrated during their offensive in the south of Somalia in June 1999.[1]

Somalia is trapped once more in a cycle of violence and fighting in which the militias of the principal clans clash over control of new territory for plunder and exploitation. Since January 2000, Kismayo, one of the main ports in the south of the country, has been the scene of clashes between the militia of the Marehan and certain Haber Gedir clans on the one hand and the Majerteen militia on the other. The Bay and Bakool regions are the scenes of frequent clashes between the Haber Gedir and Rahaweyne militias.

In the northern part of the country, the self-proclaimed states of Somaliland and Puntland enjoy some degree of stability, but these are fragile entities.

The majority of Somalis are tired of the war and want no part in it. The population suffers from the atrocities of the warlords, but people are trapped by their clan allegiance. While clans have mostly been used as a tool of division and manipulation that is shamelessly exploited by faction leaders to solidify their power, allegiance to clan also provides, at present, the only means of protection from the exactions of other militias, the only form of security, and the only way to settle disputes in a collapsed society that lacks any law other than traditional clan-based dispute settlement mechanisms.

Civilian Populations as Victims

The conflict affects the entire Somali population. The estimated life expectancy of between forty-one and forty-three years decreased in the 1990s. Infant mortality for children under five years is very high at over 210 per 1,000.[2] Maternal mortality rates are among the highest in the world. In other countries, these statistics would be considered a national emergency. But the continuation of the humanitarian crisis in Somalia means that only the most tragic situations—such as the floods of November-December 1997 or famine—are now considered to be emergencies.

The civil conflict and the deteriorating humanitarian situation constitute a vicious cycle. The conflict impoverishes the country, and the diminishing resources only exacerbate the fight for control of what is left. Furthermore, for many young Somalis, the militias represent their only potential source of "employment" and access to a minimal income from plundering and exploiting the civilian population.

The national infrastructure is damaged or shut down owing to conflicts of interest. The port of Mogadishu, unused since 1995, is a case in point. The rival militias who control it cannot agree upon the distribution of the resources that its reopening would generate.

Livestock and farming, the country's main economic activities, are plagued by instability.

The intensive and abusive exploitation of the country's natural resources, such as charcoal production (resulting in massive deforestation and thus to desertification) or fishing off the coasts by foreign trawlers in disregard of international law, also poses a serious threat to the country's environment.

In the Bay and Bakool regions, villages suspected of supporting one or the other of the warring factions have been razed to the ground, their crops burnt, and livestock seized or slaughtered. Action Against Hunger teams in Mogadishu have compiled testimonies from villagers who were victims of such atrocities and managed to survive only by escaping. The terrorized population has no choice but to leave, temporarily or permanently. Hundreds of displaced and completely destitute people regularly arrive in Mogadishu. During the months of December 1998 and January 1999, Action Against Hunger recorded the arrival of more than three thousand persons from the Bay region fleeing the conflict and the shortages of food. Similarly, in June 1999, another wave of several thousand families fled to Mogadishu to escape an offensive by the Rahaweyne militia. Some of them eventually returned to their home regions after some time to rebuild their houses and plant their farms until the next round of atrocities forces them to flee once more. In some regions of southern Somalia, agricultural production has plummeted because of the absence of over 50 percent of farmers from their land.

A major obstacle to recovery in the agricultural sector is the large number of displaced persons (more than 150,000 displaced persons live in Mogadishu in precarious conditions) or refugees living in camps in neighboring countries. The war and recurring crises have also considerably weakened the survival mechanisms of the populations and undermined or destroyed their traditional methods of coping. The collapse of the state and the virtual absence of any civilian structure mean that health services, clean water, supply systems, and education are rare in Somalia. Such services as do exist are private and must be paid for and are inaccessible to the poorest sectors of the population.

Private clinics and pharmacies, moreover, concentrate on the treatment of illnesses and show little concern for preventive action, such as vaccinations or prenatal care. Most Somali doctors have left the country to escape the war. Already far from ideal before 1991, the situation in the health sector has deteriorated markedly, especially in the south of the country. Tuberculosis is widespread, particularly among the displaced populations living in overcrowded and unsanitary conditions. Nearly a third of the severely malnourished children admitted to the feeding centers operated by Action Against Hunger in Mogadishu suffer from tuberculosis. Vaccination coverage is limited, with only 10 percent of children being immunized. Access to drinking water is limited and cholera epidemics frequent.

In 1998, a cholera epidemic claimed nearly ten thousand victims in Mogadishu. Since the water supply system was destroyed by the war, the city's population is dependent on water drawn from wells, some of which are very polluted.[3] There is no garbage collection system, and garbage therefore piles up in the streets. Camps for displaced persons are severely overcrowded.[4] In such an environment, cholera epidemics and diarrhea, a significant cause of infant malnutrition, pose a constant threat to public health.

Over four-fifths of the population is illiterate, and only one child in six attends elementary school. These grim statistics do not bode well for the country's future and are a major obstacle to its reconstruction. In Mogadishu, Koranic schools are the only ones that are accessible to the most-impoverished classes and are part of the long-term strategy of the Islamic organizations that are gradually taking root in the social and educational sectors left vacant by the collapse of the state.

The Difficulty of Humanitarian Intervention

Given these circumstances and the precarious situation in the areas of health, nutrition, and access to water, the role of humanitarian organizations should seem obvious. It is not, however. Nongovernmental organizations (NGOs) are increasingly rare in south Somalia, where the needs are greatest and most urgent.

During the massive humanitarian intervention of the early 1990s, aid was often diverted, misappropriated, and used to support the war. This is no longer true, however, for the plain and simple reason that the number of humanitarian missions in Somalia has since 1995 declined markedly. Still, humanitarian aid remains a coveted economic target. Militias are prepared to fight in order to control and profit from such resources as the rental of cars or houses to humanitarian organizations. The hiring of Somali personnel is a very sensitive issue, since each clan leader would like to see the members of his clan employed. Humanitarian organizations are thus often faced with problems of extortion and threats against which they are singularly helpless. To argue the common good and that aid is being provided to help the population is not very effective when dealing with clan leaders who show no sympathy for the victims and who are often the ones primarily responsible for their plight. Unfortunately, this state of chaos has often resulted in recent years in the murder or kidnapping of Somali and expatriate staff of humanitarian organizations. These crimes have remained unpunished and are mostly the work of militias resentful at having been excluded from the allocation of resources by the humanitarian organizations acting in concert with the local authorities.

The fighting and lack of security are also major obstacles to progress. The Bay region, one of the most populated and vulnerable parts of the country, receives only very limited assistance, since the fighting taking place there and the threats against humanitarian organizations make any intervention and follow-up action very dangerous.[5] Militias are not inclined to recognize any humanitarian law or to grant access to victims. Faction leaders do not really control their militias, and no agreement reached or guarantee given is likely to count for much in the field.

In these circumstances, the limits to the principle of the conditionality of aid quickly become apparent. On one hand, those who are against humanitarian aid in Somalia argue that the aid provided by humanitarian organizations is diverted into the war economy and is ultimately counterproductive because it only profits militias and thus helps to prolong the war. On the other hand, humanitarian organizations cannot abandon endangered populations whose survival depends entirely on the limited aid provided. To stop supporting the most vulnerable populations would punish the victims and not those who are responsible for the situation. The latter in effect are not political leaders, and the population's anger and discontent would therefore not threaten their power.

The suspension of aid is likely to result in increased population movements and thus even greater poverty. Halting aid would also deprive Somalia of the few foreign organizations working in the country, which would have two consequences. First, it would become difficult to prevent crises or even to be aware of them and thus to objectively evaluate them. Second, Somalia would risk being forgotten and would fade once again into a gray area on the fringes of Western consciousness until the next images of famine and torn bodies again attract the world's attention. But then it would be already too late.

Despite these conditions, humanitarian actors still present in Somalia succeed in creating a minimal space for intervention. By including Somalis in the decisionmaking process and by relying on the elders and local authorities, humanitarian organizations can achieve consensus within the community and prevent their staff from finding themselves "in the front line" against militia leaders. Precise and properly targeted humanitarian intervention also enables the Somali people to be more closely involved and thus minimizes the risks.

The conditions necessary to extricate Somalia from its cycle of recurrent crises and create lasting development are not yet present and can be created only if the international community has the will to work toward a political solution to Somalia's problems. Here as elsewhere, humanitarian aid could never be an adequate response to a political problem in which the fate of the majority depends on a few irresponsible faction leaders and their militias.

Notes

Michel Anglade was formerly Action Against Hunger country director in Somalia. He was then Action Against Hunger country director in North Korea until March 2000, when the organization withdrew from that country.

1. The RRA is an armed faction that since 1995 has been waging a guerilla war in the Bay and Bakool regions against the militias of Hussein Aideed, who are considered as occupiers.

2. United Nations Development Programme, *Human Development Report, 1998,* chapter on Somalia (New York: United Nations Development Programme, 1999).

3. Action Against Hunger is rehabilitating wells in Mogadishu in order to improve the quality of water. In addition, during the cholera epidemic, the organization chlorinated three hundred wells to limit the spread of the disease.

4. Action Against Hunger has built latrines in every displaced camp in Mogadishu.

5. In June 1997, a doctor from the organization Doctors Without Borders was murdered in the hospital of Baidoa, capital of the Bay region.

5

Somalia:
A Difficult Reconstruction

Roland Marchal

Since the outbreak of civil war in 1991, nearly all the political actors in Somalia, at least those with whom humanitarian organizations have been forced to deal, have been factions. A faction is an armed group led by a military or political leader. A faction is supported by a clan or subclan or subsubclan or by some families. Traditional clan leaders (elders or notable persons) are not usually the leader of a faction, although in some cases they are. The same clan can support several opposing factions.

To a large extent, however, this situation of dealing with factions is no longer true. In southern Somalia, factions have shown themselves to be weak; in the north, humanitarian organizations currently deal with administrations that demand to be treated in the same way as the government of a country at peace. This chapter will deal only with the situation in Mogadishu, both because a significant portion of the Somali population lives there and because Action Against Hunger has concentrated its efforts in that city. Without going into details, it would be a mistake to believe that the situation in northern Somalia, which is in many ways different and better, does not also raise some very important questions, especially in view of the marked discrepancy between official positions and the reality on the ground.

Breakdown of the Factional Order

Factions have been the only interlocutors of the international community for reasons that were at first inescapable. Other potential interlocutors, namely clan notables and important businessmen, had sworn allegiance to their leaders, and where a faction was not directly associated with a humanitarian organization present in the field, it was simply because other more powerful intermediaries were already at work. An easy way was sought in which to maintain a humanitarian and apolitical facade without always having guarantees about the behavior of the locals recruited as guards. It would be futile to dwell here on 1991 and 1992, a period that remains a very dark one, first for the Somalis themselves, but also for the ethics of humanitarian organizations.

While international intervention has not directly affected the way this system operates, the impact of such intervention has gradually transformed the environment in which humanitarian organizations function. Even though the failure of the United Nations Operation in Somalia (UNOSOM) has been politically devastating, the impact of UNOSOM at the social level has been more nuanced. The very strong international presence, which, it must be recalled, was more military than civilian, did not significantly alter the culture of aid that is one of the most negative legacies of the pre–civil war period. Enough can never be said about the "astonishment" caused by the composition of the majority of Somali nongovernmental organizations (NGOs), which were small, often private or family-run enterprises set up to capture a share of the humanitarian windfall, incapable of organizing the distribution of a minimum of aid to the population in need, but seeking to monopolize the provision of all the services needed by the humanitarian organizations without ever really fulfilling their proper role. In an audit of its activities in the capital, the World Food Program discovered in 1994 that it was feeding more children in Mogadishu than the total population of the city. Nor were international NGOs able to resist the temptation of easy money. Somali managers, for example, would propose projects to their local partners with the sole aim of sharing the budget, since it would be they who would supervise the project. The occasional lack of professionalism on the part of expatriate managers and the limitations inherent in the climate of insecurity, which had never really improved, created the conditions for the misappropriation of humanitarian funds.

Often in spite of itself, the international operation has nevertheless brought about more positive changes. Even though its impact was not widely felt, it genuinely contributed over a certain period to a greater sense of security over a large area of the territory in which it operated. The funds that were expended, not always in a very rational manner, contributed to an initial accumulation of capital by small businessmen who thus acquired a sufficient financial base from which to expand their activities and revive a market spurred by the demand of some eleven thousand UNOSOM employees over a period of several months. Many of the militiamen, who until 1993 had still been fighting, spontaneously disbanded to seek a solution to their poverty in business. The death in January 1994 of Siad Barre, who even from his exile in Nigeria retained a political capacity for military mobilization, brought an end to undoubtedly the most tragic phase of the civil war that was now drawing to a close. Life in Somalia was obviously still very far from returning to normalcy, even though much of the hate that existed between the principal family clans had been consumed.

Other crises have since erupted, notably the bloody clashes that took place in early 1996 within General Hassan Aideed's clan and in late 1997 within the Abgal clan. It must be said, however, that these clashes did not have the same characteristics as earlier clashes. Only the militias were involved, and it was easier to distinguish between civilians and combatants than it had been at the beginning of the war when every young man over the age of twelve was likely to be found with a rifle.

It should be noted at the same time that the international humanitarian organizations, which had paid the price for their mistakes during the 1991–1992 period and later for the errors of the international operation, before long learned the lessons of those difficult years. They did so with a particular sense of urgency as other crises (Yugoslavia, Bosnia, Rwanda, Zaire) raised similar questions about the definition of humanitarian activities and the conditions of access to victims. Among Somali NGOs, finally, the process of weeding out was equally rigorous. Only a few of them remained as genuine partners carrying out their tasks with genuine professionalism.

Although the end of the international operation was by no means easy to manage, contrary to some predictions it led neither to widespread unrest nor to economic collapse. The country's political life never saw the fulfillment of the promises made by the factions. An agreement on the reopening of the port abruptly unraveled. The airport was divided into several zones controlled by different factions and Haber Gidir subclans. The establishment in June 1995 of a government under General Aideed proved nothing but a sorry repeat of the surrealistic scene that had been played out by Ali Mahdi in the fall of 1991 when he proclaimed himself president of Somalia even though he controlled only the northern part of Mogadishu, the capital. Worse still, the crisis between the new president of the republic and one of his former financial backers, Osman Atto, escalated into an armed confrontation in the capital, even as the need for international (or at least Libyan) recognition forced General Aideed to occupy Baidoa and later the Bay and Bakool regions.

The death of General Aideed in August 1996 was without doubt one of the major turning points in the civil war. It weakened his government, which was already being widely challenged by its social base, given the string of promises that had remained unfulfilled. It also marked the end of the reign of charisma and the beginning of a moneymaking period in which his two sons, Hussein and Hassan, played a prominent role. The death of General Aideed also had another consequence: It made possible a more public (but also more violent) expression of the contradictions that existed within the Abgal clan. The clan, in fact, had to suppress its internal rivalries for fear of being weakened in its struggle against a rival who was hated as much as he was feared. The death of General Aideed also provided Ethiopia with justification for intervention once again. Indeed, by August 1996, Ethiopia had begun to intervene in Gedo, a region bordering Kenya and Ethiopia. Its intervention took a more political turn with the signing of the Sodere Accords in January 1997.

The Sodere Accords failed for three main reasons. First, they were dependent on cooperation among the various factions, even though such cooperation was already in serious crisis, especially in the Mogadishu area. Second, they underestimated the influence of Ali Mahdi within the Abgal clan before the crisis reached its peak and failed to include those groups that supported Hussein Aideed. Above all, they appeared to call into question the status of Mogadishu as the country's capital in favor of Bosaso, thus provoking a hostile reaction that transcended the factions based in the capital. For both domestic and international reasons (Egypt has never stopped considering Somalia as an Arab country and Ethiopia as its principal diplomatic rival in the Horn of Africa), the accords proved incapable of bringing about such cooperation, and a new conference of "reconciliation" was proposed.

The agreement signed in Cairo in December 1997 was also unsuccessful, since it was based on the same outdated approach to the problem. In addition to the usual rhetoric, it assigned to the factions based in the capital a key role in resolving the crisis and brought Hussein Aideed and his allies back into the international diplomatic game. In some ways, the agreement was responsible for the specific characteristics of the current situation.

After many months of internal negotiations, northeastern Somalia, which included two regions of Somaliland, in July 1998 announced the formation of a regional government whose president, Abdullah Yusuf, was none other than the principal loser under the Cairo agreement. This administration has since undergone a process of institution building not very different from the one that took place in Somaliland and may even be stronger in certain respects. It is true that its leader received more help from Ethiopia than Somaliland did and that a large measure of clan homogeneity exists in the region. Furthermore, the civil war unfolded differently in this area than it had in other regions of the former Somalia.

Meanwhile, an attempt was made in August 1998 to organize a government in the Mogadishu area following protracted negotiations between the factions, whose grassroots support had become much weaker than it had been two years previously. The failure of this attempt came as no surprise and is now manifest. When Ali Mahdi left the Somali capital in April 1999, officially for medical treatment in Cairo, he was unable to stop his own guards from pillaging his house. Hussein Aideed, who had been forced to give up his title of president in the spring in order to reach an agreement on the regional government, resumed the title in the fall of 1998. He attempted to reconstitute his base with Eritrean and Arab assistance, while importing new weapons and new bank notes to finance his strategy for reconquest and to trump Ethiopia's allies. Those allies were also receiving substantial military aid, despite the embargo on military equipment imposed by the United Nations Security Council in the spring of 1992.

Toward a Difficult Reconstruction

The reality in Somalia is much more complex and dynamic than the hastily drawn conclusions that apply to only a few hundred people in Mogadishu and to the diplomatic representations of a few countries. Since the beginning of 1998, big businessmen have assumed a role in the life of the capital that they had never played since the outbreak of the civil war.

The business class in Somalia has too often been described as a creature of humanitarian aid that exists only because of the aid. It must be acknowledged, however, that a business economy and even a service economy have now developed in the shadow of the factions. This is quite an exceptional situation, since these businessmen are not assisted by any legal or regulatory structure or even by a banking sector, which is absent from today's Somalia.

The business sector of Somalia may be divided into three quite separate groups. The first group is composed of powerful businessmen who were able to survive and prosper despite the instability of the market, the second consists of medium-sized and small businessmen who took great risks during the war and made commensurate profits, and the third consists of newcomers who have profited immensely from humanitarian aid or related activities, which provided them with an initial capital base. Of the three, the second group is dominant. The third includes a number of individuals whose names are associated with certain factional leaders. Their wealth, however real, is also inherently fragile, not unlike their easily identifiable political alliances.

For reasons too complex to examine here, these businessmen have successfully capitalized on the situation of chaos, even encouraging it at times. Their political ethos is basically no different from that of the factions' partisans, and many of them at one time or another have supported the faction of their choice with hard cash, because this was the norm within their clan and because their prestige in the clan was and remains an essential element in managing the insecurity. Indeed, if a businessman is very popular within his clan, any attack against his property is perceived as an attack against his community.

This system worked well as long as the clan was united behind a group of leaders. The business sector thus merely reflected the contradictions that existed in the political arena. These contradictions, however, were already downplayed because of the need to preserve or increase market share or to forge commercial alliances across clan lines. Such alliances were indispensable in order to operate in a market of any significant size. Taxes were paid, perhaps to the minister closest in kinship in order to avoid any payment of taxes at all if possible, as in the system still in effect in Somaliland. The system of factions thus justified itself while making it impossible to build a government or to establish a fiscal policy. In this sense, hardly any difference exists between the Ali Mahdi government of 1991 and that of the Aideed family after 1995.

These rules of the game could be seriously challenged only if the factions were similarly challenged. A double contradiction was rapidly emerging. On the one hand, as a result of political dynamics, which are not examined here, the mobilization and political centralization of the clans have been declining since 1996. This decline may be traced to individual ambitions, the inability of leaders to fulfil their promises, and the traditional tendency toward division noted in political organizations operating in a fragmented society. On the other hand, the expansion of trade and services could not come about in the absence of certain conditions, foremost among which is the existence of infrastructure and security.

Well before the rapprochement between Hussein Aideed and Ali Mahdi in the spring of 1997, the business sector had on several occasions argued for the reopening of the port of Mogadishu and the maintenance of order in the vicinity of the principal markets. At that time, the distrust was too great to permit any meaningful consensus. Even in the absence of agreement, however, the debate continued.

After giving many unmistakable signals, the business sector declared its autonomy in the spring of 1998. The majority of businessmen refused to provide the funding for the regional administration in Mogadishu on the grounds that the political process, which was welcomed by outsiders, lacked genuine grassroots support. It was finally Egypt, Libya, and a few wealthy associates of the political leaders that provided the funds. Businessmen also refused to pay taxes. After all, why pay for a government that provided no services, improved no roads, and failed to provide security in the markets?

This attitude was also more than a refusal. At the same time, businessmen were funding the establishment of Islamic courts in Mogadishu. It is interesting to note that these courts are organized on the basis of clan, which made their financing easier but reduced their efficiency. One can certainly question the role played by fundamentalist groups, if not in the creation of the courts, then at least in their management, coordination, and supervision. These groups are indeed present and active, even though they currently have no great influence over day-to-day management of the courts or over their important decisions. The great importance of clans was made clear in a number of incidents in which the courts' militias were involved. More important today, security in certain areas of the capital is at an acceptable level, and markets have become safe places.

Clearly, in comparing the divisive influence of the factions with the influence of fundamentalist groups as an emerging actor in Mogadishu, no attempt is being made to demonize one and absolve the other. While the factions with their old methods of operating no longer have anything to offer the population, the political parties, as a collective expression, remain absolutely essential to any resolution of the crisis. It would be an illusion, however, to think that businessmen who enter into politics would behave any better than the politicians who have now been somewhat marginalized. If such a development can be perceived as positive, it is because it penalizes certain methods of operation and encourages reform.

It therefore appears that mobilization at the level of the clan will not in itself resolve the existing problems. Alliances must be made on the basis of common, tangible interests and not on the basis of kinship. In order to be recognized, a government must first of all meet the basic needs of the population. Taxes make no sense unless they are used to solve problems and not to create new ones.

Of course, not everyone today fully shares this analysis. The hurdles of the past have certainly not disappeared, and foreign intervention could still lead to a return to that past. This is a challenge to which even humanitarian organizations and the international community must rise.

Notes

Roland Marchal is a researcher at the Center for International Studies and Research in Paris.

6

The Conflict in Abkhazia

Manuel Sánchez-Montero

Russian rulers have always considered the Caucasus, Russia's southern frontier with the Ottoman and Persian empires, as a bridgehead to the Persian Gulf, a strategic goal of the first importance. This border is also the line of defense for Western interests in the Middle East (Georgia, Turkey, Israel, Jordan, Egypt) against the Islamic countries represented by Iran and the "destabilizing states" (Iraq and Syria). More recently, common interests with the Western countries have reinforced this policy: Georgia and Azerbaijan have just become members of the North Atlantic Treaty Organization (NATO) Partnership for Peace, and Georgia has joined the Council of Europe.

Since the fall of the Soviet empire and the opening up to international markets of the immense reserves of Central Asia (Kazakhstan, Turkmenistan, Uzbekistan) and the Caspian Sea region (Azerbaijan), the Caucasus has been the theater of fierce conflict over control of its strategic mineral resources. The United States, the European Union, and Russia are contesting the export routes for these minerals that, because of their quality and quantity, are of vital importance for the economic and military development of the states. This contest is currently reflected in the rehabilitation of Russian infrastructural works (oil pipelines, railways, roads, and navigable waterways) in Siberia, in the Urals, and north of the Caspian Sea and in the development of multimodal transportation routes by Western countries for the regions of the Caspian Sea, Azerbaijan, Georgia, the Black Sea, and Turkey.

The conflicts in Abkhazia, Ossetia, and Nagorny Karabakh in the South Caucasus and in Chechnya and Ingushetia in the northern

Chronology

1989   Tensions develop between the Abkhazian and Georgian populations over the official use of the Abkhazian language.

1990   Georgia declares its independence from the Soviet Union. Zviad Gamsakhurdia is elected president of the republic in the first elections held in an independent Georgia.

The State of Georgia refuses to sign the treaty of accession to the Commonwealth of Independent States.

Worsening of troubles in Sukhumi; beginning of conflict in Abkhazia with an offensive by the Georgian army.

1992   Dismissal of President Gamsakhurdia; assumption of office by the ex-minister of foreign affairs of the Soviet Union, Eduard Shevardnadze, supported by a large majority of the population of Georgia and by the Western countries.

Beginning of the civil war in Georgia between supporters of the elected president (Zviad Gamsakhurdia) and those of the de facto president (Eduard Shevardnadze).

Intervention of the Russian interposition force under the auspices of the Commonwealth of Independent States.

Ratification and legitimization of the leadership of Shevardnadze, elected president of the Republic of Georgia.

1993   Abkhazian counterattack and fall of Sukhumi (capital of Abkhazia); nearly 250,000 inhabitants of Georgian origin are evacuated to the regions of Mingrelia, Imereti, and Tbilisi.

Offensive by supporters of Gamsakhurdia and fall of the city of Poti.

Accession of the Republic of Georgia to the Commonwealth of Independent States.

Death of Zviad Gamsakhurdia.

1994   End of the Abkhazian offensive; establishment of a line of demarcation in the region of Gali, between the self-proclaimed Republic of Abkhazia and the territory of Georgia, which is ruled by the government in Tbilisi.

Establishment of the United Nations Observer Mission in Georgia; dispatch of mediators to find a solution to the conflict.

1996   The Commonwealth of Independent States (at the request of the Republic of Georgia) imposes an economic and trade blockade against the territory of Abkhazia.

1997   Start of negotiations between the Georgian and Abkhazian authorities; talks are envisaged on a plan for the return of the displaced Georgian population to their homes in Abkhazia.

1998   Explosion of violence in the region of Gali; Abkhazian militias expel some thirty thousand civilians of Georgian origin to the region of Mingrelia.

First breakdown in talks and increasing tensions between the different parties.

1999   Abkhazian authorities unilaterally propose return of displaced persons.

Caucasus are rooted in an ethnic mosaic that has endured in spite of 100 years of Russification and seventy years of Sovietization. The southern Caucasus has a population of eighteen million, which for centuries has been distributed among some 100 ethnic groups speaking more than eighty different languages and subscribing to at least a dozen religious faiths. Relations between these populations have varied from alliances of interests to cruel conflicts.

The conflicts that divide the region, however, are not recent. The Russian conquest united the population of Abkhazia and Georgia within the same province from 1804 to 1917 and later in the Soviet Republic of Georgia from 1917 to 1991. The Abkhazians, native to the mountains of Caucasus, lived secluded in the valleys until the end of the nineteenth century, when they began to descend toward the Abkhazian coast, drawn by the opportunities for employment offered by the nascent tourist industry.

Georgians, Mingrelians, and Svans (originally from the plains and mountains of west Georgia) settled in Abkhazian lands with the Russian colonizers in the eighteenth and early nineteenth centuries. They were joined by Armenians fleeing the Turkish genocide of 1915 and by Greeks who had been present in the region since the period of Byzantine rule.

Starting in the early years of the Soviet era, the Abkhazians, who up until then had been a minority in the region, sought union with the Russian Soviet Republic and demanded their separation from the Soviet Republic of Georgia (1932). The Supreme Soviet, controlled by Stalin (who was of Georgian origin), found a compromise solution by creating the Autonomous Republic of Abkhazia within the Soviet Republic of Georgia. This decision fed the nationalist aspirations of the 1990s, following the collapse of the Soviet Union.

The autonomous status provided a workable solution to the problem in the sixty years that followed. During the period of *perestroika*, Abkhazian nationalist movements emerged at the same time as Georgian nationalism was reawakening (in the late 1980s). Following the declaration of independence of the Abkhazian people and other Russophile minorities (Armenians), the autonomous Abkhazian parliament (controlled by unionist Georgians) proclaimed its union with Georgia. Violent demonstrations broke out between the two communities, which culminated in the first offensive by the new Georgian army. Even though the initial months of fighting favored the unionists, the decisive support of Russian troops tilted the balance in favor of the Abkhazian separatists. The conflict reached a peak with the disastrous collapse of Sukhumi in October 1993 and the expulsion of nearly 250,000 civilians of Mingrelian origin to the regions of Mingrelia, Imereti, and Tbilisi.

54

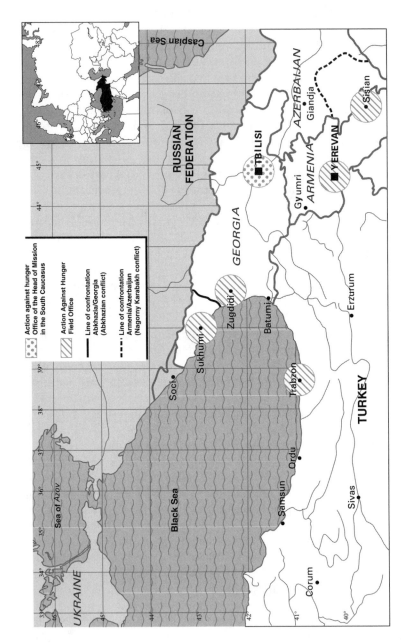

Georgia

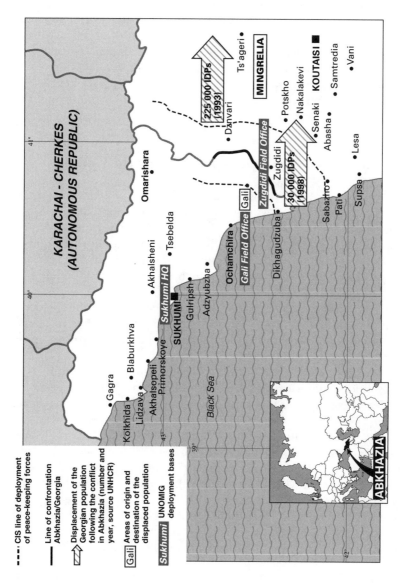

Abkhazia

CIS line of deployment
of peace-keeping forces

Line of confrontation
Abkhazia/Georgia

Displacement of the
Georgian population
following the conflict
in Abkhazia (number and
year, source UNHCR)

Gali Areas of origin and
destination of the
displaced population

Sukhumi UNOMIG
deployment bases

KARACHAI - CHERKES
(AUTONOMOUS REPUBLIC)

MINGRELIA

225 000 IDPs
(1993)

30 000 IDPs
(1998)

Zugdidi Field Office

Gali Field Office Gali

Sukhumi HQ

SUKHUMI

KOUTAISI

Ts'ageri

Potskho
Nakalakevi
Senaki
Abasha
Samtredia
Vani
Lesa
Danvari
Zugdidi
Sabazho
Pati
Supsa
Dikhagudzuba
Ochamchira
Tsebelda
Akhalsheni
Omarishara
Adzyubzna
Gulripsh
Primorskoye
Akhalsopeli
Lidzava
Kolkhida
Gagra
Blaburkhva

Black Sea

ABKHAZIA

Superimposed on the Abkhazian conflict was a more contemporary conflict between the supporters of the elected president, Zviad Gamsakhurdia (the Zviadistas), and the government forces of the de facto president, Eduard Shevardnadze. This conflict, which was waged in the regions of Mingrelia and Imereti, proved a heavy drain on the resources of Georgia and created bitterness and mistrust, particularly among the population of Mingrelia, which even today still supports the unionist and antigovernment parties (paradoxically supported by Moscow) and fosters instability by giving encouragement to armed pro-Zviadista groups.

Displaced Populations: Eradicating the Victims

The Mingrelia region (in west Georgia) is one of the areas of the Caucasus with the highest density of displaced populations. Since 1994, nearly 250,000 people expelled from the territory of Abkhazia have found refuge in the villages and towns of neighboring regions. Mingrelia was the most seriously affected by these events and received nearly 125,000 displaced persons, which increased its population by nearly 27 percent in four years.

These developments led to radical changes: first, in the socioeconomic panorama, in which sectors of the population live in conditions of extreme poverty and instability; second, in the growing insecurity and instability in the region.

The displaced population was accommodated in community centers (schools, factories, warehouses, and so on). The incapacity to absorb the excess labor that suddenly invaded the region's job market and the obstacles encountered by displaced persons seeking access to cultivable land meant that this population was excluded from local economic activity and became more dependent on food aid. More specifically, the displaced population cannot be considered inhabitants of Mingrelia, which means that they cannot enjoy the fundamental civil and social rights to which all Georgians are entitled (including the right to elect their representatives in parliament and their local representatives, access to health and social assistance services, and the right to own land before completing a one-year waiting period).

The government of Georgia has long used the existence of an expelled population concentrated along the line of confrontation with Abkhazia as a means of maintaining pressure on the Abkhazian authorities, at both the international and bilateral levels. The guarantee of the return of 250,000 persons has been used as a bargaining chip to justify its position on the territory of Abkhazia. Thus the return of the displaced Georgians was part of the strategy to attract international funds (in the form of humanitarian assistance or bilateral structural support in order to avert any potential crises that may arise from the instability of the situation). Investment, direct or indirect, of approximately $250 million during the past four years to address humanitarian problems and to meet the social obligations of the Georgian government merely increased the latter's war chest. The dependence of the displaced population on humanitarian aid merely reinforced the "client" relationship between the active Committees for the Displaced and the Georgian political cause and reduced the influence of the so-called Abkhazian government in exile; the provision of humanitarian assistance was cleverly justified by the Georgian authorities as consideration for effective government and the international credibility of its leader, Eduard Shevardnadze.

The Abkhazian government in exile, comprising unionist leaders, was formed early in the evacuation of Sukhumi and supplanted the autonomous authority in Abkhazia. In order to maintain its hold on power, it was necessary for the group to prevent the return of displaced persons to Abkhazia. To achieve that goal, the government in exile has had no hesitation in resorting to attacks against Georgian returnees in Abkhazian territory (in the Gali border region) carried out by the terrorist/paramilitary group known as the White Legion or by the efficient network of Committees of the Displaced that controls all activities in the reception centers for displaced persons. One of their main functions is to follow up humanitarian assistance, and more particularly food aid; by their presence, these committees have in effect established the following equation: Displaced person not under their control means no access to security, work, food aid, or means of food production; displaced person under their control means protection and food aid.

Blockading Besieged Populations—A New Weapon

The Autonomous Republic of Abkhazia had been one of the most privileged regions during the Soviet era. Its abundance of water resources and state investments in industry and infrastructure enabled the population to have a higher standard of living than the average in the Soviet Union. The collapse of the USSR, together with the consequences of the conflict with the government of Tbilisi, led to a virtual paralysis of economic activity.

The economic and trade blockade imposed by the Commonwealth of Independent States (CIS) further exacerbated the situation after January 1996. As a result, it was no longer possible to freely import food products and medicines except through three points of access to the territory: the Inguri bridge in Zugdidi, the frontier post with the Russian Federation at Adler, and the port of Sukhumi. At these access points goods were subject to inspection by the Georgian authorities, the peacekeeping forces, and the Russian frontier guards, who were responsible for monitoring the line of confrontation between Abkhazia and Georgia and the outer frontiers of the CIS. Fuel, medical supplies, tools, raw materials for industry, vehicles, industrial goods, and many other products were subjected either to restrictive quotas or to strict control of their destination and end use by the Russian forces (in most cases, permission to import was delayed indefinitely or even denied).

Even though the collapse of the USSR and the transfer of power from the Soviet Union's communist party to the Russian reformers might have weakened Russia's influence in the southern Caucasus, those two events—the collapse and the transfer of power—did not modify the traditional geopolitical lines. Russia does not appear to have at this time the resources to maintain the apparatus that it had used successfully over the past two centuries to control the destinies of the Transcaucasus.[1] The opening up of the *cordon sanitaire,*[2] after the fall of the Berlin Wall, enabled the Western powers to gain a foothold in an area that included the former Soviet republics. It therefore seems totally unthinkable for Russia to have a strategy of reconquest, association, or even neocolonization. The only possible issue is the destabilization of unruly states, such as Georgia and Azerbaijan. In the case of Georgia, one of the clearest examples of this strategy is Abkhazia. An Abkhazia in revolt and pro-Russia is of value as an instrument of political, economic, and social destabilization. Russian military support in the early stages of the conflict was pushed into the background when a new dimension was introduced into Russian-Georgian relations with the signing by Georgia in 1993 of the agreement to join the CIS. The economic and trade blockade therefore became an integral part of the new strategy adopted. Its consequences were the following:

1. The dramatic decline in the living standards of the Abkhazian population merely exacerbated anti-Georgian sentiment through the unchallenged manipulation of information by the authorities. This radicalization was largely responsible for the impasse reached in the 1997 negotiations between Georgian and Abkhazian authorities.[3] The ongoing mobilization at the grassroots level (forced removal of the

population and catalyzing of its frustrations) resulted in policy of conflict instead of negotiations.

2. Differences in the application of the measures imposed under the blockade on the two frontiers (Russia and Georgia) resulted in the strengthening of Russian influence in Abkhazia. The Abkhazian population, moreover, found itself isolated from the slow process of economic recovery enjoyed by the rest of the region. A government under such severe restrictions and the absence of an official status made it difficult to attract capital, import equipment, or develop local markets. At the same time, however, it led to the flight of labor (political and ethnic refugees to Georgia or economic refugees to Russia).

The population that remained was thus forced to survive by engaging in marginal agricultural activities and most of its members experienced a gradual slide into poverty (selling their jewels, clothing, means of transport, working tools, and so on). This process was accelerated by the inflationary trends that prevailed throughout the region and that were particularly acute in Abkhazia. The absence of mechanisms of control (such as a central bank to supervise monetary policy, structural support from abroad, and diversification of economic activities and markets) is the reason why the Russian crisis had a particularly severe impact on the Abkhazian economy.[4]

Control of the political or armed forces is proportional to the economic resources available. Most of the resources in the territory are generated from the transportation and trading of goods across the Russian frontier. The elite classes and the business sector are the main direct beneficiaries of the limited resources generated from illegal activity, which is regulated by the law of survival of the fittest and has resulted in the inequitable distribution of resources. Given the insecurity in the region (the source of their own power), these groups opt for investments in more lucrative markets (Moscow, Ukraine, or Western Europe), which bring no returns to the resource-starved local economy.

3. The lack of economic development and the steady concentration of power in the hands of certain pressure groups (mafia-warlords) are reflected in the lack of social development. The breakdown of families as a result of forced displacement (political, ethnic, or economic) marked the beginning of the collapse of the entire social structure that had existed before. The results were tragic: Inadequate social welfare networks at the local level left nearly fifty thousand elderly and physically and/or mentally handicapped persons (one-third of the estimated population of Abkhazia) in a state of abandonment,

dependent on the humanitarian assistance provided by international organizations.

The Future: Toward the Conquest of Eurasia

The confirmation of the failure of the Soviet ideal in its struggle against the free world encouraged a new tendency to discredit not only the socialist system but also its welfare and social assistance components. The concept of the liberalization of world markets, mitigated by the "corrective actions" of humanitarian assistance and structural support to disadvantaged countries, became the unchallenged model that has governed relations between states for over a decade. This framework has been approved by the international institutions, including the World Trade Organization (WTO), the International Monetary Fund, and the World Bank. It offers a wide range of instruments: first, support or penalize allied or enemy states; second, increase political and economic influence in the zones of interest to the powers.

The political and economic strategy of the Western powers has several thrusts, one of which is particularly concerned with the food security of the population: structural economic support and bilateral food aid programs.

The production of food staples for the Caucasian diet (local varieties of cereal, such as golden wheat, *hatchar,* and corn) is traditional in certain parts of the region. That production has experienced a number of problems that have resulted in its lack of competitiveness on local and regional markets. These problems include a scarcity of factors of agricultural production of a high-enough quality, obsolescence of the stock of available equipment, unavailability of accessible credit, absence of established markets for food products, strong influence of the interests involved in the importation of cereals, and absence of a clear legal framework governing land ownership.

To these internal factors must be added such external factors as the fall in the value of the ruble (since September 1998), which has led to a drop in the prices of goods from the Russian Federation.

In Armenia, local cereals face competition from the uncontrolled invasion of Russian cereals[5] that cross the borders of the CIS with the indulgence of the customs authorities and the connivance of local authorities.

The importation of surplus food in the guise of food aid[6] is subject to a number of conditions, set by the countries donating food aid. Food products are imported under a tax-exempt regime, the quantities sold must cover only deficits in national production, the income from the sale must be reinvested in agricultural support programs, and, above all, the criteria for the eligibility of beneficiary countries are based not only on considerations of food insecurity but also on criteria of good neighborliness.[7]

One therefore finds agricultural surpluses that are difficult to sell on international markets coming under cooperation budgets; in reality, this constitutes an indirect subsidy to the farmers of the donor country (thereby violating the principles established by these very states and set out in international agreements, such as the WTO agreements). In the meantime, subsidies to farmers in countries such as Georgia and Armenia are penalized.[8]

The immediate effects of this aid policy, such as temporary increases in access to staple foods for a part of the population, are positive. The long-term impacts are more questionable. These include changes in local food habits, drops in the prices of cereals on local markets, and a lessening of interest by the local population in the production of cereals.[9]

Nongovernmental Organizations in the Caucasus, or How to Run with the Hare and Hunt with the Hounds

Obtaining resources from international agencies and support from local actors must be accompanied by respect for human rights.

The framework for the action taken by Action Against Hunger in the Caucasus has three main thrusts.

The first of these is immediate measures. These include direct support for victims through projects for the distribution of food and/or tools and the technical assistance needed to achieve a minimum degree of food security.

The second thrust is that of medium-term actions. One of these actions is the identification and strengthening of the capacity to organize and supervise the activities of local entities. Another is the development of an organized social network that can play an increasingly active role in defending the interests of victims and in ensuring the sustainability of the activities undertaken by Action Against Hunger.

The third thrust is that of long-term actions. By these are meant identification and analysis of the human rights violated in the different conflicts and activities to promote awareness and provide information to local and international actors and organizations.

Notes

Manuel Sánchez-Montero is chief of mission for Action Against Hunger in the southern Caucasus.

1. Traditionally, the Transcaucasus was the name given by the Russian authorities to the region of the southern Caucasus.

2. This term is understood to mean the system of client states controlled by the USSR during the Cold War as a means of protecting the territories of Russia itself and particularly Mother Russia.

3. The maintenance of the economic blockade against Abkhazia was one of the principal reasons cited by the Abkhazian authorities for not resuming negotiations.

4. Between August 1998 and January 1999, the cost of the items in an average food basket rose by 280 percent.

5. The quantities of cereals imported from Russia are not recorded. The CIF (cost, insurance, and freight) price of a ton of Russian wheat from Yerevan is $190. The price of the same quantity of Armenian wheat on the local market is $230.

6. Last year, the state of Armenia authorized the acceptance of 300,000 tons of U.S. wheat as food aid for the next thirty years in order to cover the deficit in local production, which is estimated to be 10,000 tons annually. The quantity sold on local markets for 1998 alone was 30,000 tons.

7. The example may be given of the coverage in food aid for a zone such as Nagorno Karabakh in the South Caucasus, while the population of Abkhazia is excluded from this type of aid.

8. The structural support measures for the economies that emerged from the Soviet system include budgetary control and stabilization of the public treasury. In this connection, the International Monetary Fund has decided on the assessment of a tax of twenty dollars per ton of cereal produced/sold in Georgia, which in no way helps the competitiveness of local products.

9. The CIF price in Yerevan of a ton of U.S. wheat is $125. By way of illustration, in the last few years in the province of Sissian (where Action Against Hunger is undertaking food security projects), the area of land devoted to the growing of cereals fell from 22,000 to 4,000 hectares.

7

Tajikistan: What Role for Nongovernmental Organizations?

Jean-Michel Grand, Chris Leather,
and Frances Mason

The *kolkhoz* (collective farm) provided the basis for rural livelihoods in Tajikistan during the Soviet era. The breakup of the Soviet Union and the subsequent civil war in Tajikistan ultimately led to the collapse of the kolkhoz and to the political and economic marginalization of poor, rural households. This chapter analyzes the impact of the collapse on the rural poor and assesses the opportunities and constraints for nongovernmental organizations (NGOs) working to improve the food security of rural households.

Political Turmoil in the Post-Soviet Era

Following the disintegration of the Soviet Union in 1991, the independence of Tajikistan was a destabilizing factor for this country of fewer than six million people. The end of the Soviet era marked the outbreak of a struggle between the five main regionalist groups in Tajikistan: Leninabadis, Gharmis, Pamiris, Kulyabis, and ethnic Uzbeks. These communities are defined according to their area of origin. The causes of the 1992–1993 civil war are multifarious and complex, involving ideological, religious, and ethnic factors. One issue, which is given relatively little coverage in the analyses of the conflict, is the extent to which the conflict was a struggle for control of the resources of the country (land, cotton, and aluminum) and for control of the government, which remains synonymous with power and self-enrichment. The war was also motivated by a desire to control the drug trafficking network. The drug trade is a major source of

Chronology

September 1991	Independence of Tajikistan from the Soviet Union.
July 1992–January 1993	Elections. Height of the civil war.
May 1995	Introduction of the Tajik rouble.
1995	First presidential decree allocating land for household use.
August 1995	Devaluation of the national currency.
June 1996	Decree legalizing the establishment of private dekhan farms.
June 1997	Signing of the General Agreement for the Establishment of Peace and National Accord.
1997	Second presidential decree allocating land for household use.
Late 1999–early 2000	Parliamentary and presidential elections.

wealth in a country that has a low level of drug production but is the transit route for producers in Afghanistan, Pakistan, Southeast Asia, and so on and an open door to Russia.

A brutal civil war erupted in 1992, leading to the flight of approximately 250,000 people to neighboring countries (Afghanistan, Uzbekistan, Kyrgyzstan, Russia, among others) and to the internal displacement of an estimated 700,000 people. Approximately 50,000 people were killed for belonging (or on suspicion of belonging) to one of the regionalist groups. Violence between the different factions precluded the emergence of a sense of national identity and led the country into a prolonged regionalist struggle, which has lasted for eight years without any decisive military or political solutions having been found, despite the signing of a peace agreement in June 1997.

The current status quo is mainly due to pressure from a Contact Group consisting of Uzbekistan, Turkmenistan, Afghanistan, Pakistan, Iran, and Russia, which led to the signing of the peace agreement. This group, paradoxically, wants to prevent the instability in Tajikistan from spreading to the rest of Central Asia, even though the divergent national interests of the member states of the group also serve to prolong the instability in Tajikistan.

In 1992, Russia and Uzbekistan were not satisfied with the results of the elections in Tajikistan, which had given power to a democratic

Islamic majority. The two countries were therefore instrumental in the outbreak of civil conflict and were directly involved militarily through their troops on the ground. Russia and Uzbekistan could not take the risk of allowing a pro-Islamist government to become established in Tajikistan, which could have become a backyard for Uzbek Islamist opposition and could have had a domino effect on Central Asian republics and on the volatile Muslim republics of Russia.

Russia's support led to the Kulyabi group's coming to power. Consequently, the present government is fully in favor of a permanent Russian military presence on Tajik territory. As for Uzbekistan, its supporters were excluded from the peace process and from government structures. Uzbekistan is now concerned that its influence is jeopardized by the Russian military presence. The two countries clash through their support for different Tajik factions as they jostle for power and control of a country that is of major political and economic significance in the region.

Currently, Tajikistan is still engaged in the implementation of a difficult peace process, which is made all the more fragile by a lack of will to compromise and the threat of a resumption of fighting. The latter is most likely to be initiated by the parties excluded from the power structures and from the peace process, that is, the ethnic Uzbek and the Leninabadi populations. The current political scene is tripartite in nature:

- The Kulyabis supported by Russia control the governmental structures.
- The ethnic Uzbek population and the Leninabadis are excluded from these governmental structures and from the peace process but are supported by Uzbekistan.
- A democratic Islamic opposition, consisting mainly of Gharmis and Pamiris, is supported neither by Russia nor Uzbekistan but could play an intermediary role if a conflict emerges between the first two parties. This group also represents a significant armed force in the country and, following the 1997 peace agreement, has been progressively involved in the power structures.

This political situation does not favor a quick settlement of the Tajik conflict. The current balance remains extremely precarious and could degenerate into conflict, despite the combined efforts of international organizations such as the United Nations Mission of

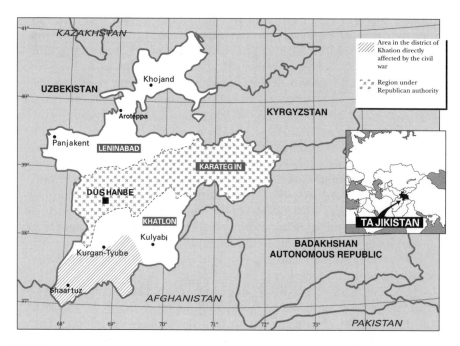

Tajikistan

Observers in Tajikistan (UNMOT), the Organization for Security and Cooperation in Europe (OSCE), and the Contact Group, which are all working toward a national and international settlement of the conflict.

The possibility of national reconciliation still exists but will require the willingness to share the power among the different regionalist factions. Parliamentary and presidential elections were held in November 1999 and February 2000, the first multiparty elections in the history of the country. Although the parliamentary elections were monitored by the OSCE,[1] there were many concerns of irregularities reported during the campaigns and voting.[2] The results showed an apparent turnout of 98 percent and the incumbent president winning by a 96.4 percent majority. However, the fear that the opposition members might lose their position in the government was at least temporarily lessened, as the president ensured that their 30 percent of seats were retained. Russia has since made it clear that were the country to descend into political turmoil once more, Russia's forces would not hesitate to undertake a military intervention.

Collapse of Agriculture and the Food Crisis

Continuing military and political tensions have served only to exacerbate and prolong the economic crisis that has resulted from the collapse of the Soviet economic system and the civil war. Tajikistan was already the poorest republic in the Soviet Union. The end of the Soviet era resulted in the cessation of subsidies from Moscow and of the supply of raw materials and inputs from other Soviet states. The rate of unemployment soared without any hope of social protection from the central government. The postcommunist and postwar period during which there has been some movement toward the establishment of democracy and a free-market economy has failed to live up to the expectations of the population, and there is a pervasive sense of nostalgia for the previous system, when the state assured the provision of food, access to free health care, education, pensions, and salaries, even if these were low.

The civil war led to the further breakdown of economic networks, a loss of confidence by investors, deterioration of the productive infrastructure, emigration of professionals, and capital flight. The absence of coherent and effective policies to address these problems causes resentment among the general population, which sees political leaders as ruling the country in their own interest and that of their region of origin. The political and economic instability of the country combined with the self-interest of the government has led to knee-jerk reactions in the form of policies providing short-term responses to long-term problems. This is particularly well illustrated in the agricultural sector.

Prior to the breakup of the Soviet Union, the main source of livelihood for rural households was the collective farm (the *kolkhoz*) or the state farm (the *sovkhoz*). Workers on these farms were paid for working as members of a brigade, which was responsible for a particular tract of land. The state told the kolkhoz what should be produced and in what quantity. The workers were paid in relation to production targets set by the farm.

Until 1995, the kolkhoz were still able to pay their members a small salary, despite the falloff in production resulting from the breakdown of the centrally planned economy and the effects of the civil war. However, the devaluation of the currency in that year led to the bankruptcy of most of the state and collective farms. Since that time, the farms have been unable to recover and usually have to sell their produce in advance to pay off debts.

The productivity of the kolkhoz has also been affected by the same range of factors, resulting in the collapse of overall economic production. The farms have suffered in particular from the

- breakdown in the system for the supply of inputs and of distribution channels;
- destruction, looting, and deterioration of buildings, irrigation systems, and assets;
- emigration of skilled professionals;
- control of the input supply and marketing by state monopolies;
- breakdown of the system for the control and monitoring of production, resulting in increased corruption and the diversion of capital and assets.

By 1995, the collapse of agricultural production combined with the poor harvest of the previous year led to a food supply crisis and to dramatic increases in the price of wheat. At this time, Tajikistan was the only country in the Commonwealth of Independent States (CIS) that had a Ministry of Grain responsible for the regulation of the price of bread. Yet even with this regulation, the price of bread increased sixfold in the first six months of 1995. The country needed to import 600,000 metric tons of wheat per year but lacked the financial resources to pay market prices.

In a country in which only 7 percent of the land is arable, access to land and food is a sensitive issue, and sound economic policies must be based on careful consideration of the most effective and efficient use of land. Strategies to meet the food requirements of the population are no longer constrained only by the limited availability of cultivable land. The country also urgently requires foreign currency to be able to acquire spare parts, fuel, and raw materials for both the industrial and agricultural sectors in order to increase production and thereby enable the payment of normal wages and the provision of social protection to the population. Cotton and aluminum were the largest foreign exchange earners during the Soviet period and remain a major source of revenue for the government. In effect, there is a trade-off between food production and foreign currency earned from the export of cotton, since wheat and cotton compete for the limited land available.

Government Responses to the Food Crisis

Faced with a food supply crisis in 1995, the government was forced to rapidly introduce policies to address the problem of food shortages in the near to medium term. Primarily, this meant increasing the production of wheat on collective farms and allocating land for the production of wheat at the household level, even if this was at the expense of cotton production.

In 1995, the first presidential decree was issued allocating 50,000 hectares of farmland for household use. This was primarily targeted at professionals and recipients of state benefits, including teachers, doctors, engineers, and pensioners. In 1997, a second presidential decree allocated a further 25,000 hectares, this time prioritizing the needs of collective farmers. The duration of use of this so-called Presidential Land allocated by the government is often not precisely defined and is left to the discretion of the kolkhoz leaders. In some instances, the kolkhoz has taken back the plot of land after two or three harvests after the fertility has improved and has allocated an inferior plot to the household.

The measures taken by the government following the food crisis of 1995 could be described as short-term decisions made to reduce the food production deficit. More recently, however, the government has started to review its policy of land reforms and wheat production in light of the need for foreign currency. The current trend in the national policy has been to increase or to at least maintain levels of cotton production. The government still asks the kolkhoz to plant a certain proportion of their land with cotton (often up to 60 percent). There has also been recognition of the need to establish a balance between the allocation of land to permit households to meet their food requirements through their own production while ensuring that farm sizes are sufficient to maximize production for the population as a whole. There is a limit to the extent to which land reform can involve the fragmentation of the land into smaller household units.

A major source of hard currency for the country is the World Bank, which offers loans on condition that the government agrees to implement the economic reforms outlined by the International Monetary Fund (IMF), among which privatization is, of course, foremost. To date, however, most of the agricultural land remains the property of the state, although there have been significant initiatives to allocate land for private use.

In June 1996, a decree legalized the establishment of *dekhan* or private farms independent of the kolkhoz. Although dekhan farmers do not legally own their land, they have full hereditary rights, are required to pay taxes, and can make their own decisions regarding cultivation and land use. In reality, however, some control has been retained over the use of the land. In fact, the utilization of dekhan land is monitored by the Agricultural Department of the district. If the department considers that the land is not being used efficiently and effectively, it can be reclaimed by the kolkhoz. The allocation of land to private farmers is clearly not in the personal interests of the leaders of the kolkhoz, who would ultimately lose a part of their power, influence, and ability to profit from the diversion of capital and produce. However, a variety of attitudes is apparent among chairmen, ranging from pure self-interest to a genuine concern for the social and economic development of the members of the kolkhoz and their region.

Despite pressure from international financial institutions, such as the World Bank and the IMF, or from donors, such as the European Union and the United States of America, to promote privatization of the land, the government is still reluctant to do so. One of the reasons could be the risk of losing control over the economy, especially in cotton production, which is one of the major sources of revenue for the Tajik government. The government is still able to exert firm control over the kolkhoz by determining the levels of cotton production and controlling the supply of inputs and the distribution channels.

Government agricultural policy since the end of the civil war may be characterized as short term and lacking in coherence and consistency. To some extent, it has been necessary to address the immediate problem of ensuring an adequate supply of food for the population. However, there has been little progress in implementing the reforms that would enable longer-term increases in agricultural production. The uncertainties of the government and the lack of a coherent national economic policy have affected the most vulnerable households in particular. The brief analysis presented above reveals the marginalization of the majority of rural households from the benefits of large-scale agricultural production.

Analysis of the Food Security of Rural Households

Impact of the Collapse of the Kolkhoz at the Household Level

The most significant impact of the economic collapse on collective farmers was the low level or nonpayment of salaries. There is no obligation for people to work on the kolkhoz. However, a number of factors "encourage" families to "offer" their labor. These factors vary in the extent to which they can be considered as coercive and verging on forced labor. The kolkhoz do offer various forms of remuneration for work beyond cash payment: for instance, collection of fuel wood and the allocation of low-quality land. Most often these incentives are just sufficient to attract workers while being kept to a minimum by the kolkhoz to reduce production costs. Many workers continue their labor in anticipation of future payment. Circumstances have been reported in which people are forcibly made to work on the kolkhoz and threatened if they refuse.

Alternative Sources of Cash Income

The possibility of earning cash outside of the kolkhoz is also severely limited. The government cannot afford to pay, on a regular basis, the salaries of public sector workers or the benefits of those classified as being vulnerable, such as pensioners and disabled people. The economic crisis has had the same result on the industrial sector as on the agricultural sector, resulting in high rates of unemployment. Trade is controlled by the mafia to the exclusion of small businesspeople. As a consequence of these limited opportunities, household members adopt coping strategies such as involvement in the drug trade, migration to towns and other countries, and temporary contract labor in construction or as market carriers.

Household Food Production and Its Determinants

In the absence of income from the kolkhoz and because of the lack of alternative income earning opportunities, rural households are heavily dependent for their food security on their own production from small plots of land. Owing to the low levels of production, the amount of surplus food available is limited. The household economy revolves around constant trade-offs between the consumption of sufficient food and the sale of produce to purchase basic necessities such as oil, sugar, salt, medicines, and clothing. Food and cash income are often insufficient to cover all requirements, thus threatening the nutritional, health, and educational standards of the population. The capacity of households to meet their food requirements through their own production is determined by a range of factors.

Access to land. Despite the restrictions placed on the use of Presidential Land and the uncertainty of tenure, there is no doubt that its allocation has made a significant difference to the food security of both urban and rural households. In the absence of sufficient cash income, such land is often the most important source of food for many families. Ultimately, however, the access of households to land for their own production is limited by the lack of cultivable land, the priorities of the national economy, and local political relationships.

Irrigation. The method and capacity of irrigation are the most significant factors and may account for up to 50 percent of the shortfall in potential yield. Irrigation systems have ceased to function because channels have become broken or clogged by sediment, pumping systems have broken down, and capital and spare parts to make repairs are lacking. In many cases, the system of organization that used to ensure their maintenance and management no longer functions. Without irrigation, households are unable to harvest a second crop of cereals in the same year, thus reducing significantly the quantity of food acquired from their own production.

Access to inputs. Another important factor that determines household output is access to inputs, such as high-quality seeds, fertilizers, tools, pesticides, fuel, and spare parts for machinery. Farm machinery is either unavailable, inoperable, or unsuitable for use by individual farmers on small plots of land.

Climatic conditions. Climate plays a highly significant role and can account for marked variations in productivity from year to year, particularly in rain-fed areas. In Khatlon Oblast in the southwest of the country, the length of the growing season decreases by about one month from west to east, mainly as a result of the increase in altitude.

Livestock. The capacity of households to keep livestock is determined by the extent of their access to pasture, fodder, and veterinary services. Most households cannot afford to purchase high-quality feed for their livestock, which could increase milk yields and improve the health of the animals and hence the cash income of the family.

Availability of labor. To some extent, all of the above factors are influenced by the availability of labor within the family. Over the past seven to eight years that availability may have been reduced as result of deaths (from war or disease) and economic migration. The returnee population has been particularly affected in this respect. In some "returnee villages," over 25 percent of households are headed by women. However, even those households less directly affected by the war may have experienced a loss of agricultural labor as members (particularly young men) have migrated to the capital, Dushanbe, or to other countries in the CIS to seek work. This circumstance not only has an impact on agricultural productivity but has significant social costs due to the breakup of the family unit.

Vulnerabilities and Capacity to Cope of Poor, Rural Households

A final factor to take into consideration in analyzing food security is the capacity of households to cope with ad hoc events that further reduce the productivity of the household, such as the death of a family member or poor rainfall resulting in a poor harvest. If in a bad year the household experiences a drop in food income from its own production, it may be forced to sell some of its assets, notably livestock, in order to acquire food and other necessities. The risk is that the capacity of households to withstand the effects of further setbacks will gradually be exhausted. This is particularly true for the returnee population, which experienced almost total loss of its capital and assets during the war. Despite the fact that the majority of refugees have been resettled in their former villages for at least two to three years, most have still not been able to rebuild sufficient assets and capital to see them through periodic hardship without jeopardizing their ability to cope in the longer term.

Geography as a Determinant of Vulnerability

Analysis of geographical variations in the influence of some of these factors suggests a pattern that may be useful to understanding the differences in the food economies, risk levels, and vulnerability of different geographical areas.

Key characteristics that can be used to distinguish between different food economy areas are altitude and relief as well as proximity to commodity and labor markets. Areas may be divided into four categories: (1) mountainous, (2) accessible rural lowland, (3) remote rural lowland, and (4) urban industrial.

The principal economic activities in mountainous areas are animal husbandry and grain and fruit production. Even though households have been affected by the collapse of the kolkhoz, they have been able to cope much more easily than those in other areas owing to fewer restrictions on access to and use of land and to a greater diversity in food sources through the sale of fruits, livestock, and wild products.

Analysis suggests that the most vulnerable of all rural households are those in the remote lowlands that depend almost exclusively on their own production to meet their food requirements, which they are the least able to satisfy owing to the small size and poor quality of their plots, the lack of irrigation, poor access to inputs, and low labor availability within the household. These households are most likely to be found in remote areas, where cotton is the main product of the kolkhoz and cereal production is low. Where the influence of these economic factors is compounded by the impact of the war on household assets, the highest proportion of vulnerable households is likely to be found.

The situation of poor families in urban areas is thought to be even more desperate than that of rural dwellers. Despite the range of income-earning activities (e.g., wage labor, petty trade, contract labor) available in the cities, these are accessible only to a minority of people on a temporary and irregular basis. Competition is strong, and returns on labor are low.

Opportunities for and Constraints on Humanitarian Assistance

Trends in Humanitarian Assistance

As might be expected, humanitarian intervention began in Tajikistan to address the effects of the war through the provision of material assistance to meet the urgent basic needs of the population. As the situation has changed, the nature of humanitarian assistance has evolved away from direct relief strategies to approaches that seek to build the capacities of households, civil institutions, and government structures to be more productive and self-sufficient. While this transition takes place, interventions have tended increasingly to address the impact of the economic collapse and transition rather than the consequences of the civil war. It is important to emphasize that it is the breakdown of the previous political and economic system and the structural problems inherent in this change that are the fundamental causes of the poverty of so many households. The civil war was a consequence of these changes and exacerbated their effects, but it should not be seen as the sole determinant of the economic crisis facing the country.

Increasing Household Food Production

Beyond the free distribution of material inputs, such as food, to meet the needs of the population for survival, the intervention of Action Against Hunger is usually geared toward increasing the capacity of vulnerable households to sustainably produce their own food. In Tajikistan, the potential for increasing household agricultural production is quickly reached owing to the limited availability of land and inputs. Furthermore, increasing food production at the household level is a short-term strategy and may not be desirable from a macroeconomic perspective.

Organizations can work within these constraints to increase production from lands already under cultivation. Unfortunately, this measure may not be sustainable on a long-term basis, since, apart from the small plots around individual houses, land allocated to households could be reclaimed at any time by the kolkhoz. Some organizations that have facilitated the lease of land from kolkhoz to households have already experienced this problem. In these circumstances, it is difficult to encourage a community approach to farming. The objective of any intervention often has to remain the development of farming on individual plots.

Improved access to agricultural inputs is an objective that NGOs may be able to achieve. Clearly, many households are unable to afford the cost and overheads of high-quality inputs. However, the constraints are such that, even if inputs were distributed free of charge or at subsidized prices, individual families would still have difficulty in acquiring the products they need. NGOs could therefore encourage cooperative purchases and supply inputs to groups of households.

There is still an important role for international NGOs to play in providing direct assistance and in increasing the agricultural output of families. Organizations might try to contribute in the following areas:

- Assist family farms and collectivities in increasing their food production, having regard to the macroeconomic and political constraints;
- Support private initiatives for the creation of small businesses to supply agricultural inputs and to process and market agricultural produce;
- Provide "emergency assistance" for the most vulnerable households during the difficult transition period;
- Monitor on an ongoing basis the food security situation of families so as to be able to identify any worsening of their vulnerabilities or loss of their ability to cope and to be able to target assistance with greater accuracy.

However, the current situation in Tajikistan is such that food production from family plots cannot be the only resource on which rural dwellers can rely to meet their needs. Investment in large-scale agriculture and industries is needed in order to create jobs for those unable to produce enough on their own plots to meet their needs.

Conclusions

Since the breakup of the Soviet Union, rural households in Tajikistan have become increasingly marginalized from the means of improving their access to food and cash income. The breakdown of the former economic system has led to high rates of unemployment and to the nonpayment of wages without the possibility of receiving any unemployment benefits from the state. In the absence of alternative sources of income, the majority of households have been forced to turn to the land in order to meet their food requirements. Yet, their capacity to do so is limited in a fundamental way by the scarcity of cultivable land and by political decisions on access to land. Dysfunctional input-supply networks and irrigation systems further limit the capacity of households to produce sufficient food for consumption or market exchange.

The government is faced with major dilemmas if it is concerned with improving the food security of the population through reforms of the agricultural sector. These dilemmas require choices or trade-offs to be made between

- food crop or cash crop production;
- collective or private production; and
- small-scale or large-scale production.

The nature of government policies will be determined by personal, economic, national, and international political considerations. Currently, change is infrequent and slowly implemented. Agricultural policy appears to be caught in an impasse between liberalization and state control, as the *apparatchiks* seek to hold on to a system in which they have powerful vested interests, while concessions are made to free-market reform in order to maintain international financial support. It is often these same *apparatchiks* who derive the benefits from the liberalization of the economy as they utilize their financial power and political influence to increase their control over the means of production and the trading networks. It is in this chaotic economic "system" that poor rural households become increasingly marginalized from access to economic and political structures.

The ability of international NGOs to provide assistance in such a context is constrained by macroeconomic and political factors that they are not well placed to address. However, they do still have an important role to play in improving household food security. This can be achieved by promoting household food production and income-generation while providing a safety net for vulnerable households as the country proceeds through an unpredictable and complex political and economic transition.

Notes

Jean-Michel Grand is Action Against Hunger's head of mission in Tajikistan. Chris Leather is the Action Against Hunger officer in charge of food security in Tajikistan. Frances Mason is head of the Nutrition and Food Security Department of Action Against Hunger–London.

1. Organization for the Security and Cooperation in Europe.

2. Confirmed by the Joint Election Observation Mission to Tajikistan in a press release issued 27 February 2000 on the parliamentary elections.

8

Colombia:
A People Displaced by Violence

Pablo Alcade Subias

Paz con hambre no dura. La lucha el pan nos asegura.
[Peace with hunger cannot endure. Only by fighting can we survive.]
—Painted in the streets of central Bogotá

Forced internal migration in the aftermath of violent events is the most serious consequence of the present armed conflict in Colombia. Its worrying increase is the result of regular attacks on the civilian population, and its immediate consequence is the victims' loss of citizenship. More than 3 percent of the Colombian population is directly affected by this phenomenon, which forces its victims to abandon their property and their region and, in the majority of cases, to join the expanding belts of poverty around the towns.

Some 308,000 people are estimated to have been violently displaced during 1998 by the climate of terror, death, and exodus created by the massacres, assassinations, and threats by the various armed groups. In 1999, approximately eight households per hour were driven from their homes in Colombia.[1]

The civilian population is the main victim of this endless situation of crisis. As a general rule, confrontations between factions do not spin out of control. It is rare for these factions to reach the point of actual fighting or to engage in direct clashes. In contrast, they prey with impunity on the innocent population and on the groups of isolated farmers who live in conflict zones. Thus, taking their scorched-earth strategy to its height, guerillas and paramilitaries launch extremely violent attacks on families and their property for no reason other than the fact that they happen to live in areas through which

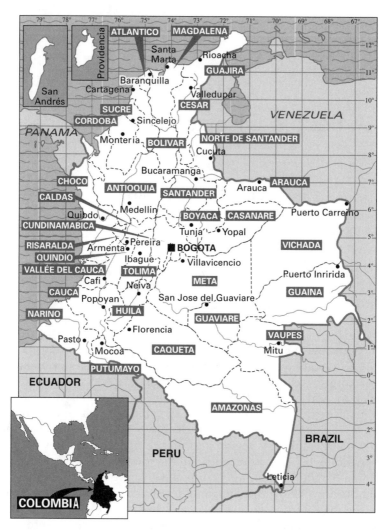

Colombia

either of the two factions pass. These attacks sometimes take the form of atrocious massacres or selective killings. Anyone who is suspected of having given so much as a glass of water to a combatant finds himself immediately in the line of fire of the enemy. The civilian population has become a military target and must consequently "submit, die, or flee," according to the code imposed by the rule of arms.

Carlos Castaño, leader of Autodefensas Unidas de Colombia, a paramilitary group that emerged out of the movement founded by stockbreeders and landowners to protect themselves against guerilla incursions, declares:

> In the present irregular war, a civilian population that finds itself caught up in military operations necessarily becomes a participant. The difference is that the aim of the guerilla group is to make sure that its militancy passes unnoticed within the civilian population so that it can conceal its terrorist actions. The civilian population is therefore dragged into a conflict of which it is the primary victim.[2]

The book *La Guerra Moderna* states the following: In modern warfare "it is difficult to define the enemy. ... The dividing line between friends and enemies exists within the nation itself, within the same town and sometimes within the same family. Every individual who in one way or another favors the intentions of the enemy must be considered a traitor and treated as such."[3]

Faced with the repression and ruthlessness of the guerillas, paramilitary groups, and even the army, Colombians—approximately one and a half million of them at the present time—have been forced to pack their bags and leave with their families, abandoning crops and homes.[4] The path they follow is always the same: They head to the nearest suburbs and settle in a marginal space between the trash cans and the sewers where they set up small makeshift homes known as *cambunches,* made of cardboard and plastic, from which they hope to begin a new life. Most of the time the change from farming a fertile plot of land to existence in this new and hostile environment ends up cutting people off from everything and leads to lives of poverty, small-scale selling,[5] prostitution, alcoholism, and family violence.

The majority of these migratory flows are concentrated in areas on the fringes of urban centers where people attempt with little success to satisfy their immediate needs for health services, food, and water and later their need for housing and work. The fundamental consequences are the rupture of the social fabric, collapse of rural economies, and the breakup of rural communities and family units. The population density in the areas on the fringes of Colombian towns continues to rise. These populations do not seek to return to their former lands on which they grew yucca, bananas, or corn, but to survive at all costs in the face of the hardship of the urban environment, which is so hostile to the newcomer from the countryside.

The government, however, has repeatedly refused to assume its real responsibilities and deludes itself when it argues that return is the only possible option, the only solution worth considering. It seems unaware that this return means an implicit mortal risk, which few families are willing to take. The trauma caused by the sight of razed villages and of relatives or other farmers who have been killed prevents the majority of displaced persons from returning to their land. A few months later, the family will attempt to build a new life with its makeshift home and its possessions now reduced to a minimum.

In his speech delivered on 7 January 1999, during negotiations with the Armed Revolutionary Forces of Colombia (FARC), President Andrés Pastrana declared that "Colombia could not continue to be divided into three irreconcilable countries of which the first kills, the second dies and the third, terrified, lowers its head and averts its gaze."[6] But, in this speech, the president forgot to mention a fourth country: this Colombia in flight, the victim of barbarity, which has no other option than to abandon everything and to wander in search of shelter. Indeed, the Colombian government has paid little attention to the displaced. Unofficially, for a long time, the exodus has always been associated with deliberate disruptions of public order, and those involved have been suspected of maintaining connections and supporting insurgent movements. The Colombian state never ceases to prove its inability and/or lack of desire to find solutions for the underlying causes, provide humanitarian aid to the displaced, and alleviate the social consequences of displacement. Under Ernesto Samper's government, legal means to support the displaced were hesitantly created by means of Act No. 387 of 1997, which provides for protection in the case of forced displacement: support, protection, assistance, and socioeconomic stability for those displaced by violence within the Republic of Colombia. But these provisions are merely theoretical and are rarely put into practice. Similarly, the creation of a Presidential Council for the Support of Displaced Persons had few achievements during the previous presidency and has remained inactive under the new administration.

The Geography of Violence

While the Colombian conflict extends to the whole country, scenes of war are witnessed mainly in the rural areas, from north to south and from east to west. FARC guerillas control large areas of the Amazonian region and the Orinoco basin as well as its traditional bastions in the Urabá, along the Andes cordillera, and on the Atlantic Coast. The National Liberation Army (ELN), although weakened in recent times, remains active in certain parts of Magdalena and Cauca, in the south of Bolívar, Santanderes, and Arauca. On the other hand, the Autodefensas and other paramilitary groups are rapidly extending their control to an ever-increasing number of regions across the country. Based initially in the northwestern regions, their presence is now stronger all along Magdalena, on the Atlantic coast, and they are steadily advancing toward the principal strongholds of the FARC situated in the east of the country. Meanwhile, the government's army has been on the defensive against relentless and skillful guerilla attacks.

This conflict area coincides with the geographical location of illicit crops in a country that has become the world's top coca producer and one of the main producers of marijuana and poppy. The armed struggle is very often a struggle for control of these zones of cultivation. In other cases, the fighting conceals a fierce battle for control of regions rich in mineral resources (gold, oil, and emeralds). The sources of Colombia's wealth are the root cause of conflict in one of the most biologically diverse places on the continent.[7]

From a socioeconomic perspective, the most striking contrast in Colombia is precisely the very visible gulf between extreme wealth and extreme poverty. Economic differences between social groups, so common in all of the Latin American countries, are particularly glaring in Colombia. Unequal and inequitable distribution of wealth in a fragile state in which for decades governments have relied on patronage, political interests, and corruption creates an explosive cocktail of problems that transforms the road to peace into a painful dead end. As a result of these intractable problems, it is always the same groups of families that are displaced by violence and forced to share space with the poorest classes, the marginalized masses in the poverty belts around the villages and towns. When all is said and done, given the state's incapacity, the displaced are the final link in the chain, which only worsens their situation and sows the seeds of future conflict.

The Geography of Displacement

From the geographical location of the conflict, a zone of displacement has emerged that covers the country from one end to the other. Regions such as the south (Meta, Caquetá, Guaviare, Vaupés, and Putumayo), Urubá (Chocó, d'Antioquia, and Córdoba), southern Bolivar, Cesar, and Santander are the scene of confrontations, victims of the State's helplessness and passivity. Floods of terrified emigrants are on the move daily, and the map of displacement currently shows large concentrations of displaced people in the main Colombian towns (particularly Bogotá and Medellín, spilling over into Cali, Barranquilla, Bucaramanga, Villaviciencio, and Cartagena). Smaller towns such as Montería and Sincelejo on the Atlantic coast, Barrancabermeja in Magdalena Medio, or smaller municipalities (Magangué, El Carmen, Río Sucio) receive even more new families that arrive silent and unaided, crammed together and melting into the anonymity, poverty, and indifference of the urban environment. Yet other groups remain refugees in administrative centers or small villages near the conflict zones, waiting for a truce that never arrives to allow them to return or at least to recover their property or the remainder of their harvests.

One of the characteristics of Colombia's displaced population is its individual and silent character. Unlike other exoduses in other parts of the world that become real movements of wandering crowds, in Colombia such massive mobilizations are unusual. There are important exceptions, some of them significant, but the majority of the displaced are made up of an endless trickle of lowly families whose fear of violence eventually prevails over their attachment to their land and life's work.

For this reason, we do not see large concentrations of these united but isolated populations, despite the overall size of the population movement. In Colombia, few camps are set up for the displaced. On the contrary, those who flee prefer to do so discreetly and anonymously. They avoid forming groups with other displaced persons in order not to leave any trace and to prevent violence from pursuing them in their exile, as has very often occurred. Temporary camps or refuges are specific examples of exceptions to this rule (though insignificant in terms of the number of people they accommodate). The best known among them is that of Pavarandó (Urabá d'Antioquia), although mention should also be made of the coliseum of Quibdo or that of Turbo, the dangerous refuges of Barrancabermeja, and the precarious camp for displaced people at Tierradentro (in the south of Córdoba).

The steady exodus to towns and villages has resulted in an inordinate increase in the population density of the suburbs as new residents join the impoverished population already living there. Consequently, large urban areas are converted into "districts of the displaced" where the heavy concentration of people has a great effect on the family groups fleeing the conflict zones. Displaced by violence or poverty, each person struggles to survive in surroundings of general degradation in the new citadels of the displaced such as "Nelson Mandela" in Cartagena, the district of Cantaclaro in Montería,

Ciudad Bolivar in Bogotá, the communes of Medellín, and many others.

The Arduous Road to Peace

It is clear that the solution to the tragedy of which a million and a half Colombians are victims must be through peace and a return to normalcy in the vast rural stretches of the country. But pending the advent of a peace that will be difficult to achieve, the administration, municipalities, regions, and government should act forcefully. A clear policy of social support and an emergency plan are urgently needed to relieve the dire situation to which these groups are condemned. This effort also requires greater sensitivity from Colombian citizens, who should establish pressure groups in reaction to the state's failure to assume its responsibilities. The solidarity shown after the tragic earthquake that occurred along the coffee-growing belt, or *Eje cafetero,* on 25 January 1999 has proved the capacity of Colombians to help the most needy people in rural areas. For weeks on end, earthquake victims in the Quindío region and in parts of the neighboring regions received support from all corners of the country. A humanitarian tragedy of such scale and severity as that of the displaced population should provoke a greater reaction from the society. It is unacceptable to see the relative indifference and insensitivity shown by various sectors in Colombia in the face of the tragedy of those fleeing violence. It is also unacceptable that this very violence has been historically prolonged by the fragility of the state and by the gross negligence and incompetence of the political class.

Armed groups have taken up positions with impunity throughout the national territory and are seriously threatening the stability and future of present-day Colombian society. The civilian population is constantly in their line of fire. Forced to participate silently in the war, the rural population is condemned to an unjust and brutal destiny of hunger and uprooting. Once again, the people's hunger is one of the motives for the fighting. The hunger of the displaced, often stripped of their rich and productive lands, is the best proof of the state's failure to resolve a conflict that has been a fixture of Colombian life for decades. From a rich and varied diet, displaced farmers have been reduced to a bowl of rice, infant malnutrition, and unhealthy conditions near sewers and garbage dumps in a country where vast and prosperous cattle farms, fabulous ore deposits, and abundant natural reserves contrast with the daily struggle for survival of a million and a half people.

Notes

Pablo Alcade Subias is the Action Against Hunger head of mission in Colombia.

1. Information System on Forced Displacement and Human Rights in Colombia (Sistema de Información sobre Desplazamiento Forzado y Derechos Humanos en Colombia; SISDES).

2. Letter from the Autodefensas Campesinas of Córdoba and Urabá to the director of the Office of the United Nations High Commissioner for Human Rights, Almudena Mazarrasa, dated 23 May 1998.

3. *La guerra moderna* (Bogotá: Army Library, 1963), pp. 32–33.

4. According to the bulletin of the Agency for Human Rights and Displacement (CODHES) of July 1998, the army is the cause of 6 percent of displacements, the guerillas 22 percent, and the paramilitaries 54 percent.

5. The resale activity (of water, fruit, and vegetables) constitutes the main resource of the informal economy.

6. Release of the Press Agency of the Office of the President of the Republic.

7. Colombia possesses natural sites of exceptional beauty. The Sierra Nevada of Santa Marta, Chóco, Amazonia, the "Llanos Orientales," Sierra de La Macarena, and a great variety of national parks are a few examples of Colombia's diversity.

Bibliography

Action Against Hunger. *Análisis del desplazamiento en la Costa Atlántica*. Madrid: Action Against Hunger, 1997.

Action Against Hunger. *Análisis del desplazamiento en el departamento de Córdoba*. Madrid: Action Against Hunger, 1999.

Action Against Hunger. *El sur de Córdoba y Montería: áreas de conflictos, pobreza y desplazamiento*. Revista interacción. Bogotá: Cedial, 1999.

Aldana, Walter, et al. *Conflictos regionales. Atlántico y pacífico*. Bogotá: IEPRI et FESCOL, 1998.

Castaño, Berta Lucía, et al. *Violencia política y trabajo sicosocial*. Bogotá: Corporación AURE, 1998.

Codhes informa. *Boletín de la Consultoría para los Derechos Humanos y el Desplazamiento* (October 1998; December 1998; February 1999).

Fundación Revivir. *Estudio de la realidad para transformarla*. Bogotá: Fundación Revivir, 1995.

Memorias del encuentro Colombo-español Paz en conflictos de baja intensidad: el caso colombiano. Bogotá: Colección Ejemplos de Paz, 1996.

Negrete, Victor. *Los desplazados por la violencia en Colombia. El caso de Córdoba*. Antillas: 1995.

Negrete, Victor, et al. *Urabá, conflictos y educación rural*. Bogotá: Corporación Universitaria del Sinú, 1998.

Reyes Posada, Alejandro, et al. *Pacificar la paz*. Bogotá: Commission to Combat Violence, 1992.

9

Guatemala:
Inequality and Food Security

Carmelo Gallardo

Do not expect foreigners to remind you of what you owe them because you must have a conscience and the wisdom to do so. All of your good deeds must come from your own initiative.

—Popol Vuh[1]

Guatemala is a country of contrasts. I can still remember my first impressions upon arriving in Guatemala in January 1999. These were based mainly upon amusing visual contrasts: the colorful blouses of the indigenous women contrasting with the sad, monotonous blue of the Pepsi Cola logo that, like a threat, can be seen on school walls and on road signs; the buses, which never stop but which pollute non-stop, loaded with a hodgepodge of merchandise and dangerously overtaking the bicycles ridden by the indigenous people of the high plateaus; the numerous, well-stocked supermarkets in all the large municipalities, in particular those of the capital, which compete against itinerant street vendors, the most visible part of the country's informal economy.

Guatemala is also a country rife with internal divisions. In terms of ethnicity, the indigenous population accounts for 60 percent of the total population. Since the beginning of the Spanish conquest, this group has been excluded when not exploited by the mixed-blood population.

From the ideological point of view, the spirit of confrontation and resistance remains, even though the armed conflict has ended. This was clear in the May 1999 referendum when the constitutional reforms intended to provide a legal structure for the 1996 peace accords were rejected. In terms of access to goods and services,

Chronology

1524	Spanish conquest led by Pedro Alvarado. Two-thirds of the indigenous population killed.
15 September 1821	Guatemala achieves independence.
1871	Beginning of the open market period with Justino Barrios. German influence. Land held by the church and indigenous peoples is confiscated and distributed to large property holders for coffee production.
1914–1918	World War I. Decline of German influence and rise of U.S. influence.
1931	Jorge Ubico, a conservative and Nazi sympathizer, is elected president. Laws banning vagrancy are introduced.
1944	Faced with popular opposition, Ubico resigns. A military triumvirate takes power. The October revolution introduces democracy.
1950	Jacob Arbenz is elected president.
1951	The Guatemalan Labor Party (PGT) is legalized.
1952	The Agricultural Reform Law is passed.
1953	Confiscation of uncultivated lands, which are distributed to 100,000 families.
1954	Counterrevolution led by Castillo Armas and supported by the U.S. Central Intelligence Agency. Installation of a military government.
1962	Birth of the Revolutionary Armed Forces (FAR). Talks begin with the guerillas, but the antiguerilla crackdown is rapidly intensified.
1968	Rupture between the PGT and the FAR.
1975	The Poor People's Guerrilla Army (EGP) gains prominence by assassinating the "Tiger of Ixclán," a landowner with a reputation for cruelty.
4 February 1976	Earthquake leaves twenty-five thousand dead.
1979	The People's Armed Organization (ORPA) emerges by assassinating thirty-nine people.
3 January 1980	The police set fire to the Spanish Embassy.
November 1981	Beginning of the "scorched earth" policy.
7 February 1982	The PGT, FAR, EGP, and ORPA organize the URNG (the Guatemalan Revolutionary National Union).
23 March 1982	Rios Mont leads a coup d'état and intensifies the scorched earth policy. An estimated 150,000 peasants flee to Chiapas; others form the Popular Resistance Movement (CPR).
14 January 1986	Vinicio Cerezo of the Christian Democrats is elected president.

(continues)

Chronology Continued

30 May 1987	The National Reconciliation Commission (CNR) is formed.
7 October 1987	Talks begin between the government and the URNG.
9 October 1987	Talks broken off at the request of the army.
27 December 1987	Creation of the CCPP (Permanent Commission for Refugees) in Mexico.
1990	Meetings are arranged between the guerillas and various sectors of the country in El Escorial (with the political parties), Ottawa (with the business sector), Quito (with religious leaders), Pepetec (with the workers' union), and Atlixo (with scholars, supporters, professionals, and small business owners).
25 July 1991	Conclusion of Framework Agreement on Democratization for Peace through Political Means.
8 October 1992	Agreement between the government and the CCPP for the return of refugees to Guatemala.
20 January 1993	First organized and collective return of refugees. The community of the "January 20th Victory" is founded.
29 March 1994	Comprehensive Agreement on Human Rights.
17 June 1994	Agreement on the resettlement of populations uprooted by the armed conflict.
23 June 1994	Creation of a commission to investigate human rights violations and acts of violence perpetrated against the Guatemalan population.
31 March 1995	Agreement on the Identity and Rights of the Indigenous Population.
5 October 1995	Xamán massacre: The army assassinates eleven peasants.
7 January 1996	Arzú·Irigoyen is elected president.
6 May 1996	Agreement on socioeconomic and agrarian issues.
19 November 1996	Agreement on the strengthening of civilian authority and on the role of the army in a democratic society.
4 December 1996	Definitive cease-fire agreement.
7 December 1996	Agreement on constitutional reform and the electoral system.
12 December 1996	Agreement to legalize the URNG.
29 December 1996	Agreement for the broadening, implementation, and fulfillment of the Agreements for a Firm and Lasting Peace.
26 April 1998	Assassination of Monsignor Girardi.
25 February 1999	Submission of the report "Guatemala Report: Memory of Silence" by the Comision de Esclarecimiento Historico (commission investigating the events).
16 May 1999	Referendum to ratify constitutional reforms.

Guatemala, like Brazil, has the widest gap in Latin America: Twenty percent of the population is rich and 20 percent poor.

This internal division between rich and poor has its roots in the extreme inequalities in consumption levels and above all in land ownership. A mere 2.56 percent of the population owns 65.1 percent of the land. What is the relationship between this inequality in land distribution and the food security of the population?

This chapter attempts to provide two responses to this question:

- To highlight the inequality in the nutritional standards of the population in a country in which chronic illnesses (diabetes, heart disease) have increased by 100 percent in this decade and are accompanied by nutritional deficiencies and infant malnutrition (INCAP 1998).
- To show how inequality creates the food insecurity with which the majority of Guatemalans live. Indeed, access to land influences the availability of food resources, while uneven income distribution affects in turn the possibility of access to land.

Widespread Poverty

During the period from 1960 to 1996, Guatemala experienced one of the most tragic armed conflicts in Latin America, resulting in more than 100,000 dead, an equal number of wounded and maimed, thousands of disappearances, over a million displaced persons, and 120,000 refugees.

Since the December 1996 Agreement for a Firm and Lasting Peace, stability has returned to Guatemala. However, even though peace has been achieved, it must still be consolidated. Justice and peace must be strengthened and refugees and displaced persons resettled.

Guatemala is the most populous country in Central America, with a population estimated in 1996 at 10.92 million. Population density is 100.4 persons per square kilometer,[2] and annual population growth (projected at 2.6 percent for the period 1995–2015) is the highest in Latin America. Sixty-five percent of the population lives in rural areas and 22 percent in the capital.[3]

The adult illiteracy rate is 44 percent, the highest in the region. Nicaragua, at 34.3 percent, has the second highest rate; Costa Rica, at 5.2 percent, has the lowest rate. In Guatemala, this lack of education directly or indirectly exacerbates the country's principal problems.

Persons with little education are more likely to be unemployed, and most of them are poor. Socioeconomic and cultural exclusion sometimes prevents citizens from exercising their civil and political rights in a nation that is in the midst of a transition toward peace. Moreover, the weakening of the institutions that contribute to an individual's emotional stability and identity (school and family) explains much of the crime in Guatemala.

Guatemala has the highest mortality rate of any Central American country (6.7 percent per thousand in 1995) due to the inadequate health care system and the high crime rate.[4]

The United Nations Development Program (UNDP) has developed multidimensional indexes, such as the Human Development Index (HDI).[5] Of the 174 countries studied, Guatemala ranked 111th in the 1995 HDI (UNDP 1998b).

The index of unmet basic needs (UBN) is generally used to measure levels of poverty.[6] If a basic need is not met, an individual or family is considered to be poor. Paradoxically, with this method, food is not considered to be essential to the individual.

In Central America, thanks to the work of the Economic Commission for Latin America and the Caribbean (ECLAC), the United Nations Food and Agriculture Organization (FAO), and the Institute of Nutrition of Central America and Panama (INCAP), among others, a basket of basic goods and services that provides 100 percent of the calories needed by the average individual is the method most widely used to determine the threshold of extreme poverty. An individual who does not have access to all of these goods is considered to be indigent. Guatemala's National Statistical Institute uses another basket of basic goods and services in which food accounts for 42.25 percent of the total weighting. An individual who lacks access to this basket of goods and services is placed in the category of poor Guatemalans.

This method of baskets of basic goods and services was used by the World Bank in Guatemala for its 1995 study. The main conclusions of that study are as follows:

- Seventy-five percent of the population is poor, meaning that they do not earn enough to purchase essential goods and services.
- Fifty-eight percent of the population is indigent, that is to say, below the threshold of extreme poverty. They thus do not have enough buying power to purchase the basket of basic goods to meet their needs.

- In comparison with other countries with identical incomes, Guatemala exhibits a very high level of poverty relative to per capita Gross National Product.
- Poverty mainly affects rural areas (principally the high plateau regions), the least educated (79 percent of uneducated heads of households are poor as opposed to 48 percent for those with a secondary school education), and the indigenous population (90 percent are poor as opposed to 66 percent for the nonindigenous population).
- A poor resident of Guatemala City, the capital, has a mean income that is 19 percent below the poverty threshold, whereas a poor person living in a rural area has an income 54 percent below the threshold.

Article 118 of the Constitution of the Republic of Guatemala (1985) provides as follows: "The economic and social system of the Republic of Guatemala is based on principles of social justice. It is the obligation of the State to direct national policy in such a way as to make full use of the State's natural resources and human potential, to increase wealth and to try to achieve full employment and equitable distribution of the national income."

Seventy-five percent of the population of Guatemala, Honduras, and Nicaragua is poor. How is it that Guatemala, with a per capita income twice that of Honduras and Nicaragua, has the same level of poverty?[7] Is the Gross Domestic Product (GDP), the most important index used to measure economic production, unevenly distributed among the population? The World Bank is clear on this: Of the forty-four countries used in the comparison with the same per capita GDP (between $2,000 and $4,000 per annum) adjusted to reflect purchasing power, Guatemala is ranked first on the poverty indexes (World Bank 1995).

Historically, inequality already existed in Mayan society during the classical period (from 150 A.D. to the tenth century). It was based on a system of classes in which an elite class held religious and political power. Spanish colonization altered the ethnic composition of the hierarchy and raised problems of access to land. These problems were exacerbated by the market-oriented reforms of 1870, which distributed communal and municipal land to coffee producers.

A political and social analysis of the current situation reveals inequities in the exercise of civil rights. Indeed, in past elections, no more than 18 percent of registered voters have ever voted.

From a geographical point of view, the HDI shows a difference that is more than double between Guatemala City and one of the northern departments.[8] Moreover, expenditures are unequal, since Guatemala continues to be one of the countries on the continent with the lowest level of social spending.[9] A graphic illustration of this inequality is the fact that in 1990, the spending on the two largest hospitals in the capital was more than the amount spent on all the other health centers in the country.[10]

A comparative analysis of the various official agricultural surveys carried out in Guatemala between 1964 and 1979 (the last year for which figures are available) reveals disturbing trends in land owner-ship patterns: The size of properties owned has increased by 20 per-cent. This means that the agricultural frontier has "claimed" 700,000 hectares from the forest in fifteen years.

More recent studies reveal that the distribution of land is extremely uneven: Some 2.56 percent of landowners own 65.1 per-cent of the land. In reality, the concentration of land is even more pronounced, because 1,335 farms, or 0.02 percent of landowners, control more than one-third (34.1 percent) of the land (1979 agricul-tural survey). To support these data, Guatemala's Gini index for agri-culture is 0.85, one of the highest in the world[11] (INCAP 1998).

The agricultural sector contributes over 25 percent of Guate-mala's GDP. Rural dwellers account for 60 percent of the total popu-lation, and the unemployment rate in rural areas is 47.5 percent.[12] A person who has no land, therefore, has to scramble to survive. In short, a consensus exists that the uneven distribution of land is the primary cause of the extreme poverty in the rural areas of Central America (IDB 1998).

Inequality and Food Security

The rural population represents 60 percent of Guatemala's total pop-ulation. The total area under food cultivation is 45 percent of the productive land, and the agricultural sector accounts for 25 percent of GDP. Based on these data, the national agricultural sector should easily meet the population's needs. Over the last twenty years, howev-er, Guatemala has reduced its per capita production of staple grains, while agricultural production for export has increased (UNDP 1998a).

The last national child health survey, which was carried out in 1995, showed that half of all Guatemalan children under the age of five suffer from chronic malnutrition (which made it possible to iden-tify children with stunted growth by comparing the actual size of the child with its age-appropriate size).

Agriculture has traditionally been the main source of income for most Latin American economies. At present, in countries such as Guatemala, Bolivia, Nicaragua, and Haiti, agriculture accounts for more than 25 percent of GDP. However, even though agriculture in Guatemala is the main contributor to GDP, this is not necessarily a sign that the sector is thriving.

- Commodity exports are subject to fluctuations in international prices, resulting in lower employment levels among the population.[13]
- The shift in commodities produced for export over the last few years (sugarcane has replaced cotton) has mainly affected poor peasants employed as day laborers. Mechanized harvesting techniques used in sugarcane harvesting have reduced the need for workers, and day laborers are forced to migrate to the northern agricultural frontier or to emigrate.
- The limestone soils of the tropical ecosystems found in the northern lowlands are extremely fragile and vulnerable to degradation. They therefore cannot guarantee sustained development and are farmed for only a few seasons before new land must be found. Land that is no longer fit for farming is, in most cases, bought by livestock ranchers, who use it for grazing, thereby precluding any possibility of forest regeneration. The expansion of the agricultural frontier is threatening the Mayan biosphere, one of the world's great forests.
- The farmer who still farms his small plot of land is tending more and more toward crops that deplete natural resources in an unsustainable way. In many cases, farming is increasing in hilly areas that have low productive capacity and that are subject to severe erosion. A study carried out by Action Against Hunger in Jutiapa and Jalapa has shown that the lower the land's fertility, the greater the family's income from activities linked to migration or day labor (Action Against Hunger 1999).

The crisis in the agricultural sector limits access to land and to employment for the majority of the Guatemalan population, even though increasing numbers derive their principal source of employment from this very sector. This leads to a vicious circle of poverty, deforestation, land degradation, and malnutrition. As long as the model of development favors export crops, consolidates the best land, and offers few opportunities for employment, food insecurity will continue to be the primary reason for the depletion of the country's natural resources.

Traditionally, the diet of the rural population has lacked variety and has consisted mainly of staple grains. This contrasts with the varied dietary intake of the urban population, which has easy access to imported products. The processes of urbanization and advertising for food products alter consumer habits and influence current health and nutritional standards. Throughout Central America, the epidemiological model has changed with death from nontransmissible chronic diseases (diabetes, heart disease), one of the primary causes of mortality, increasing by 100 percent over the last ten years. These diseases, which are typical of industrialized countries, coexist with widespread dietary deficiencies and infant malnutrition (INCAP 1998).

It is possible to scientifically calculate the optimum calorie intake for each country. In Guatemala, it is 2,250 calories daily, but studies done by INCAP have revealed that the actual intake was 2,075 calories; that number, moreover, was not attained by all citizens. While physical fitness is becoming fashionable in the capital just as it is in Western countries, with gymnasiums and health-food stores that cater to a minority, women in the high plateau regions expend 700 calories each day, or a third of their total calorie intake, fetching water and performing other necessary household chores.

In addition to providing needed calories, the intake of nutrients is necessary for childhood development. Studies done by INCAP beginning in 1969, under which the typical diet of a group of Guatemalan children was supplemented from birth to age seven with calories, protein, vitamins, and minerals, have shown that in adolescence and early childhood, these children were taller, stronger, and more intelligent than those who had not received supplements. Improving nutritional and health conditions represents an effective strategy for the economic and human development of Guatemala.

Which noneconomic factors can influence nutrition? In some cases, diet depends on such external factors as the aggressive marketing of soft drinks, which targets the younger generation in particular. These commercial practices explain, for example, why in El Salvador, the red Coca Cola color is found in all the country's cafés, whereas Pepsi Cola's blue predominates in Guatemala. But this aggressive marketing strategy is not only a U.S. phenomenon. Guatemala, as further evidence of its many contrasts, exports franchises of the fast food chain Pollo Campero (Country Chickens) to other Central American countries even though chickens in its own rural areas are dying from a poultry disease.

Geographical frontiers sometimes determine differences in consumption, although this phenomenon may be difficult to explain. For example, Nicaraguans and Salvadorans consume red beans, while over the border in Guatemala black beans are preferred. Moreover, even within the country, a large and opaque variety of the same black bean is preferred in the highlands while in the east a small, black, shiny variety is cultivated. This concept of taste is not frivolous. The latest variety of bean developed by the Guatemalan Institute of Agrarian Science and Technology (ICTA), called "Icta Ligero," which was developed to resist disease (in particular the tobacco mosaic virus), is the variety of seed that was distributed on credit to a few families in Jutiapa who had lost their second harvest in 1998 from the damage caused by Hurricane Mitch. In addition to undergoing strict biological and agronomical tests prior to marketing, it underwent a cooking test for housewives to evaluate its cooking time and approve its consistency and taste.

For farmers, food security depends on access to land. In Belize, a family wishing to farm receives permission from the state to use the land. Other Central American countries have launched land redistribution and land reform programs. In Guatemala, Central America's most populous country, agricultural reforms introduced in 1952 by the government of Jacob Arbenz, who had been democratically elected with the support of 65 percent of voters, were overturned in 1954 by a military coup d'état. Nearly all the redistributed land (883,615 hectares among 100,000 poor farming families) was returned to its former owners, the large landholders. Moreover, between 1955 and 1992, 765,393 hectares were distributed among 116,239 people. According to the United Nations Verification Mission in Guatemala, large landowners were favored in this distribution along with high ranking military officers and professionals (MINUGUA 1998).

In Guatemala, INCAP studies have shown that in 1985 one hectare of land and the necessary factors of production distributed in farming and ranching regions should produce food of sufficient quality and quantity to provide a balanced diet at minimal cost for a family of five. During the 1979 census, 240,000 of the 605,000 farms surveyed were less than 0.8 hectares in size. Most small farmers neither possess nor have access to a hectare of cultivable land. If they do own a hectare of land, then its yield is very poor.

The rural family has therefore been forced to develop coping strategies, which have allowed it to overcome its food insecurity. However, environmental, economic, and biological factors of an internal nature can weaken the ability of families to use these coping mechanisms. In Guatemala, this is frequent in regions susceptible to drought (the El Niño phenomenon), floods (Hurricane Mitch), and the recent experiences of armed violence (INCAP 1998).

For families buying food, food security depends above all on money income earned in most cases from work in the informal sector. In particular, from the point of view of nutrition, it is important to distinguish between in-kind income (food grown by individuals) and money income. In terms of money income, a minimum wage exists in Guatemala.[14] Its buying power determines the relation between income and food security since, given Guatemala's high rates of underemployment, the minimum wage is often the maximum amount earned.

For a family of 5.38 members, the daily cost of the basic food basket (twenty-six items) was 31.98 quetzales in November 1994. During the same period, the minimum daily agricultural wage was 14.5 quetzales and 16.5 quetzales in the city. The minimum wage bought only half of the basic food basket. In February 1999, the cost of the same basic basket for the same type of family was 38.88 quetzales (INE 1999), and the minimum agricultural wage was 17.86 quetzales compared to 19.71 in the city. The buying power of the minimum wage in Guatemala has therefore not risen since the signing of the Peace Agreements.

Even the implementation of the Peace Agreements, which provide for increased social spending and a more equitable redistribution of taxes, will not eliminate poverty from Guatemalan homes. The uneven distribution of national wealth leaves the majority of the population on the brink of food insecurity. This affects mainly the rural population (65 percent of the total population) and unemployed or undeclared workers (47.5 percent of the working population.)

This economic gap also creates a cultural gap. Differences in consumption patterns are developing. A minority of the population is consuming increasing amounts of packaged and imported foods (and producing 70.75 percent of the solid wastes) while a majority continues to consume staple crops.

Notes

Carmelo Gallardo is Action Against Hunger head of mission in Guatemala.

1. The *Popol Vuh* is the sacred book of the Kiche, one of the principal Mayan groups in the country. It is the Book of the Councilor of the Community, also known as the Manuscript of Chichicastenango. It was orally transmitted from generation to generation. In the early eighteenth century, a

copy written in Kitche but with Latin characters was discovered by the Dominican father Francisco Ximénez. Who wrote this copy and when remain a mystery. Ximénez translated it into Spanish, but it was not made available to researchers until 1930.

2. El Salvador, the Dominican Republic, and Cuba have higher population densities.

3. Statistics in this paragraph and the next paragraph are from UNDP 1998a and UNDP 1998b.

4. In 1995, 66 percent of the population had access to health services and 60 percent to potable water. These rates drop to 25 and 43 percent for the rural population (IDB 1998). In regard to the crime rate, in 1994 the primary cause of death among Guatemalan teenagers and adults was firearms (UNDP 1998a).

5. The HDI is based on the following criteria: longevity (defined as expected life span), level of education (defined as the adult illiteracy rate and school registration rates), and quality of life (defined by per capita Gross Domestic Product).

6. The UBN is a weighted index used in Guatemala by various institutions. It permits an evaluation to be made of the level of poverty using six criteria: rate of growth, quality of life, health services, access to drinking water, primary school enrollment levels, and income level.

7. In 1995 the real per capita Gross Domestic Product (that is, PPP, or purchasing power parity in dollars) was as follows: Guatemala, 3683; Honduras, 1977; Nicaragua, 1837 (UNDP 1998a).

8. The internal evaluation of the HDI in 1995–1996 in each district highlighted the glaring inequalities between the district of Guatemala (HDI = 0.829) and the rest of the country (the HDI in Alta Vera Paz was the lowest in the country, at 0.355). This difference in level of development is similar to the difference between Brazil (HDI = 0.809) and Tanzania (HDI = 0.358) (UNDP 1998b).

9. During the 1994–1995 period, social spending was 3.7 percent of GDP, the lowest in the region. The percentages in El Salvador, Nicaragua, and Costa Rica were 5.3 10.6, and 20.8, respectively (IDB 1998).

10. Seventy-two percent of the expenditure of the Ministry of Health was allocated to hospitals and only 19 percent to basic needs centers (World Bank 1995).

11. The Gini index is one of the indexes of equality. It may range from 0 (where land is evenly distributed among all landowners) to 1 (an extreme case in which one landowner owns all the land).

12. In all Latin America, only Haiti has a lower urbanization rate than Guatemala. This percentage includes both real unemployment and underemployment rates. The main reason for this high percentage is that industrial growth is not rapid enough to absorb surplus agricultural workers.

13. In May 1996, Guatemalan engineers decided to halt production of sugarcane when sugar prices dropped by 50 percent. Entire fields were left unharvested.

14. According to Article 103 of the 1971 Guatemalan Labor Code, "Every worker has the right to a minimum wage that permits him to meet his material, moral and cultural needs and to discharge his responsibility as head of household."

References

Action Against Hunger. 1999. *Study of Food Security in the Departments of Jutiapa and Jalapa.* Madrid.

ASC [Assembly of Civil Society]. 1996. *Peace Agreements.* Guatemala: Commission for the National Public-Awareness Campaign.

ASC. 1997. *Guía para le estudio de los Acuerdos de Paz.* Guatemala.

Cadesca [Committee for Action and Support for Economic and Social Development in Central America]/CEC [Commission of the European Communities]. 1990. *Macro-economic Policy and Its Impact on Agriculture and Food Security—The Case of Guatemala.* Panama: Central American Training Programme in Food Security.

CEH [Commission for Historical Clarification]. 1999. *Guatemala, Memory of Silence.* Guatemala: United Nations Operations and Procurement Service.

Centro de Estudios de Guatemala. 1995. *Así vivimosá: las condiciones de vida en Guatemala.* Guatemala: Nuestra América Publishers, collection "Guatemala Hoy."

ECLAC [Economic Commission for Latin America and the Caribbean]. 1998a. *Balance preliminar de las economías de América Latina y El Caribe, 1998.* Santiago, Chile.

ECLAC. 1998b. *Centroamérica: évolución económica durante 1997.* Mexico: ECLAC Regional Office.

ECLAC. 1998c. *Guatemala: evolución económica durante 1997.* Mexico.

FAO [United Nations Food and Agriculture Organization]. 1996. *Food Security and Nutrition.* Guatemala.

IDB [Inter-American Development Bank]. 1998. *Las economías deálos países centroamericanos.*

IDB/IFPRI [International Food Policy Research Institute]. 1998. *Agriculture, Environment and Natural Poverty in Latin America.* Washington, D.C.

INCAP [Institute of Nutrition of Central America and Panama]. 1998. *La iniciativa de seguridad alimentaria nutricional en Centroamérica.* Guatemala.

INE [National Institute of Statistics]. 1999. *Consumer Price Index.* February 1999 Bulletin. Guatemala.

INE, MSPYAS [Ministerio de Salud Publica y Asistencia Social], USAID [U.S. Agency for International Development], UNICEF [United Nations International Childrens Emergency Fund], and DHS. 1995. *National Maternal and Child Health Survey.* Guatemala.

INE [National Institute of Statistics]/UNFPA [United Nations Population Fund]. 1989. *Perfíl de la pobreza en Guatemala, Encuesta Nacional Sociodemográfica 1989.* INE and UNFPA Guatemala.

Laure, Joseph. 1996. *Minimum Wage, Food Security and Poverty in Central America.* Guatemala: INCAP.

MAGA [Ministry of Agriculture, Livestock and Food Production]. 1998. *Marco de funcionamiento de políticas.* Guatemala: UNDP.

Microempresas de Centroamérica. 1999. "Política econmica y problemas sociales en América central." *Cortos económicos*, no. 24.

MINUGUA [United Nations Verification Mission in Guatemala].1998. *Suplemento sobre la verificación del Acuerdo sobre Aspectos Socioeconómicos y Situación Agraria.* Guatemala.

PAHO [Pan-American Health Organization]. 1998. *Health in the Americas.* 1998 Edition. Guatemala.

PRISMA [Salvadoran Research Program on Development and the Environment]. 1997. *Evaluación Nacional de la Sostenibilidad. El caso Guatemala.* Project "Strengthening the Prospects for Sustainable Development in Central America." Guatemala: World Wildlife Fund and Central American Commission on the Environment and Development.

SEGEPLAN [General Secretariat of Planning]. 1994. *Necesidades Básicas Insatisfechas en la República por Departamentos.* Guatemala.

SEGEPLAN/GTZ [Gesellschaft für Technische Zusammenarbeit]. N.d. *Hacia la seguridad alimentaria y nutricional de la población guatemalteca.* Guatemala.

Sichar, Gonzalo. 1998. *¿Guatemala: Contrainsurgencia o contra el pueblo?* Collection "Gnarus." Madrid.

Sum, David. 1998. *Perfil socioeconómico de Guatemala.* San Marcos, Guatemala: University de San Carlos de Guatemala.

Termes, Rafael. 1998. *Capitalismo y ética,* Web page of Francisco Marroquín University, Guatemala.

UNDP [United Nations Development Program]. 1998a. *Guatemala: los contrastes del desarrollo humano.* Guatemala: United Nations system in Guatemala.

UNDP. 1998b. *Human Development Report 1998.* Madrid: Mundi-Prensa Libros.

URNG [Guatemalan National Revolutionary Union]. 1998. *Cumplimiento de los Acuerdos de Paz. Enero-Septiembre 1998.* Guatemala.

USAC [University of San Carlos de Guatemala]. Various issues. *Economía al día.* Guatemala.

World Bank. 1995. *Guatemala, An Assessment of Poverty.* Regional Office for Latin America and the Caribbean.

10

Nicaragua:
No Way Out of Rural Poverty?

Jorge Pereiro Piñon

Hurricane Mitch caused the most dramatic increase in poverty ever recorded in Nicaragua. It had a negative impact on the food economy of the populations in those villages in which Action Against Hunger administers its programs. The consequences of Hurricane Mitch are closely linked to the current trends toward increasing poverty in the country's rural areas, trends that the hurricane exacerbated but did not create. This fact should therefore be taken into consideration by the government and donor nations (although it is unlikely that it will be) in planning for Nicaragua's reconstruction.

Aftermath of the Disaster—
Heightened Social Inequalities

During the last week of October 1998, Hurricane Mitch, the century's worst hurricane, reached the coastlines of Nicaragua and Honduras. It passed over the countries from northeast to southwest, and with its intensity diminishing to that of a tropical storm, it headed toward El Salvador and the south and east of Guatemala before spending itself in the Caribbean Sea. The hurricane's impact was severe, and it left the region in chaos in the days following its passage: Homeless families crowded into shelters, there were threats of epidemics, communications were cut, and contradictory statements led to confusion about the scale of damage. As the days went by, the real extent of the damage wrought by the hurricane became clear. Although Hurricane Mitch affected the entire region, not all countries were impacted to

Chronology

1933–1934	The United States army leaves Nicaragua after twenty-one years of occupation. In February 1934, Anastasio Somoza, head of the national and military guard and an ally of the United States, emerges as the country's strongman after ordering the assassination of his main rival, Augusto César Sandino (commander of the Las Segovias army, who had successfully fought against the American occupation).
1956	The poet Rigoberto López Pérez assassinates Anastasio Somoza in León. Somoza's sons, Luis (r. 1956–1963) and Anastasio (r. 1967–1979), succeed him.
1963	On 13 December, Nicaragua joins the Central American Common Market. Rising agricultural exports bring strong economic growth to Nicaragua.
1972	Managua is destroyed by an earthquake on Christmas Day. Much of the international assistance received is diverted by Somoza to himself and his supporters. The government begins to lose the support of the middle class.
1978	Pedro Joaquim Chamorro, editor of the opposition newspaper *La Prensa,* is murdered by hit men on the orders of Anastasio Somoza. Chamorro had been a longtime opponent of the Somozas' dictatorship and the most brilliant member of the "Government of 12." He had been preparing to propose an alternative to Somoza, and his assassination left the guerilla force of the Sandinista National Liberation Front (FSLN) as the sole possible opposition force by strengthening support for the FSLN among moderate parties.
19 July 1979	The Sandinista revolution triumphs. The FSLN is integrated into a provisional government composed of various political forces. A few days earlier, the dictator Anastasio Somoza had left the country to seek refuge in Paraguay, where he is assassinated soon after.
1981	Break in relations with the United States. The provisional government is overthrown, and the FSLN seizes power. The United States trains and arms in Honduras the opposition guerilla group known as the Contras.
1984	Intensification by the government of the war against the Contras. Nicaragua devotes 40 percent of its economic resources to the war. The United States mines the port of Corinto and declares an economic embargo against Nicaragua.

(continues)

	Chronology Continued
1989	The FSLN loses the presidential elections to a coalition of opposition parties known as the National Opposition Union. Violeta Chamorro (widow of the assassinated journalist) succeeds Daniel Ortega as president of Nicaragua.
1990	Violeta Chamorro signs cease-fire agreement with the national resistance guerilla group, the Contras. However, groups of former Contra members, known as Recontras, and of former members of the FSLN, known as Recompas, remain active in the north and east of the country until 1997.
1993	The Nicaraguan government signs the first structural adjustment agreement with the International Monetary Fund (IMF). The partial reduction of Nicaragua's foreign debt is made conditional on the achievement of the ESAF targets, and compliance is monitored by the IMF.
1996	The Liberal Alliance of Arnoldo Alemán narrowly defeats Daniel Ortega's FSLN in presidential elections, which are marred by accusations of massive electoral fraud.
26 October 1998	Hurricane Mitch (through 1 November).

the same extent. Honduras and Nicaragua were the hardest hit, whereas Guatemala and El Salvador were only partially affected.

In Nicaragua, the damage caused by Hurricane Mitch was spread over many regions. There were both human loss (nearly four thousand persons died or disappeared) and material losses: roads, bridges, homes, school equipment, partial destruction of the electrical and water supply systems, loss of crops and livestock, and damage to agricultural land and forests. According to civil security officials, 867,752 persons, or 20 percent of the country's total population, were affected. The government and humanitarian organizations described them as disaster victims, but people in rural areas invented the more appropriate term *huracanados* (hurricane victims).

The entire world saw these *huracanados* on television, trying to survive the flooding of their villages or, in more dramatic cases, as in Posoltega, searching through the mud for the bodies of dead family members. International solidarity in the face of the situation in

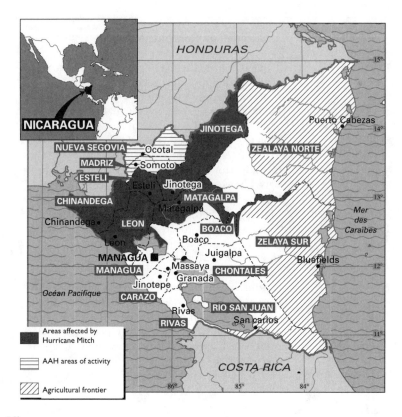

Nicaragua

Central America exceeded all expectations and was so strong that it surprised many observers. In Spain, material and financial assistance were collected in unprecedented amounts. Other European countries, such as France, which had fewer historical ties to Central America but whose citizens were moved by the disaster that occurred, mobilized significant amounts of donations for humanitarian aid. Foreign governments and international institutions funded immediate assistance and began planning for the funding of a reconstruction program for the region. This was discussed in late May 1999 in Stockholm by the four affected countries and the principal international donors.

In examining the aftermath of Hurricane Mitch, as in looking at all natural disasters, one can identify immediate consequences of the hurricane's passage and the medium- and long-term consequences.

These consequences, and in particular those of a long-term nature, relate to the structural poverty in which most of the Nicaraguan population lives.

In analyzing the immediate consequences, it can be seen that during the weeks following the hurricane, three categories of the population found themselves in an extremely vulnerable situation. These were the homeless families with no access to communication, those housed in temporary shelters (generally schools or other community buildings), and those without access to potable water.

The first two groups lost not only their homes but also the possibility of pursuing any economic activity (generally agricultural) and thus found themselves dependent on outside assistance to feed themselves. It was therefore essential to provide them with water, food, and proper sanitary conditions.

The population in the third group lost access to potable water on account of the destruction of the water systems or wells on which they relied. This group was therefore exposed to the risk of epidemics, since dead animals and mud slides increased pollution of the surface water, their sole source of supply after the hurricane. The water distribution systems for these families thus needed to be repaired urgently in order to prevent the spread of diseases and to provide prompt medical care as a means of preventing both the spread and risk of fever.

The medium- and long-term consequences of Hurricane Mitch were more complex. Villagers in the dry northern, central, and western areas of the country, where many *huracanados* live, comprise the poorest sector of Nicaragua's population. Since 1996, Action Against Hunger has been working with these villagers, developing water and food security projects in the districts of Madriz and Nueva Segovia.

The Nicaraguan economy has always been dependent on the agricultural sector, which accounts for over 25 percent of the Gross Domestic Product (GDP). Nonetheless, this sector has always been the country's least developed, both during the 1960s and the 1970s, when Nicaragua's exports rose thanks to increased agricultural production levels, and later, during the Sandinista regime and under the current neoliberal governments of Violeta Chamorro and Arnoldo Alemán.

Under the regime of the Somozas, neither small nor medium-sized farmers benefited from the income generated by the rapid expansion of the agricultural sector.[1] The wealth earned in the rural areas was pocketed by the land-owning middle class whose ties to the ruling classes allowed it to benefit from favorable treatment in exchange for its political support. Later on, because of economic difficulties and the greed of the Somozas, it was impossible to guarantee sufficient distribution of wealth to the middle class, which reacted by supporting the Sandinista revolution.

The Sandinista government did not consider small farmers to be participants in the nation's economic development. After its victory, agricultural reform policy was based on collectivism, and the government established people's property zones consisting of property that had belonged to Somoza supporters and was now administered by the state. When peasants grew disillusioned by the regulation of domestic commerce and began to lend support to the guerilla resistance forces (the Contras), the Sandinista government reacted by launching a program of genuine agricultural reform. Some 320,000 hectares of state-owned land were distributed to communal groups of farmers. This second phase of the reform, which provided opportunities to landless farmers and to those with very little land, created the most equitable system of land ownership in Latin America. Wartime policies, the embargo, and poor management on the part of the government, however, gradually led to a deterioration in the country's economy, which virtually collapsed by the end of the 1980s.

All of the above factors contributed to the defeat of the Sandinistas and the victory of Violeta Chamorro in the 1989 elections. Chamorro, supported by loans from multilateral organizations and massive amounts of international aid to finance the revival of the country's economy, swiftly introduced neoliberal policies. Her government, like that of Alemán, who was elected in 1996, based the development of the agricultural sector on a policy of support for agrofood industrial complexes (Sebaco valley), coffee exports (Matagalpa and Jinotega), and livestock farming (large ranches in Rivas and in the country's dry regions). Small and medium-sized farms did not benefit from these agricultural support policies, although medium-sized farms, in particular, were the most efficient producers in the rural areas. Eleven years of neoliberalism have not sufficed to launch a process of national development. This is especially true in the rural areas where, on the contrary, neoliberal policies have accentuated social inequalities.

Poverty in the rural areas led to continued emigration, not only to urban centers but also abroad (mainly to the United States and Costa Rica) and to the agricultural frontier. Nicaragua's agricultural frontier is located in the area known as the Atlantic coast (administratively, this corresponds to the autonomous districts of the north and south Atlantic and to the Río San Juan district). Although this area covers over 50 percent of the national territory, it contains only 10 percent of the population. Originally, it was an undeveloped region covered with tropical rain forests, but since the 1940s, it has attracted an increasing number of immigrants from Nicaragua's central and western regions. Peasants emigrating to the Atlantic coast were drawn either by the gold mining industry, which thrived in the region until the 1970s, or by the possibility of acquiring more land or owning land if they did not already have any. These immigrants moved onto the land, which until then had been preserved as forest, planted basic seed crops and coffee (in the higher altitudes), and raised livestock.

Those who began with some capital obtained good harvests and managed to improve their economic situation. They were thus able to play a meaningful role in the nation's agricultural development. However, the abundant harvests depleted the already fragile soil, which was unsuitable for the traditional farming methods used in the dry regions (slash-and-burn techniques). Thus the areas where the first immigrants arrived more than twenty years ago are now completely deforested. The land yields poorer and poorer harvests and is used as pasture for cattle. Farmers who were unable to acquire enough land or livestock while yields were good or to settle on land that offered comparative advantages (such as coffee growing) were forced to sell their land and emigrate east to undeveloped land on which they began the process all over again. Poor farmers from the Pacific coast therefore had a chance to improve their situation, but at the price of mortgaging the resources of future generations. Moreover, the rate of depletion of undeveloped land is accelerated by the uncontrolled activity of the large lumber companies that, in the absence of political will to protect the area's resources, are destroying the forest much more rapidly than the peasants have done.

Small farmers in the central and western regions who did not emigrate were forced to become wage earners. Lacking any government support, they were unable to feed their families from the crops they grew. As a result, a farmer's sons cannot survive on their father's subdivided land. The farmer (with no credit, technical assistance, or access to the main markets) is unable to increase his income in order to buy more land or animals, much less to afford to educate his children so that they could enter other economic sectors. The children therefore become wage earners and work as servants or tenant farmers for the large landowners of the region. This worsens their situation and makes it virtually impossible for them to lift themselves out of poverty.

At the same time, the land owned by their father falls into the hands of a large landowner. Only those small farmers who are able to compensate for the subdivision of the land by increasing its productivity (market garden crops) are able to escape this process. However, increased productivity is not possible unless the produce can be marketed. In view of the inadequate infrastructure in Nicaragua, many small farmers do not have this possibility.

Through the processes of emigration and proletarianization, land ownership in the rural areas has become increasingly unequal. More land is concentrated in the hands of a smaller number of individuals. The policies pursued during the last few years have not created wealth and have instead increased the levels of poverty among people in rural areas. Action Against Hunger's 1997 survey of household poverty in the district of Madriz showed how the level of poverty had increased since 1993, when the Nicaraguan Institute for Statistical Studies (INEC) conducted a survey using the same criteria (Unmet Basic Needs Index). In contrast, the level of poverty in urban areas has declined.

In the country's dry regions, the food economy of disaster-stricken families depends on corn, beans, and sorghum, planted in small parcels of land (which they own or rent) not exceeding 4 hectares. The crops are planted for the family's own consumption (corn and beans) and for farm animals (sorghum). Families supplement their household income through sale of the surplus production of beans (allowing them to buy cooking oil, salt, coffee, and household utensils) and through seasonal work harvesting coffee on large farms. These practices place farmers on the edge of food insecurity, since they barely cover the daily caloric intake needs for one family. Not only does such a modest economy prevent farmers from acquiring more land or livestock, but it is also extremely vulnerable to any drop in the family's income.

The hurricane caused the loss of a good part of the second annual harvest (the last in the year), thereby depleting the food reserves that should have enabled affected families to survive until the first harvest of 1999 in July and August and leaving them without reserves for the planting season. The loss of their crops is not a new phenomenon for these families. Aware of the precarious nature of their economic base, they have developed a number of coping strategies over the years: lengthening the time spent or increasing the number of family members who help to harvest the coffee; permanent emigration of some or all family members to Costa Rica, the United States, or the Atlantic coast of Nicaragua itself. In addition to these survival strategies used by farmers, the World Food Program (WFP) now distributes food aid, seeds, and farming implements through the assistance programs of certain countries or humanitarian organizations. In the short term, a combination of these solutions has made it possible to prevent the famine that some had predicted. Up until May 1999, no significant rise in severe malnutrition rates (as measured by weight/height ratios) had been observed. It is not known what the medium- and long-term consequences will be. The damage to crops, homes, and arable land will accelerate the processes of emigration and proletarianization that, in turn, increase poverty and inequality.

The question is one of how effective the free distribution of food, seeds, and other factors of production will be once the emergency phase is over. Analysis of the situation on which these programs are based takes no account of the fact that the root cause of the vulnerability of these families is not Hurricane Mitch but the fragility of their economy. Nor do these programs take into account the fact that the most serious problem created by the hurricane, apart from the loss of human life, was not the risk of famine or epidemics, but the accentuation of the trend toward impoverishment among farmers, which is becoming increasingly difficult to control. These programs do not address the structural causes that are at the root of this process, but simply replace what Mitch destroyed. The disadvantage of these aid programs (free distribution of supplies) is that they work against local initiatives that for years have been trying to improve conditions for small farmers through loan programs, the gradual introduction of improved farming techniques, or soil protection. Preoccupation with the next harvest leads to more serious problems, namely, a slowdown in the rural development process and lack of motivation on the part of farmers (if food and the factors of production are distributed for free, why not take advantage of them?).

A Program of Reconstruction for Nicaragua: Beyond Hurricane Mitch

This chapter does not claim to offer recipes for the reconstruction of Nicaragua. It will therefore add nothing very new to what has already been suggested by numerous organizations.[2] We would simply like to underscore certain key factors that should be taken into account in the planning of reconstruction programs.

Meeting the Real Needs

Donor countries and organizations should not accept that the reconstruction program should be limited to simply paying the bills for the damage caused by Mitch without any matching contribution from the Nicaraguan government. The structural adjustment agreements signed with the International Monetary Fund appear to be the best policy for development. The role assigned to international aid is limited to covering the costs incurred by Mitch. The Nicaraguan government has proposed a variety of programs that include much more than a mere long-term reconstruction strategy. However, we have seen how eleven years of massive international aid, provided on the basis of the same criteria (instead of compensating for the shocks caused by Mitch, international aid substituted for the state in the social sector), have not contributed to the meaningful development of the country or given any hope of such development. A sound program of national reconstruction should take account of the failure of previous policies and of the opinions of political parties and civil organizations. It should also facilitate rather than prevent the involvement of all social classes in future development programs.[3] The involvement of the rural sector in these processes and protection of the natural environment should be the highlight of the program.

Reduction of the Foreign Debt[4]

The complete cancellation of Nicaragua's foreign debt, or at least its reduction to bring it down to a manageable level, is an indispensable precondition for the country's development. On 31 January 1999, the nominal value of Nicaragua's foreign debt was $6,271 million. Compared with other national economic indicators, one sees that Nicaragua's debt is unsustainable relative to its economy. It is among the highest in the world on a per capita basis ($1,315 per capita) and also one of the highest relative to GDP ($280). Moreover, debt servicing in 1998 represented over 60 percent of the value of exports and two-thirds of the government's resources. A large part of international aid funds thus goes toward debt payment, to the detriment of the social sector, which sees money initially earmarked for social programs disappear. Nicaragua's foreign debt is therefore the major obstacle preventing the country from breaking out of the vicious circle of poverty. Cancellation of the debt should not be automatic, however. It should be granted on condition that the extra funds generated by debt cancellation be used in the social sector to launch development programs for the benefit of the entire population and in particular the most vulnerable sectors.

Rigorous Oversight of the Reconstruction Program

The planning of a coherent reconstruction program and discussions about it between the government and donor countries are not enough to guarantee its implementation. It is imperative to secure the political commitment of the current government and its successors in office to see the program through to completion. During the consultations held in Geneva in 1998, the Nicaraguan government submitted to the donor countries a rural development program that received unanimous support. This program based the country's development on increased production in the agricultural sector, which would be used for either domestic consumption or for export, thereby reversing the trade deficit (one of the causes of Nicaragua's foreign debt). Through loans, technology transfers, and training, small and medium-sized farmers were to have been integrated into the process of rural development. However, when the time came to make these loans available to villagers, the government allocated the funds through large national banks. Since these banks do not have branches in certain parts of the country, they are not in contact with this sector of the population and are reluctant to run the risk of working with people who do not have sufficient collateral. Consequently, most of the loans earmarked for small farmers were granted to large agricultural landowners, thereby undermining the initial strategy.

In order to avoid such practices, clear follow-up indicators must be established to ensure compliance with reconstruction policies that are put in place in the same way as structural adjustment agreements are monitored. The donors must also affirm their commitment to monitoring compliance with the terms of the agreements. The international community is currently attempting to reach an agreement on the distribution of funding by sector of activity (the International Development Bank is funding the reconstruction of roads; the European Union is responsible for health care and education) without supporting any particular intervention strategy. Since the early 1990s, this same scenario has been endlessly repeated ... and has always failed.

Notes

Jorge Pereiro Piñon is Action Against Hunger head of mission in Nicaragua.

1. For more on the historical exclusion of the Nicaraguan peasant, see the study by Maldidier and de Marchetti, *Le paysan propriétaire terrien* (Managua, Nicaragua: UCA, 1996).

2. For an example, see the document by the Civil Emergency and Reconstruction Coordinator, *Transforming the Tragedy of Mitch into an Opportunity for Sustainable Human Development in Nicaragua* (Managua, 1999). For an overview of the position of the European nongovernmental organizations, see the document by VOICE, *Document de Bruxelles: proposition des ONG*

européennes lors de la réunion de Stockholm pour la reconstruction et le développement de l'Amérique centrale (Brussels: VOICE, 1999).

3. The cities of León and Estelí illustrate this strategy for reconstruction. The development program was already in place before Hurricane Mitch. The original plan has been adapted to the new situation in order to integrate reconstruction into the long-term strategy for the cities.

4. Data used here were taken from the economic indices for January 1999, published by the Central Bank of Nicaragua.

11

Honduras: Supplying Water to Victims of Hurricane Mitch

Eric Drouart

In October 1998, Hurricane Mitch, which devastated Honduras from the Caribbean to the Pacific coast, caused a major disaster whose scale even today is difficult to evaluate precisely. The main figures announced by the authorities following the hurricane indicate that the damage was enormous:

- in terms of human cost, the best estimates are 7,070 dead, 12,303 injured, 9,014 missing, 1,960,000 people affected, and 645,201 people living in temporary shelters;
- in terms of economic cost, 169 bridges were destroyed, 15 main roads and 60 towns were damaged, one town was totally destroyed, and 15 municipalities were partially destroyed;
- in the agricultural sector, the loss of crops was estimated to be between 60 percent and 80 percent of national production (a loss of $600 million in all sectors combined, according to the World Food Program).

Total rainfall over a three-day period was 911 millimeters (mm); normal annual rainfall is between 1,400 and 2,000 mm. The average rate of flow of the Choluteca River, which flows through the towns of Tegucigalpa and Choluteca, is 55.5 cubic meters per second (m³/s), with peaks capable of reaching 1,000 m³/s at times of flooding. During Hurricane Mitch, the rate of flow was estimated to be between 5,000 and 6,000 m³/s.

The low-lying town of Choluteca and the villages along the river were submerged by a sheet of water several meters deep and of

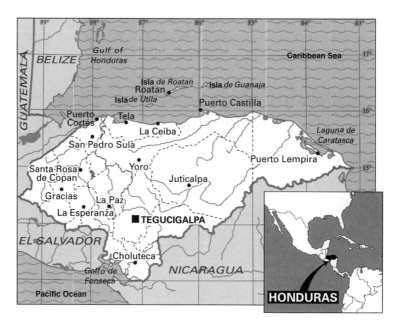

Honduras

unprecedented violence: bridges and warehouses swept away, river banks eroded over several hundred meters, houses and buildings destroyed, vehicles and containers swept away by water. A warehouse containing drums of pesticide was swept away across the plain by the flood.

An evaluation mission was led by a multidisciplinary Action Against Hunger team. The evaluation report established a priority area of operations and identified the major damage done and its medium-term consequences in the context of a difficult economic situation.

Priority Area of Operations

Although the whole country was affected by Hurricane Mitch, Action Against Hunger identified a priority area of operations, along the Choluteca River starting from Villa San Francisco (in the department of Francisco Morazan), passing through El Paraíso and up to the mouth of the river in the Gulf of Fonseca (department of Choluteca).

The authorities listed several thousand direct victims of the hurri-

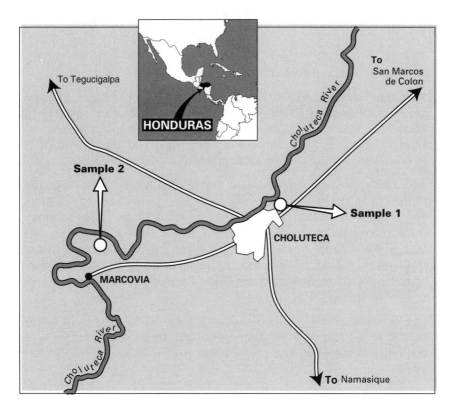

Locations of sites: Choluteca plain

cane in the department of Choluteca. Some of the affected population described an ordeal lasting several days, which they spent cling-
ing to trees or taking refuge on the roof of a house on solid ground.
In the municipalities of Choluteca and Marcovia (downstream from
Choluteca), the most severely affected towns (40 percent of the population), the authorities reported the relocation of 7,797 people in the
hurricane's aftermath.

This area was particularly hard hit because of the many rivers and
streams that flow into the Choluteca River and the large number of
villages along its course. It should also be noted that those who were
most affected in these villages were primarily the most vulnerable
(those living in fragile homes) and the owners of small agricultural
plots (melons, corn, sorghum, and so on) often situated along the
river and thus completely destroyed. Not only were crops lost, but
much of the land was rendered unsuitable for any farming at all.

Damage to Infrastructure and Other Major Damage

The major damage caused by Hurricane Mitch in the three departments may be classified as follows:

Road infrastructure and bridges.   Part of the population living in isolated
areas was beyond the reach of the main roads: in the municipalities of
Morolica, San Isidro, Liure, and Soledad in the department of
Choluteca; Trojes, Teupasenti, and Yuscarán in the department of El
Paraíso; and Malaíca in the department of Francisco Morazan.

Public infrastructure (schools, health centers) and individual homes.   Because of the
destruction, the population had to be accommodated in shelters.
Some of these shelters were quickly closed in some villages, others
remained open longer, such as the one in the town of Choluteca that
housed some 6,000 people. Emergency rehabilitation operations are
in progress thanks to civil security organizations, in collaboration
with the population and with the "food for work" program sponsored
by the World Food Program.

Crops and food distribution.   Destruction of up to 70 percent of crops
meant dependence on food distribution. The next planting season
was in April-May 1999 and the next harvest the following July-August
1999.

Medium-Term Consequences

In terms of nutrition, some moderate cases of malnutrition were
reported by the monitoring system. These led to fears that the situation might worsen for the most vulnerable groups, in particular children, if the general distribution of food failed to cover all needs in
certain at-risk zones.

The risk of a regional epidemic existed in the zone adjoining the
Fonseca delta, where 264 cases of leptospirosis were identified in the
provinces (Chinandega and Estelí) on the border with Nicaragua. In
the department of El Paraíso, there was an increase in cases of diarrhea, an illness usually most widespread during the rainy season. The
numerous bodies of stagnant water and the contamination of wells
and surface water led to fears of the outbreak of disease, in particular
cholera. An effective epidemiological monitoring system was established within the health services and its decentralized community network, but greater vigilance was still needed.

In the area of water supply, the problems were both the serious disruptions in the services provided by the small urban water supply systems of the municipalities and the destruction of or damage to wells in rural areas, making rapid action necessary. Work to restore the networks and to provide emergency supplies (purification units, transportation of water by trucks, pumps, and chlorination) was soon in progress but needs were difficult to meet, given the current problems of access. These emergency supplies had to be followed up by more long-term actions focusing on preserving the gains already made.

In response, the state, with massive assistance from civilian relief organizations and the national armies of other countries (Mexico, the United States, and some states of the European Union), immediately provided emergency relief: The government cleared roads, rebuilt metal bridges (within a few days for the Tegucigalpa bridge), and assisted people in remote areas. This was the first time that we have witnessed on this scale such a mobilization of states whose armies and civil organizations have provided emergency relief. A few months later, the Kosovo crisis confirmed the growing humanitarian involvement of states in certain very visible humanitarian crises, unfortunately to the detriment of others that were less visible.

A few months after the disaster, Choluteca was a town under reconstruction. It was invaded by dust from the silt deposited by the flood and had a displaced population of several thousand residents. They were housed first in schools and public buildings and later in temporary shelters along the road to the airport as they awaited the permanent reconstruction of their homes on a new adjacent plot. A new town, New Choluteca, was rebuilt with international assistance. What will be its future? Its economic viability is questionable.

The process of allocating plots of land for rehousing Choluteca families under the authority of the town council was a long one. Uncontrolled scrambling to obtain a plot came as no surprise, and identifying needy families was very difficult. By early 1999, a story making the rounds in Choluteca testified to the complexity of the situation. According to this story, tents were springing up like mushrooms along the road leading to New Choluteca, put up by families who claimed to be victims and installed one of their members in the roadside shelters. In this country where land is scarce, one can easily imagine what might be done by unscrupulous speculators in order to rent out later a house that they had acquired through scheming or other arrangement.

Farther upstream, the river valley was destroyed. The rare very fertile areas cultivated by the inhabitants were completely eroded. Numerous landslides and mudslides claimed many victims, and here too, the material damage was considerable: roads, homes, water conveyances, water pipes, and fittings all swept away (90 percent of the installations). Nevertheless, the number of victims was much lower, since only 2 percent of the population of the department of El Paraíso were estimated to have been directly affected by the hurricane.

Action Against Hunger concentrated its efforts on providing and protecting water resources along the Choluteca river valley by developing three specific responses: (1) undertaking long-term rehabilitation of gravity-based drinking water supply networks for disaster victims in rural areas, (2) drilling deep wells in the Choluteca plain, and (3) carrying out a hydrogeological analysis of the department and monitoring water quality.

Before the long-term rehabilitation of gravity-based drinking water supply networks was started, emergency steps to restore water supplies to villages were carried out; in 80 percent of the cases these steps were taken immediately after the hurricane by villagers with or without outside help. These repairs were temporary, however (a plastic hose referred to locally as a *manga* placed on the ground with no protection, landslides stabilized, springs redirected), and we proposed long-term solutions that would enable these villages to regain the same degree of autonomy they enjoyed before Hurricane Mitch. Villagers genuinely and effectively assumed responsibility for this work. A complete rehabilitation of service, from catchment to distribution of the water, took between ten and fifteen days of community work, with a single technician from Action Against Hunger on site.

Drilling deep wells in the plain will protect water supply points from pollution, particularly at relocation sites for disaster victims (New Choluteca and Marcovia). The Choluteca plain suffered from water pollution from two sources: agriculture (in an area of intensive cotton farming and today melon farming) and accidents, following the spillage of pesticides from containers swept away by the floods. The "drilling" option that allows protected, deep underground water to be tapped is all the more important because of the pollution. Action Against Hunger was the only nongovernmental organization to propose this technical approach, which had significant success in alleviating the problem.

Carrying out the hydrogeological analysis of the department and the monitoring of water quality involved development of remote sensing to estimate damage and to evaluate hurricane-related risks. In partnership with a Thai company (Promotion of Appropriate Technologies), Action Against Hunger has developed light percussion and rotary drilling equipment able to pierce compact and other soil formations and has gained considerable experience in this area as well as in the area of water research. The ACF/PAT401 rotor-percussion drill in stock in Paris is a machine that can be transported by pickup truck, thereby permitting quick drilling in any type of aquifer at an exploratory depth of approximately 100 meters.

The drilling equipment was transported by priority air freight to Choluteca in late November 1998, after the first test results had been confirmed by the on-site hydrogeologist. In hydrological terms, the potential aquifers of the Choluteca department are the alluvial, somewhat coarse deposits and the fractures in hard volcanic formations.

Use of the appropriate tools is vital in the search for subterranean water. These include the development of a structural satellite image, aerial photographs, and geoelectric soundings. A geochemical and hydrogeological analytic capability (piezometric and water-quality maps, extensive pump testing) of the Choluteca plain has also been developed.

Nearly a dozen successful drillings (output of 1 to 30 cubic meters per hour) were initially completed on the relocation sites, and a well was sunk to supply the town of Choluteca, since the pumping station, located in the main riverbed, was totally submerged by the floods and destroyed. These wells are equipped with either hand pumps or submersible pumps, depending on their characteristics.

In addition to the normal bacteriological analyses of the water that were required because of the risk of chemical pollution, caused mainly by agricultural activities in the plain and aggravated by spillage from warehouse stocks, we carried out systematic monthly analyses of organophosphate and organochloric pesticides at each new drilling. These chromatographic analyses are performed by a Tegucigalpa laboratory that is certified by the U.S. government for the export of food.

During the hurricane, metal barrels of pesticide from the storage depot were swept away by the floods. Information concerning the number of barrels in storage before the hurricane was either unavailable or unclear. Only a list of the types of product in stock was provided by the storage company's officials. A number of these barrels were found downstream on the riverbanks and retrieved by villagers. It is highly likely that some of these barrels were carried to the mouth of the river and into the sea during the flood. Others are likely to be buried in the sediment, which is very deep (several meters) in this area.

No cases of poisoning were reported in the short run. The major risk was certainly from direct contact when the barrels were found by the residents just after the hurricane. Public awareness campaigns were carried out on the radio by civil security officials.

Drillings at four sites revealed the presence of pesticides, all of them organochlorides: lindane, benzene hexachloride, and endosulphates. Drillings at two sites revealed concentrated amounts of pesticides that were above safe drinking levels (endosulphates in one case and benzene hexachloride in the other).

The test results at Marcovia that revealed a concentration of endosulphates (1.32 ppm [parts per million]) far above the acceptable norm of 0.01 ppm were reviewed after pumping was done for a longer period and at other water supply points in the immediate vicinity.

For wells containing benzene hexachloride, which is not considered to be a highly toxic chemical, the authorities decided to dilute the water to ensure that it was of acceptable quality for drinking.

Given the limited scope of testing and the constant risk of chemical pollution (buried barrels, pesticides), follow-up action on an ongoing basis is essential.

Mapping of Damage and of At-Risk Zones

Radar images taken before and after Hurricane Mitch and a spot image taken after the hurricane were used to identify areas affected by the floods.

The first phase of the study was carried out by a geoscience consultancy based in Paris, and a field survey was conducted by on-site Action Against Hunger teams. Images were provided free of cost by Spot Image and by the European Geoscience Space Agency.

These images revealed the extent of the flooding and the movement of the river beyond its main bed. Eroded areas and areas where sediment was deposited and cultivable land destroyed were all easily identifiable. Areas that are vulnerable to accidental pollution, such as that caused by pesticide spills, were also easily identifiable. For example, the damage to the town of Marcovia, half of which was under water, was clearly visible. As part of this study, the geoscience consultancy also showed the erosion of the shore caused by the powerful waves that lashed the Caribbean coast in northern Honduras during the hurricane.

Though limited in scope, this study confirmed the need for remote sensing equipment in the aftermath of a major natural catastrophe such as Hurricane Mitch in order to assess and identify the main damage caused within a short period of time (about ten days).

Honduras, like all of Central America in general, is a region that is very vulnerable to hurricanes. The situation in Honduras continues to cause concern. The landslides caused by Hurricane Mitch have not stabilized; the level of riverbeds has been raised in certain areas by deposits of sediment; and the next flood will encounter significantly shallower channels, which is likely to result in extensive overflowing. The population residing along the rivers has returned, as might be expected, given the fertile farming land and the shortage of land in the country, and at-risk zones therefore continue to be inhabited.

It is now urgently necessary to prepare a precise map of the at-risk zones along the Choluteca River and to classify them into categories (habitable, crop-farming, or cattle-rearing areas).

Such a risk map will clearly also be a tool for the development of a land use plan, and only the strict adherence to that plan in the medium term will enable Honduras to limit the loss of human life and the damage caused by hurricanes like Mitch in this region.

Notes

Eric Drouart is a hydrogeologist.

Bibliography

Drouart, Eric, and Jean-Michel Vouillamoz. *L'Alimentation en eau des populations menacées*. Paris: Hermann, 1999.

12

The Tragedy of Kosovo

Frances Mason and Kathryn Ogden

Throughout the 1980s, accusations grew within the Serb community in Kosovo of a "physical, political, juridical, and cultural genocide" by the Albanian majority. This gave excuses for the Serb leadership to add further to the repression forced upon the Albanian majority. One person, Slobodan Milosevic, whose initial interest in Kosovo had been distinctly lacking, knew how to make use of this growing Serb nationalism and used Kosovo as his catapult to power. The economic and political sanctions imposed by Belgrade on the Kosovars following their loss of autonomy gradually led to the splintering away of the Kosovo Liberation Army (KLA) from the initial nonviolence policies of the Albanians, policies that were led by the president of the Albanian-declared independent Kosovo. Hunger was again, as in many countries, being used as a weapon.[1] Access to land was reduced, unemployment rose to 70 percent, and the economic sanctions resulting from the Bosnian war imposed by the international community on Serbia and Montenegro had detrimental repercussions on the Kosovars; worse was to come. In February 1998, a sudden escalation in fighting began, and in May 1998, the Serbian authorities banned twenty-seven of the most essential items (such as flour, meat, vegetables, fuel, and soap) from all Albanian shops. This chapter exposes the ways and methods employed by the authorities in manipulating the food economy as a weapon of repression.

Chronology

1989	Slobodan Milosevic strips Kosovo of its autonomy.
February 1990	The Federal Republic of Yugoslavia sends troops, tanks, warplanes, and 2,000 more police into Kosovo.
July 1990	Ethnic Albanian legislators in Kosovo declare independence. Serbia dissolves the Kosovo Assembly.
May 1992	Ibrahim Rugova elected president of the self-proclaimed republic of Kosovo.
October 1992	Serb and ethnic Albanian leaders in Kosovo hold face-to-face peace talks for the first time in three years.
July 1995	A Serbian court sentences sixty-eight ethnic Albanians to imprisonment for allegedly setting up a parallel police force.
August 1995	Serbs settle several hundred Croatian Serb refugees in Kosovo. The Kosovo Liberation Army emerges for the first time, claiming responsibility for a series of bomb attacks.
January 1998	An ethnic Serb policeman is killed in retaliation for the reported killing of an ethnic Albanian by the police.
February-March 1998	Serbian police operations in Drenica. Dozens are killed, houses burnt, and villages evacuated; protests and street clashes in Pristina. Rugova demands outright independence for Kosovo. Ethnic Albanians vote for a president and a parliament in elections that are considered illegal by Belgrade.
April 1998	Ninety-five percent of Serbs vote against intervention in Kosovo. The contact group for the former Yugoslavia, with the exception of Russia, agrees to impose new sanctions against Yugoslavia over Kosovo.
May 1998	U.S. envoy Richard Holbrooke begins a round of shuttle diplomacy, which results in Milosevic's inviting Rugova for peace talks. The fighting continues.

Demographics:
The Key to Power and Economic Strength

The birthrate of the Albanian population in Kosovo, despite its apparent reduction since the period following World War II, remains the highest in Europe. Almost half the population (48.2 percent) is under eighteen years of age. The population density of 200 per square kilometer (km²) is twice that of Serbia at 104/km², creating a serious problem of access to land in a province in which more than 60 percent of the population live in rural areas. Urban areas have been expanding, moreover, encroaching on rural areas. It has been estimated that between 1960 and 1970, the area of cultivable land diminished by 1,000 hectares per year.

Migration: An Economic
Coping Strategy for the Kosovars

Social organization within the Albanian community is based on clan and family structures that are maintained by a code of honor. Strong solidarity exists among families of the same or neighboring villages, manifesting itself in economic terms in the form of loans and the sharing of food.

In forcing large numbers of Kosovar Albanians abroad, the Serb authorities inadvertently paved the way for an improved coping strategy for those remaining in the province. As is the case with other Muslim communities, many ethnic Albanians from the diaspora contribute a 3 percent income tax (the Zakhat), which has helped to fund the medical and educational institutions within the province. Sending a member of the family abroad has been one of the principal means of survival for many families. The great solidarity between families is such that the member abroad will send all the money he (or sometimes she) has available after meeting his or her basic needs. The money enters Kosovo with visa holders or through travel agencies that offer a transfer service for a 10 percent commission.

The situation was similar in the Serbian areas of Kosovo. With the closure or reduction in output of metallurgical mines in the northern municipalities and other manufacturing industries, there had been an increase in unemployment and a subsequent move into Serbia to seek work, especially by young people. But jobs found in Serbia have generally been low paid, and Serbian workers have faced more difficulties than Kosovar Albanians working in the European Union in sending any money back for relatives.

A History of Two-Way
Accusations of Ethnic Cleansing

Accusations by the Kosovo Albanians

There is nothing new in Kosovars having to leave their homeland in search of work abroad. In the 1970s, Germany, then suffering from labor shortages, had an agreement with the former Yugoslavia as a result of which nearly 15 percent of the present-day population were issued with permanent visas allowing free travel between the two countries.

Before the mass exodus of refugees in March and April 1999, those working and living abroad could be grouped into three broad categories:

- long-term emigrants who had spent twenty or more years abroad;
- those who had left since 1989;
- those who had left since the mid-1990s.

It is the latter two groups, however, whose departure from Kosovo was mainly triggered by the imposed economic strife and fear of persecution. The Serb policies of the 1990s demonstrated a will to render the life of the Albanians so intolerable as to force them to leave. In this they were more than successful: Between 1990 and 1995 an estimated 350,000 Kosovars moved out of the province.[2] Estimates at the end of 1998 were that since 1989, 500,000 to 600,000 Albanians had moved as a result of the economic and political crisis.[3] Furthermore, the authorities "Serbianized" the province by changing names of streets, imposing the Serb language, suppressing the Albanian media, and destroying Albanian cultural institutions.

There are certain more sinister accusations, some say evidence, by the Albanians of the attempts to empty Kosovo of its majority Albanian population. In March and April 1990, thousands of children were taken to the hospital with mysterious headaches, stomach pains, and nausea. Rumors spread rapidly that the children were being deliberately poisoned at school. Most observers at the time believed this to be mass hysteria, but a UN expert on toxicology argued to the contrary. Tests showed that the substances Sarin and Tabun (used in chemical weapons) were found in urine and blood samples. In 1995, evidence emerged that the Yugoslav army manufactured Sarin. The Albanian uproar over this episode gave Serbia an excuse to transfer 25,000 policemen from Serbia to the province.

In 1990, within a Yugoslav Programme of Measures to be Taken in Kosovo, family planning was introduced for the Albanians. (According to one Serbian gynecologist, out of every one hundred babies born in the whole of Serbia, sixty-four are non-Serbs. It has been predicted that by the middle of the next century the Serbs will be a minority in the entire Serbian Republic.) Albanians were "encouraged" to seek work in other parts of Yugoslavia, and sales of property to Albanians by departing Serbs were retroactively annulled.

Attempts to change the balance between Serbs and the Albanian majority were also manifested in a form of "colonization." In 1991, a law was passed giving Serbs and Montenegrins who returned to Kosovo the right to 5 hectares of land, to be supplied free of charge out of municipal land holdings. Furthermore, during the Bosnian war, Serb refugees were willingly welcomed by the authorities in Belgrade to settle in Kosovo. However, both these attempts by the Serb government to change the Kosovo ethnic imbalance were unpopular with the respective Serb populations in question. One busful of Serb refugees leaving Bosnia, on learning that their destination was Kosovo, held the bus driver at gun point and demanded that they head for Belgrade instead.

Accusations by the Kosovo Serbs

The 1980s saw an increasingly fervent campaign of complaint from the Kosovo Serbs, manifesting itself in several ways. In the autumn of 1985, a petition was organized demanding protection for the Kosovo Serb population and claiming the presence of 300,000 Albanians who had crossed into Kosovo from Albania since 1941 (the implication being that they should all be sent back).

Serb nationalism was clearly growing. In 1985, a memorandum was drawn up that claimed "physical, political, juridical and cultural genocide" of the Serb population (the full text of this was only published in 1989). However, the objective of the memorandum was its claim that 200,000 Serbs had emigrated during the previous two decades and its advice that the government should establish "objective and lasting conditions for the return of [these] exiled people."

Seven years later, with the launching of Serbia's war of territorial expansion against Bosnia in April 1992, the position of the Albanians in Kosovo worsened greatly. Serbian nationalism concentrated rhetoric on the "Islamic threat," alluding to the Muslims in Bosnia right down to those in Kosovo. However, it is widely recognized that the role of religion in Kosovar politics is negligible (an example of this can be seen in the fact that no one questions the existence of a

Christian Democratic party in which the overwhelming majority is Muslim).

Political Upheavals:
Kosovo Launches the Career of Milosevic

This rise in nationalism shocked the majority of the senior communists in Belgrade. However, one member of the Serbian Central Committee, namely Slobodan Milosevic, knew how to use the nationalism to his advantage. In April 1987, his moment came. Ivan Stambolic, the Serbian party president, was called upon by sixty thousand Serb and Montenegrin activists to give a speech in the town of Kosovo Polje in preparation for a large protest in Belgrade to warn that the Kosovo Serbs could no longer endure the "genocide" being inflicted on their community by Albanian irredentists and to demand the purge of Kosovo's Albanian leadership. Already bruised from past experiences (in which he had spoken against Serb nationalism), Stambolic asked his deputy, Slobodan Milosevic, to take his place. Stambolic since recalls that before this moment, Milosevic had shown no interest in Kosovo. Milosevic had once told Stambolic to forget about the provinces and get back to Yugoslavia. However, at the meeting in Kosovo, carefully preplanned fighting broke out between Serbs and the police. Milosevic broke off the meeting and spoke out, "No one should dare to beat you." Fortunately for Milosevic, this was on camera, leading to an eloquent speech on the sacred rights of the Serbs. By the end of 1987, Stambolic was dismissed from power, and Milosevic took over as president of the Serbian League of Communists. In November 1988, Milosevic held a rally of 350,000 in Belgrade in which he declared, "Every nation has a love that eternally warms its heart. For Serbia it is Kosovo."

The Buildup to the Loss of Autonomy for Kosovo

Accusations and demands from the Serb nationalists contributed greatly to Belgrade's review of the status of Kosovo. Early in 1989, the Kosovars detected clear signs of a far greater transfer of power to Serbian control. Kosovo's police, courts, and civil defense were to be put under Serbian control, together with social, economic, and educational policies. Serbia assumed the power to issue "administrative instructions." Rapidly diminishing rights led to a series of protests, strikes, and mass demonstrations by the Albanians. Serbian leaders responded by sending in troops to Kosovo and declaring a state of emergency. Final amendments to the constitution were adopted on 28 March 1989, whereby Kosovo's "autonomy" was reduced to a mere token. More protests were answered with more troops and police.

Kosovo: "An Equal and Independent Entity Within the Framework of the Yugoslav Federation"

The reactions of the Albanian members of the Provincial Assembly appeared, initially, to be submission under pressure.

However, in July 1990, 114 of the 123 Albanian members of the assembly met in the street outside the locked assembly building and passed a resolution declaring Kosovo "an equal and independent entity within the framework of the Yugoslav Federation." Intellectual circles were the very core of the Albanian move, which established a party called the Democratic League of Kosovo (LDK), whose leader was a specialist in literary history and aesthetics, Dr. Ibrahim Rugova. In response, the Serbian authorities dissolved the assembly and the government, thus destroying the last threads of Kosovo autonomy. On 24 May 1992, the Kosovars held elections throughout Kosovo, using private houses as polling stations under the noses of the Serbian authorities, to create a new republican assembly and government.

The basic policy of the LDK and Rugova was threefold: to maintain nonviolence, "internationalize" the problem, and systematically deny Serbian rule by boycotting elections and censuses and creating at least the outlines of the state apparatus of a Kosovo Republic.

International recognition of the independence of Croatia and Slovenia in June 1991 gave further hope to the leaders of the LDK that their dreams would become reality.

Strict adherence to nonviolence was ordered by the Kosovar leaders, and because of the importance of the clan structure and the resultant respect for leaders, this order was smoothly followed, at least initially. In order to further understand the apparent belief in and optimism about the prospect of independence and of imminent support from the international community, the prevailing political climate must be understood. In 1989, political change through nonviolent means had been demonstrated: The Berlin Wall had fallen; in Poland the strictly nonviolent movement around the trade union Solidarity enjoyed worldwide support and brought down the totalitarian communist regime; previously dependent territories such as the Baltic states were regaining their independence and even imposing their own language on their former master; Czechoslovakia gained a new president—a dissident writer. Hence, within this context, the idea appeared plausible that a Kosovo led by an intellectual who advocated nonviolence would become an independent republic.

Changes in the Kosovar Strategy of Nonviolence

The Albanian population increasingly lost faith in Rugova. After his prognosis of the impact of the Bosnia war on Kosovo, Rugova lost credence when the Dayton Agreement of November 1995 left Kosovo in a position that was no different than before. The only recognition it received was the Security Council's decision to continue sanctions against Serbia until its human rights record in Kosovo was reformed. Beyond that, the recognition by the West that Milosovic was a key player in the implementation of the Dayton Peace Agreement only reinforced the Kosovars' enemy.

Rugova was criticized within Kosovo for refusing to negotiate with Belgrade. When he eventually began talks with Milosevic, the agreement under which school and university buildings (but not state salaries) would be made available to the Albanian parallel education system was later totally ignored by Milosevic, thus furthering Rugova's loss of face.

For years, the Kosovar "terrorism" referred to in the Serb media had been little more than stone throwing. However, the growing discontent within Kosovo resulted in an increase in more serious activities such as bombings and shootings. By the summer of 1997, a spokesman for a body calling itself the Kosovo Liberation Army was giving interviews from Switzerland in which he announced, "This is the movement people support now."

Economic Sanctions as a Weapon

Despite sizable deposits of lead and zinc in Kosovo (especially in the region of Trepca and in the Kopaonick range) and abundant reserves of lignite and chromate, the province of Kosovo has for many years been considered among the poorest regions in Europe. Even before the current crisis, many sanitary and electricity installations were rudimentary and the unemployment rate extremely high.

Agricultural Subsistence Economy

Agriculture plays a central role in the economy of Kosovo. However, it is constrained by a number of factors:

- Access to cultivable land is limited, owing to demographic pressure and the scarcity of land. Approximately two-thirds of the land is mountainous and composed of forests and pasture-land (on which only limited cereal production is possible). The remainder consists of plains, which are used for growing cereals.
- The size of family plots is small, the result of historical circumstances. Unlike many former socialist or communist countries, Tito's Yugoslavia did not have a system of state farms or agricultural cooperative systems. Land privatization started in 1946 and quickly averaged 90 percent of all available land. Originally, families possessed several hectares, but over the years demographic pressure has led to subdividing. Today the average family plot is rarely more than 5 hectares (50 percent of plots are between 1 and 5 hectares).
- The provision of agricultural inputs is dependent on supplies from Serbia and Vojvodine.
- Productivity is low, owing to poor seed quality, lack of access to hybrid varieties that yield better results, outdated planting techniques, limited use of fertilizers, poor irrigation techniques, and slow harvesting of grains caused by the lack of agricultural machinery.

Under "normal" conditions, agricultural and livestock production covers about two-thirds of the food needs of the population of Kosovo, with the rest being imported, particularly from Serbia and Vojvodine. The chronic deficiencies are in wheat (35 percent) and animal protein (30 to 60 percent). Shortfalls in wheat production usually occur in June and July.

1990: Loss of Jobs for 70 Percent of Albanian Kosovars and Prosperity for Serbs

In response to Kosovo's "declaration of independence" in 1990, the Serbian Assembly passed a special law on "labor relations" in Kosovo, which made possible the subsequent expulsion of more than 80,000 Albanians from their jobs. Some 70 percent of Albanian state employees in Kosovo were dismissed from their jobs. The larger food manufacturing factories in Kosovo closed or reduced their capacity.

Kosovar unemployment is estimated at 70 percent (the number of unemployed having risen by 130,000 since 1990). According to the Kosovar Pristina Economic Institute, earnings from regular employment accounted for 10 percent of total Kosovar income in 1996, compared to 49 percent in 1988. Emigration is generally viewed as the only way to make a decent living. Any remaining employment for the Kosovars is mainly in the service sectors, small businesses, international organizations, and black market trading.

At the same time, a Programme for the Realization of Peace and Prosperity in Kosovo was launched by the Serb authorities. This included the creation of new municipalities for the Serb population and the building of new houses for Serbs who returned to Kosovo.

Economic Sanctions During the Bosnian War

In the 1980s, Kosovo experienced an economic boom in mining and food production. However, the international economic sanctions that were eventually imposed on Serbia and Montenegro had an equally detrimental effect on Kosovo, leading to the closing of the Kosovo-Macedonia border to most forms of direct trade. This came on top of an already chaotic economy (by simply printing more money to pay his soldiers, Milosevic had created a spiral of inflation). However, the forced reliance of Kosovars on self-subsistence through agriculture and private trade rendered them, in some ways, less vulnerable to economic sanctions than were the Serbs, whose income was dependent on salaried state employment.

An additional reason for the economic disarray within Serbia was the emergence of Mafia-style gangs that took over the market in foreign goods and hard currency.

Economic Strengthening of the Kosovars: Impact of the Fighting and International Interventions

Despite the heavy dependence of households on money from family members abroad and the support of the diaspora for the parallel Albanian education and health system, Kosovar authorities have generally had problems raising money in the last five years. Since the Drenica violence in early 1998, however, the inflow has exceeded all expectations. Substantial funds were mobilized, particularly in Aachen, Germany. Many Kosovars are choosing to contribute to the fund of the Kosovo Republic rather than to that of the largest political party, the LDK with its government and its leader, President Rugova, in exile.

Evidence toward the end of 1998 showed furthermore that the growing economic strength of the Kosovars could also be attributed to the presence of the Organization for Security and Cooperation in

Europe (OSCE) and, to a certain extent, of humanitarian organizations. Rental prices for properties tripled within a few weeks of the arrival of the OSCE, while market prices increased and salary demands far exceeded previous levels.

Control of Goods: Using Hunger as a Weapon

Financial resources are of no use if access to goods is prohibited. The greatest effect on the circulation of essential food and nonfood items within Kosovo began with those items whose trade came under the control of the Serbian authorities just after the start of the present conflict in May 1998. This resulted in Albanian shopkeepers, who are the core of market activity, being refused permission to stock certain basic items in their stores.

Initially, twenty-seven items were banned from sale at Albanian stores. The food items to which the population was being denied access included flour, the key to their staple diet of bread. Replacement starches such as rice, pasta, and potatoes were also banned. Salt, sugar, oil, butter, and margarine were banned, and some of the most protein-rich foods, such as meat and fish, were also included in the list. When Action Against Hunger assessed the situation in January 1999, controls had been lifted on milk, yogurt, and cheese. The population was further deprived of an essential source of minerals and vitamins through the inclusion of canned fruit and vegetables on the list of items banned from Albanian shops. Nonfood items on the list included soap, shampoo, detergent, drugs, sanitary items, engine fuel, diesel, engine oil, and gas.

At the beginning of the summer of 1998, a complete ban was imposed for a three-week period, immediately after which the heavy demand for certain items resulted in long queues. A crisis ensued until traders began the black market trade, easing the situation but far from addressing the root problem.

The remaining items became available only on the black market. Individuals with private cars or warehouse owners with trucks may have attempted to travel outside Kosovo to Serbia and buy the items, finding ways and taking severe risks to bring back the goods. Suppliers from Serbia with whom they dealt may also have delivered directly, but many warehouse owners preferred to be in direct control of their goods. Heavy fines or bribes were more often than not demanded by the border police and at checkpoints to get passage for the goods.

Village stores either bought directly from Serbia using the method described above or from a store in the nearest larger town.

Previously, they would have obtained supplies from different towns, but since they were subject to stops by police, there was greater risk in traveling and therefore supplies were restricted to goods available in the nearest town. The items were concealed in the vehicle and brought directly to the village shop. During the most serious times of conflict in 1998, it was extremely difficult to supply the shops, partly on account of roadblocks that forced some to drive tractors through mountain roads to get supplies. Some shops had to close temporarily while others have never reopened.

As a result, village stores stocked far fewer items than they had before the conflict, and with the rise in prices villagers were unable to afford a wide range of goods, hence often purchasing only the most essential items needed for daily use. Certain shops offered credit to the customers (one week to three months), but others suffered such huge losses through this system that it was no longer an option for the customer.

Conclusion

A few landmarks were of particular importance in influencing and furthering the cause of the Kosovars. Initially, the atmosphere within Europe in the 1980s suggested that a fight for independence through nonviolent means might succeed. The increased economic support from the diaspora countered the Serb objective of creating such economic hardships that Kosovars would be forced out of the province, and the increased insecurity that led to greater international awareness of and presence in Kosovo led in turn to a sudden and sharp increase in the funds raised by the KLA in 1998.

This has been accompanied, however, by escalating terror against the Albanian population: the "Serbianization" of the province, suppression of Albanian culture, and denial of the rights of Kosovars to their property. Despite the hopes of the Kosovar leaders, the Bosnian war did nothing to support their cause and only brought further economic hardship and a missed opportunity for Western mediators to avoid the horrors being observed today. As greater opposition was shown by the Albanians, particularly through the formation of the Kosovo Liberation Army, so too did the clampdown by the Serbian authorities increase. The most recent manifestation of this in economic terms is perhaps best demonstrated in the "control on trade," which reduced the Kosovars to a state of insecurity in terms of access to their basic daily food and nonfood needs, to say nothing of the deliberate destruction of assets during the fighting.

In all this stands a man who only twelve years ago proclaimed a total lack of interest in the province and who has used the land and its peoples to expand and consolidate his own power. In human and population terms, Yugoslavia has already lost Kosovo. The Serbs who live in Kosovo are a minority. The majority of the rest of Serbia has no wish to join them. The whole concept of creating an "ethnic" balance in an area with a population of 200,000 Serbs and nearly two million Albanians remains an illusion.

Notes

Frances Mason is head of nutrition and food security, Action Against Hunger. Kathryn Ogden is a nutritionist at Action Against Hunger.

1. See Action Against Hunger, *Geopolitics of Hunger, 1998–1999* (Paris: PUF, 1998).

2. *Kosovo Spring Report*. Brussels: International Crisis Group Kosovo, 1998.

3. Information from the Council for Human Rights, Pristina.

Bibliography

Economic Activities and Democratic Development of Kosovo, Research report. Pristina: Riinvest, 1998.

Ferrand, Cyril. *Agricultural Study: Province of Kosovo, Federal Republic of Yugoslavia.* London: Action Against Hunger, 1998–1999.

Kosovo Spring Report. Brussels: International Crisis Group Kosovo, 1998.

Malcolm, Noel. *Kosovo: A Short History.* N.p., 1998.

Ogden, Kathryn. *Food Security Assessment in Kosovo, Federal Republic of Yugoslavia.* London: Action Against Hunger, 1998–1999.

13

A Survey of Kosovar Refugees in Macedonia, May–June 1999

Michael Brewin

Background to Assessment

The oppression of the ethnic Albanian majority in Kosovo, which began when their autonomous status was revoked in 1989, reached a head in 1999, forcing the migration of over 750,000 people from the province. Nearly 222,000 of them sought refuge in Macedonia, where Action Against Hunger and other aid agencies were stationed in anticipation of an influx of refugees.[1] In the weeks that followed the arrival of the first refugees, in addition to carrying out emergency relief programs, Action Against Hunger worked to collate information on the conditions that the refugees had faced in Kosovo prior to their arrival in Macedonia, focusing particularly on issues pertaining to their ability to procure, grow, and harvest food.

There were three main reasons for carrying out the survey. First, it was important to get an idea of the extent to which denial of access to food or the means to produce food was used as a tool of war by Serbian forces. We attempted to ascertain whether there was a deliberate attempt by the police and paramilitaries to starve Albanians out or to force them to move and not return through a kind of "scorched earth" policy. Denial of food to civilians contravenes a number of human rights conventions, so evidence of such activity is important to the authorities responsible for investigating war crimes.

A second area of interest was the coping mechanisms of the refugees during the period of the conflict and the level to which the populations of different areas were prepared for possible food shortages. We tried to build up a picture of the survival strategies employed by the Kosovars during their displacement.

Third, we were keen to establish what people's priorities would be upon their return home in order to pre-plan Action Against Hunger's strategy when return to Kosovo became possible.

Methodology

During May and June 1999, 233 families (a total of 1,675 individuals) living in the Stankovac and Cegrane camps were surveyed, using a combination of interviews, written testimonies, and questionnaires. Refugee families living in camps were chosen in preference to those in host families because they were easier to access. We experienced no difficulty in getting people to answer questions. Indeed, nearly all were thankful that their stories were being recorded.

Families to be surveyed were selected on the sole criteria of being farmers as opposed to urban dwellers but were otherwise chosen at random. We focused on farmers for two reasons. First, as was evident when we eventually returned to Kosovo, the people in the rural areas bore the brunt of the persecution; second, most Kosovars depend on farming for a living. Any plans to rebuild the area after the conflict must therefore be based largely on an accurate assessment of the extent to which rural livelihoods have been rendered unsustainable.

Because the Kosovar refugee population in Macedonia was composed largely of people from only certain regions in Kosovo (see Figure 13.1), for example, Ferizaj, Gjilan, Obiliq, and Gllocovc, it would be inaccurate to claim that the survey is representative of the population of Kosovo as a whole. Other organizations working with refugees in Albania and Montenegro have conducted similar surveys that confirm that the abuses suffered by Macedonia-based Kosovars were by no means unique to them.

Most of the data used in this report were gathered using a questionnaire that asked for information in five areas.

1. Respondents were asked for general information, the number of people in their family, and where they were from.
2. Respondents were asked the ways in which families obtained food during the period of the conflict and while they were internally displaced.
3. Questions were asked about damage sustained to food or property used in the production of food, such as tractors. We also asked whether they were prevented from accessing their land, and if so, why. Questions determined whether they had had food stolen or poisoned and whether they had been prevented

Figure 13.1   Regions of Origin of Surveyed Population

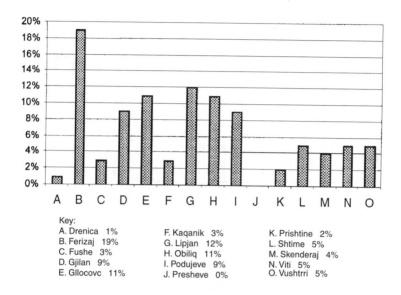

Key:
A. Drenica 1%
B. Ferizaj 19%
C. Fushe 3%
D. Gjilan 9%
E. Gllocovc 11%

F. Kaqanik 3%
G. Lipjan 12%
H. Obiliq 11%
I. Podujeve 9%
J. Presheve 0%

K. Prishtine 2%
L. Shtime 5%
M. Skenderaj 4%
N. Viti 5%
O. Vushtrri 5%

from buying food and from farming their land. The testimonies given also provide a valuable source of information on this subject.

4. In an attempt to give focus to the planning of future relief activities, respondents were asked to rank their needs upon their return in order of priority.

5. Refugees were asked to write down their personal testimonies, detailing their experiences and giving names of persons responsible for perpetrating human rights abuses against them. The main objective here was to collate evidence for use in any judicial proceedings that might ensue from the conflict, but the information given was also useful as a way of illustrating the more quantitative findings of the survey.

Causes and Immediate Effects of Displacement

The average time spent as an internally displaced person (IDP) was forty-one days. As is apparent from Figure 13.2, time spent as an IDP ranged from over 301 days to under one day. Some people arrived in Macedonia on the same day on which they left their homes in Kosovo. The testimonies of refugees reveal that many were forced to move from their homes by the police and paramilitary:

Figure 13.2   Duration of Internal Displacement in Kosovo Before Arrival in Macedonia

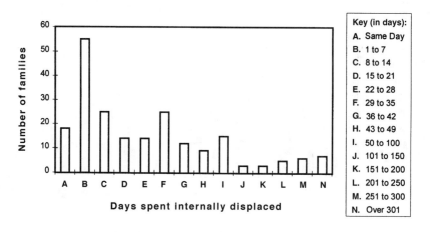

At 6 P.M. on the 5th April 1999, police came from [Serbian] Babush telling us to leave the village because it was dangerous as the military were coming. We didn't want to leave but at around 11 P.M. they came to the village shooting and shouting so we escaped to the mountains and slept there. ... The next morning we returned to Crnilla but the police came again at about 10 A.M. and told us to leave so we went to Gadime. —Farmer from Crnilla, Ferizaj

I declare that at about 10 P.M. on the 24th of May 1999, three Serbian policemen and two paramilitary gypsies, all armed, ordered us to leave our house. ... We had to leave our house or else they would have killed us. —Farmer from Vodice, Obiliq

We left our house on the 27th March because a lot of army came to Millosheve. They took over the school buildings. We stayed with our cousins until the 1st of April when the police came with masks and snipers and gave us two hours to leave the house before they set it on fire. —Farmer from Millosheve, Obiliq

In some cases a shortage of food within the household or in the local area was the catalyst for internal migration. Figure 13.3 shows that people's access to food and to the means of producing food was severely affected as a result of the war, although the extent to which destruction or theft of food and property was a deliberate "scorched earth" policy of the Serb forces is unclear. The means of food production (tractors and tools) and livestock were among the most valuable and easily transportable possessions of the farming families and therefore primary targets for thieves after money and gold had been taken. Indeed, the testimonies collected indicate that gypsies (the Roma minority who make up about 5 percent of the population of

Figure 13.3   Abuses Suffered by Kosovar Refugees While in Kosovo

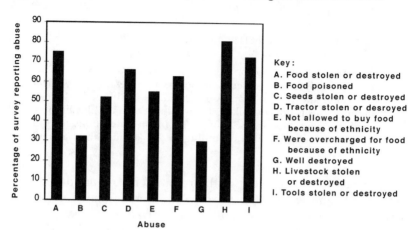

Key:
A. Food stolen or destroyed
B. Food poisoned
C. Seeds stolen or destroyed
D. Tractor stolen or desroyed
E. Not allowed to buy food
   because of ethnicity
F. Were overcharged for food
   because of ethnicity
G. Well destroyed
H. Livestock stolen
   or destroyed
I. Tools stolen or destroyed

Kosovo) were responsible for a significant amount of the stealing that took place. Food was an inviting target, especially for troops whose supply lines were being disrupted by North Atlantic Treaty Organization (NATO) attacks, so it is important not to confuse opportunism with a deliberate attempt to starve Kosovar Albanians out of the country.

Notwithstanding the need for caution before making accusations of ethnic cleansing, and taking into account the many *Schindler's List*–type stories about how Serbs tried to help Albanians, there is plenty of evidence to suggest that an Albanian-free Kosovo was the desire of at least some non-Albanian civilians and military/paramilitary units. The virtual 100 percent destruction of some towns and villages demonstrates that the Serbs did not want the Albanians to return. Also, for example, many Kosovars reported that non-Albanian shopkeepers either refused to sell them food (55 percent of respondents) or sold them food at an inflated price on the basis of their ethnicity (66 percent of respondents).

Evidence of a policy of destroying the means of survival is also found in the testimonies of those surveyed. A farmer from Feronikel reported:

> I was prevented from farming my two hectares of land for two years through a combination of my tools being stolen, snipers, and my land being mined. In Feronikel and Gllogovc, there were many police and every day we suffered abuse, rape, robbery and destruction of houses and property. The Serbs killed two cows, destroyed 1,000 kg of flour and 4,000 kg of wheat and burned my animal fod-

der, stole my Yugo 45 motor car, destroyed my house and stole my tractor, plough, trailer and harrow.

Another farmer from the Ferizaj area wrote:

We were pushed from our houses; we were shot at and shelled. They killed our animals and abused us in our own houses. People wearing masks came and our children were afraid. They shouted "Go away from here, this is not your place. Go to Albania, go to Bill Clinton— he will give you chocolates." We stayed in the mountains for one week with nothing to eat and nothing to drink and with small children.

The fact that 30 percent of the respondents reported that their wells had been destroyed or in some way contaminated to prevent their using them is another indication that attempts were made to ethnically cleanse Kosovo. These reports were corroborated when, on return to Kosovo in June, some wells were found to have been contaminated with rubbish and even corpses, and others had been booby trapped or mined.

One of the biggest problems the Kosovar Albanians faced in obtaining food was access to their land. As Figure 13.4 shows, the threat of being shot by snipers while working in the fields posed an obstacle to growing and harvesting crops for 88 percent of the families interviewed. Mines were also a problem, although these were laid both by the Kosovo Liberation Army (KLA) and the Serbian army. Seventy percent of the population surveyed reported that, even if they did not face the threat of mines and snipers, they still could not

Figure 13.4   Reasons Why Kosovars Could Not Farm Their Land

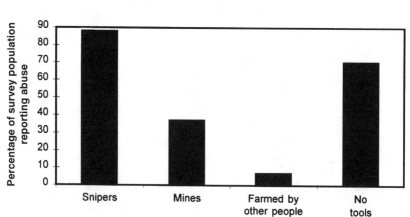

have farmed the land because their tools had been stolen or destroyed.

Although food and the means of producing food formed the main focus of our survey, respondents were anxious for us to record the physical abuse and theft of money and jewelry that they had experienced. In many instances, this was as much a reason for leaving Kosovo as the lack of food. Being robbed meant that they no longer had the means to buy food if the opportunity arose, and some refugees we spoke to said they were extremely worried about how they would provide for themselves in Macedonia without money. They did not realize that food and shelter would be provided to them free of charge.

Many of the families we questioned had witnessed beatings or the detention of family members by the police, and nearly all who wrote testimonies had had items of value stolen from them or had had to pay bribes to secure their passage out of Kosovo (although it is probable that the people who had suffered were more likely to write testimonies than those who had not). What is clear, as is illustrated in the quotes that follow, is that the Serbian forces and gypsies were very much aware of the cash economy that had operated in Kosovo since the collapse of the Bank of Yugoslavia and knew that many people would be traveling with all their wealth in cash (Deutschmarks [DM]), jewelry, or gold.

> After three weeks staying in the mountains we traveled to Ferizaj via Mirosala. We were stopped by two soldiers—Serbs in a civilian car—who asked us for money. When I said no they stripped me naked and found 200DM which they took. After that they beat me, shooting near my legs and then released me. —Farmer from Ferizaj
>
> The police took our money, our gold and all the things from the house and then burned the house. On the journey to Pristina they stole everything, even shoes; they asked for money while we were on the train and threatened to kill us if we didn't give it to them. We gave them the money we needed for bread. I can't tell you everything which happened to us in such a short time. —Farmer from Lupe I Eperm, Podujeve
>
> The paramilitary group came to our place. I had my daughter 17, some other girl 23, my mother-in-law, the son of my brother in law and the others and I was so scared. They came swearing and shouting in Serbian "Give us money, give us money or I will kill you with this machine gun." I had some money that I had saved, about 300DM and I gave them 100DM. Then he started shouting again saying "more, more" and I had to give him everything. He then insisted on gold and jewelry. I told him I have nothing but said to him take this ring—I took the ring off my finger just to save my life. He then

turned to the girls—my daughter had some money and she gave it all and the rest of the women had to do the same—give everything.—Woman from Cirez.

Coping Mechanisms of IDPs in Kosovo

Anecdotal evidence suggests that people from certain areas were better prepared for food shortages than others. Urban populations, for example, were often worse prepared than those in rural areas, as they thought that the conflict would not reach the larger towns. Some refugees told us that, prior to their evacuation, the Organization for Security and Cooperation (OSCE) warned them to prepare food stocks. This is reflected in Figure 13.5, which shows that 45 percent of families had put emergency rations of flour aside. (Flour was cooked in ovens that IDPs either took with them if they had transportation or borrowed from other people living in the areas where they were seeking refuge; yeast was cultured locally from existing supplies. Most refugees entering Macedonia had to surrender their vehicles at the border and therefore lost all the domestic equipment they had tried to bring with them—another consideration for aid delivery to returnees).

It was not always possible to mill or bake flour. One respondent reported: "We were eating boiled corn and boiled wheat, we didn't

Figure 13.5   Sources of Food for IDPs

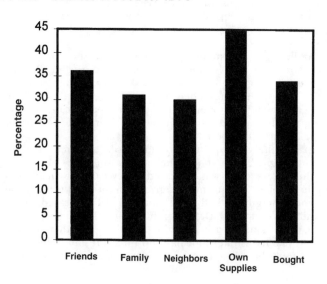

have mills." Another refugee (a woman from Drenica) told us of people eating raw, unmilled grain and wild edible grasses that they found in the forests when their food supplies had run out.

If they were not forced out of their homes under the threat of violence, Kosovar Albanians lived off stocks they had prepared beforehand. However, insecurity or the lack of food often forced Kosovars to move to the urban areas where food could still be bought or to rely on friends, relatives, and neighbors. Figure 13.5 illustrates the fact that often a combination of these survival strategies was used, with people relying on friends, family, and neighbors at different stages.

The survey demonstrates the strength of ethnic and family bonds among Kosovar Albanians. In the majority of cases families in hiding together would share any food they had. One refugee in Stankovac II recalls:

> The first time we were in hiding for five days I managed to buy 100kg of flour; I took 50kg and left it with the people [with whom I was staying] in case I had to return. ... When I returned I used it for five days. As we were 12 people together, we had to keep the usage as low as possible. Then it was finished, but fortunately we had some friends and relatives who really helped us. They brought us some buckets full of flour and I must say they really helped us.

It is probable that without the strong sense of Albanian ethnic identity that cut across national boundaries, as evidenced by the support given to the refugees by Macedonian Albanians and the financial support provided by remittances from Kosovars abroad, the food aspect of the emergency would have been far more severe. Food prices rose during the crisis—partly because of scarcity but also because non-Albanian shopkeepers overcharged Albanians. Hard currency sent by relatives living overseas was an important safety net for many Kosovars, not only through the crisis but during the preceding nine years when many Albanians were unemployed as a result of Serb discrimination.

Priorities for and Actions on Return

At the time the survey was executed, it was still unclear how long the refugees would remain in Macedonia and Albania (the United Nations High Commission for Refugees [UNHCR] was making preparations for winter accommodation), so it was deemed useful to try to identify what the refugees' priorities would be upon their return to Kosovo. This was done by asking them to rank five things in order of priority: shelter, food aid, repairs to their wells, new seeds, and new tools. Most refugees indicated that they would not feel safe with anything less than a NATO protection force, many citing the ineffectiveness of UN-led peacekeeping missions in other countries. Many respondents either did not answer this question or misunderstood the need for ranking; for those who did answer, most refugees saw shelter as their major concern once basic safety issues had been dealt with. Some 69 percent of respondents claimed that they would need their homes rebuilt, with food aid, refurbished wells, new tools, and new seeds following in descending order of importance.

It would be wrong to place too much emphasis on this aspect of the survey, for two reasons. First, because of the low response rate we got to this question; second, because some refugees did not fully know what had happened to their property once they left. Some of them based their perception of future needs on speculation and rumors rather than on concrete evidence.

When refugees did actually start to return to Kosovo in June 1999, no longer threatened by snipers, one of the first things they did was to check their houses for booby traps and to de-mine their land, either by hand (after some basic training from the KLA) or by driving livestock across it. The next priority was to harvest whatever crops remained and to clear the land for the planting of winter wheat—a task aid agencies were working to assist with through the provision of scythes and other tools. Provision of food aid was vital to the returnees' survival. Aid agencies did respond relatively quickly to people's needs, though the emergency phase of the operation ended within a few weeks of the start of the refugees return.

Conclusion

The Kosovo crisis is the latest in a series of post–Cold War conflicts characterized by internecine hostilities, ethnic cleansing, civilian displacement, and the need for large-scale humanitarian intervention. While it is beyond the scope of this chapter to go into the issues behind the profusion of these civil-style wars, it is clear that nationalism is emerging along with poverty or disenfranchisement of particular ethnic/political/social groups as the catalyst of conflict in many countries. Often, as in Kosovo, the military and police are controlled by one ethnic group, so abuse of a particular grouping appears to become a state-sanctioned activity.

One of the principal messages that the Kosovo crisis reinforces is the importance of adding value to traditional humanitarian activities by bearing witness to and recording human rights abuses. It is central to the reconciliation and rebuilding process that victims of human rights abuses should know that their grievances will be recorded and acted upon. The perpetrators of crimes must also be made aware that the atrocities they commit will not be forgotten or ignored.

Acknowledgments

The data on which this report is based could not have been collected without the hard work and dedication of Fatmir Selimi.

Notes

Michael Brewin worked with Action Against Hunger in Macedonia.

1. Statistics in this section are from the UNHCR web site, www.UNHCR.org, July 1999.

14

Are There Still "Natural" Famines?

Sylvie Brunel

At the end of the twentieth century, do people still die of hunger because of nature? The question is worth asking: Never have natural catastrophes seemed so numerous, from floods in China or Bangladesh to Hurricane Mitch in Central America, droughts in the Sahel region, and earthquakes in Colombia.

Most catastrophes strike in the tropics. Although natural disasters, including avalanches and floods, do occur in the temperate zone, the magnitude of the damage and the violence of the cataclysms seem less severe. Why is this so? Is the tropical world by nature more exposed, more "violent" than the temperate world?

Because It Is Poor, the Tropical World Is Particularly Exposed to Natural Disasters

The two principal characteristics of the tropics, which gird the earth straddling both sides of the equator, are the absence of winter and the abundant rainfall.

The absence of winter means that there is constant heat throughout the year. The average temperature in the coldest month is at least 18 degrees Centigrade (65 degrees Fahrenheit). The difference in temperature between day and night is greater than the difference in temperature between the coldest day of the year and the hottest. (In climatic terms, the diurnal thermal range is greater than the annual thermal range).

Abundant rainfall, greater than 500 millimeters (20 inches) per year, represents the point at which agriculture is possible without irrigation and rivers flow all year round (in contrast with arid and semi-arid zones). Except in the equatorial belt, rain in the tropics falls only during one part of the year, the rainy season, which is characterized by destructive rainstorms, notably in those regions of Asia that are affected by monsoons.

On the surface, it would appear as though the tropical world is especially favored: The absence of winter prolongs the period during which plants can grow (the growing season), in contrast with temperate countries. Tropical soils are rich (but they are fragile, because the heat and humidity cause rapid demineralization of the surface humus layer, which is therefore very thin).

Yet, nearly the entire humid, tropical region consists of poor and underdeveloped countries. Is this linked to the very nature of the climate, its unhealthiness, its heat that favors the proliferation of insects, its parasites and molds, which together prevent the countries from developing? Such was the view of writers in the past. Montaigne wrote that "hot air relaxes the fibers"; Littré evoked the "furious delirium that seized Europeans upon contact with the tropical world."

It is easy to forget that, in reality, there are developed areas in the tropics, such as Florida, parts of Japan and Australia, and the French Antilles. There the environment is as healthy as that of temperate countries: no malaria, no parasitic or intestinal diseases.

The real reason for the unhealthiness of the tropical world stems from the fact that the industrial revolution made its appearance in the temperate world, more precisely in England in the eighteenth century, because of the problem of the overpopulation of limited spaces. At that time, the temperate world was at least as unhealthy as the tropical world today: Drinking water, often polluted, spread cholera; epidemics of measles, diphtheria, even of influenza, were deadly; "swamp fevers" decimated children in the most humid areas (which have often kept their old name of "the marshlands"). It is medical and scientific research that has made it possible to clean up the temperate world and improve the health of its inhabitants as standards of living improved (hygiene, vaccination, health regulations, and medical care for the population).

But the inhabitants of the tropical world have not benefited from these gains because research has not been (and still is not) directed toward this world, which at the time of the industrial revolution was sparsely populated and viewed as backward.

Moreover, the soils of temperate countries have been worked for decades in order to improve their quality and fertility. Thanks to the addition of lime, fertilizers, and all sorts of products, the formerly hardscrabble Champagne region has become a great agricultural region, and the Landes and Camargue areas have become great producers of wine, fruit, and so on. In contrast, the soils of most tropical countries have not been changed: No one has tried to enrich them. In many cases, the only means of replenishing their fertility is to leave them fallow. Today, as the population increases, the length of the fallow period can no longer be maintained, and the soil becomes exhausted. Increased clearing of land for planting allows the rain to wash through the earth, leaving a denuded, demineralized soil that hardens and becomes unsuitable for cultivation. Many African villages are ringed by "dead" patches of land that have been exhausted from overcultivation, thereby forcing farmers—in reality women because it is they who produce the food—to go farther and farther away from the village to find fertile land.

The sudden and rapid population increase in the Third World has thus created problems for many population groups, which have grown rapidly in size while trying to live from the produce of land that has not been improved or that has been degraded by overcultivation.

The large populations of today are much more exposed to risks than in the past. Because their density is increasing and their production techniques have remained the same, many of these populations are confronted with the terrible challenge of having to feed larger numbers of people on less fertile soil. Because of this, they have taken more risks. Traditional societies carefully guarded the memory of natural disasters and learned to live with risk and to guard against it; for example, the villages of the Sahel used policies of collective grain storage as a means of combating drought. The new populations, disorganized by their increasing numbers and lured by city life, which is perceived as more modern and easier, have lost this memory of natural disasters. They settle on high-risk lands in order to feed themselves, despite the difficulties. These include the slopes of volcanoes or the floors of valleys, where the land is more fertile. In the Sahel, farmers have gone too far north into semiarid zones formerly reserved for nomadic livestock farming. In the Andes, they have settled on steep slopes because the best lands were taken over by large landholders, descendants of the colonizers.

This increasingly dense settlement of marginal lands has left the populations much more vulnerable. Too many people living in difficult places: All the conditions are in place for tragedies to occur.

Only Developed Societies
Can Effectively Prevent the Risks

The big difference between rich countries and poor countries as they face risks of natural disasters is that the rich countries have the means and the will to implement disaster-prevention policies.

Today, the earth is being continuously surveyed: Satellites study the movement of air masses and oceans and can predict any type of climatic catastrophe (droughts, hurricanes, tidal waves) days or even weeks in advance. Earthquakes and volcanic eruptions are detected and announced by monitoring stations, large numbers of which are located in all the sensitive parts of the globe. Global warming, for example, or the hole in the ozone layer are the subjects of detailed analysis, and even if experts disagree among themselves over the exact causes, they are in agreement about the reality of the natural phenomena registered.

In response to these observations, certain societies have the financial means and the will to take effective measures: In earthquake-prone areas, such as in Japan and California, the state enforces compliance with very strict codes for the construction of public buildings. In India, the government keeps up-to-date and very detailed descriptions of the early warning signs of drought and of the methods to be used to prevent them from devastating entire regions. Dikes keep rivers in their beds in China in order to prevent floods.

But some states are weak and therefore incapable of putting in place prevention and early-warning mechanisms. In others, governments attach no importance to protecting their population from these risks, because they know that those who will suffer in the event of disasters are the poor, who live on marginal lands and have no political influence. When a state lacks the power or the will to truly manage the whole of its territory, it neglects entire regions and populations, which are not taken into account in national land use policies.

The same hurricane may therefore cause thousands of victims in the poor regions of Central America and only material damage in the rich and protected regions, such as the French Antilles. The same drought can ravage the Sahel region of Africa and cause a human tragedy, then hit India, killing only a few heads of cattle. And African families that lose all their possessions in a natural disaster will endure hunger over an extended period, while the Indian families will very quickly receive from their government seeds and cattle to enable them to restock their herds and plant their fields, and so resume a normal life.

The big difference between developed and developing countries is this capacity to conceive, finance, and implement the three components of a risk-management policy:

- Disaster prevention through the adoption of measures to strengthen the population's ability to cope;
- Protection of the population during the disaster (evacuation plans, organization of food and medical assistance, and so on);
- Rapid reconstruction after the disaster to permit a return to normalcy in the shortest possible time.

Of course, for such policies to work, there must be at least a minimum of infrastructure: If the country has no roads, if the population is illiterate and therefore cannot read newspapers and does not have radios, if the state's finances are drained by the repayment of excessive debt, then it is impossible to respond effectively to the risk of natural disasters. The poorest states therefore do not always have the means to put into place such responses: Prevention, protection, and reconstruction require considerable financial and logistical resources. Sometimes, however, the states also pursue other strategies.

Famines Due to Nature
Alone Have Become the Exception

Famine never strikes out of the blue. When disaster strikes somewhere on the globe, when a food shortage threatens certain populations, it does not happen from one day to the next. The warning signs of famine are well known: disappearance of food stocks, recourse to gathering or hunting, men abandoning their families, children who begin to show signs of acute malnutrition, and so on.

Although it is rare, there are still some regions that are truly isolated from the rest of the world—for example, in certain mountainous regions of central Asia or in the isolated savannas of Africa. There it is possible for drought to cause populations to die because of the total disappearance of food.

But such famines have become the exception since, more often than not, aid organizations are alerted by the early warning systems put in place by the Food and Agriculture Organization (FAO) and by the governments of the countries concerned, which appeal for emergency aid. Journalists disseminate the terrible images of hunger. Food aid is mobilized to offset the deficit, and food is distributed to the stricken population, while children are cared for in feeding centers.

From the time that aid organizations intervene to help the victims, it takes only a few weeks to halt a famine: Cared for in a specialized center, a skeletal child can regain normal weight in less than a month, if unaffected by other illnesses.

The problem with this food aid is that it sometimes takes time to arrive on the scene: Months can go by from the moment the government gives the alert to the moment when the effective decision is taken to dispatch aid. Humanitarian organizations react more swiftly. But their capacity for action, while very effective, is more limited than that of the United Nations: If famine threatens an entire region, then assistance must be mobilized on a massive scale.

But the United Nations is slower to mobilize than are nongovernmental organizations because it is more cumbersome and more subject to often-complicated bureaucratic procedures. The United Nations sometimes also has difficulty in convincing the donor states of the North that the situation is urgent: Certain states, such as those of the Sahel, for example, appeal for aid every year. How can one identify those years when a disaster will really occur unless massive aid is dispatched as rapidly as possible from those years in which the state needs food aid mainly for resale on the open market or to distribute to its supporters?

The problem is that, while donors seek to ascertain whether a request is motivated by a genuine emergency, people are in danger of dying, especially children, who are the most vulnerable sector of the population. Unfortunately, there are situations in which aid does not arrive in time to save the populations suffering from hunger. This is so either because the government appealed for help too late or because the United Nations took too long to react. But sometimes also because, while help did indeed arrive, it was not properly distributed to hunger victims: A portion was diverted for the benefit of other populations closer to the regime than the starving population, another portion was resold to enrich certain merchants, while still another portion was simply distributed to the army.

Therefore, while the initial disaster was certainly caused by nature, the famine itself is the result of human actions: There is nothing "natural" about it since, if the aid had indeed reached the victims, they would never have died of hunger. Unfortunately, for certain governments, a natural disaster is a windfall, as long as it strikes populations that do not count politically in that country: The disaster allows the governments to justify an appeal for massive amounts of emergency aid. The goal, then, is not to help the starving but to extract a portion for the government's own benefit.

When drought struck the nomadic peoples of the northern Sahel in the early 1970s and then again in the early 1980s, the tons of aid dispatched did not reach these people. They were considered second-class citizens, always in revolt against the power of the states in question, rebels against the sedentary life. Instead, the aid piled up in the cities, where much of it was misappropriated.

In the northeast of Brazil, drought helped to consolidate the power of the large landholders, who took the opportunity to make famine victims work on improvement projects on their property in exchange for food aid: The landholders even appeared to be genuine benefactors, since it was they who coordinated the distribution of food!

To ensure that assistance reaches those in need of relief and those alone is therefore the challenge that faces the aid agencies if they truly wish to avert famine.

Notes

Sylvie Brunel is strategy adviser, Action Against Hunger.

PART TWO

CONFRONTING UNJUST FOOD DISTRIBUTION: WHICH STRATEGIES FOR HUMANITARIAN INTERVENTION?

Today, humanitarian organizations realize that they have become pawns of a new geopolitical game that seeks to use them as an instrument, be it in the North or in the South. Therefore they must relentlessly struggle to reaffirm their relief mission, their impartiality, and their independence when confronted by governments trying to make them tools of political interests. How to have efficacy and justice together? How to find a right way to avoid becoming marginalized or becoming a purely technical service provider? How to secure an enhanced protection for the victims both in the short and long term? These are issues and questions raised in Part 2.

15

Humanitarian Action in North Korea: Ostrich Politics

Christophe Reltien

Is North Korea becoming the grim theater of the most disastrous human tragedy of the turn of the century while the humanitarian movement remains helpless to respond? As signs of a famine on a scale reminiscent of the worst periods of the Great Leap Forward in China from 1959 to 1961 or in Ukraine in the early 1930s appear with greater frequency, the relevance of the humanitarian aid programs in place in the country poses a number of ethical and practical problems.

Introduction

This chapter was written in the fall of 1999. During the winter months, Action Against Hunger attempted negotiations with the North Korean authorities in order to gain better direct access to the population. Convinced that humanitarian aid does not reach the most vulnerable and is completely controlled by the government for its own benefit, Action Against Hunger decided to withdraw from the country in March 2000. A complete report as well as a testimony before the U.S. Congress can be found at www.aah-usa.org.

A Ruined Economy with Serious Humanitarian Consequences

North Korea's economy appeared to continue its decline in 1999. In the absence of reliable statistics, it is impossible to determine precisely the extent of the economic disaster. However, observations made by the Action Against Hunger team during their travels to the country were quite revealing: large factories now abandoned, massive population movements along the roads to collect firewood or gather herbs and roots, hospitals without heat, denuded hillsides, absence of tractors in the fields ... all signs of the country's economic collapse.

North Korea's Gross National Product is estimated to have declined by half since 1996. The abrupt end of the system of preferential trade with the socialist countries, especially the USSR, in the early 1990s was a severe blow to the North Korean economy. This highly industrialized nation found itself deprived of energy, which inevitably led to a sharp drop in industrial production. Chongjin, a large city in the north of the country, where Action Against Hunger maintains a presence, is a vivid example of this industrial disaster. Economic activity has virtually disappeared from the city, and the great chimneys of the factories no longer belch smoke.

The country is also deeply in debt, which it has no means of paying. Foreign countries are therefore very wary of expanding their economic ties. North Korea appears increasingly isolated, cut off from the rest of the world. The last foreign airline to serve Pyongyang stopped its flights in April 1999. Two weekly flights by the national carrier Koryo Air between Beijing and Pyongyang are one of the last links to the outside world. The Chinese have closed three of their five border posts along the Sino-Korean border due to the lack of traffic.

Despite its economic difficulties, North Korea continues to spend large sums of money on its military in order to maintain a massive army and to pursue its weapons research activities. This situation is evidenced by the firing of a missile in August 1998 and by the nation's attempts to build a nuclear weapon.

The country's agricultural potential is limited, since only 20 percent of the land is fit for farming. In the past, this land was intensively cultivated, and fertilizers and pesticides were widely used. The sharp drop in fertilizer production led to a major decline in agricultural production, a process aggravated by farming techniques that damaged the soil. Deforestation is also a major problem, causing serious erosion and making fields even more vulnerable to natural disasters that, like the floods of 1995 and 1996, are frequent in the country.

Action Against Hunger's agronomists in North Korea have observed on their regular visits to collective farms how agricultural production remains low owing to the lack of fertilizer and of fuel or tires for tractors and to inefficient farming techniques.

Some observers nonetheless claim to see signs of positive developments. The Supreme National Assembly, which was newly elected in

1998, has introduced constitutional changes and allowed the use of a new vocabulary in official political and economic discourse: the notion of the "village market" where private individual produce may be sold and the notion of plots of land for private use. Other developments are also noteworthy, given the country's notorious rigor and isolation. These include sending North Korean managers abroad under the auspices of United Nations programs to study and learn the concept of the free market or the attempts made to approach international financial institutions.

These attempts are limited, however, since the country's economic liberalization still faces obvious ideological hurdles. Will the liberalization policy advocated by the South Korean government and supported by some of that country's largest industrial conglomerates lead to significant change? No one can say for sure.

Korean officials continue to blame the 1995 and 1996 natural disasters for all of their country's economic difficulties. It is significant to note in this regard that the government body that serves as the liaison for humanitarian organizations is called the Committee to Repair the Damage Caused by the Floods. According to the official Korean line, all of the country's ills are attributable to these floods, since any acknowledgment of economic errors would lead to criticism of the system as a whole, which is unthinkable under the current Korean regime, based as it is on a highly developed cult of personality.

In 1999, North Korea's food deficit was estimated to be approximately 1.3 million tons.[1] This figure no doubt hides conflicting realities. The food shortage has a greater effect on the deficit northern provinces, which have more limited agricultural resources. Traditionally, the surplus from southern provinces was shipped to the northern provinces. This "redistribution" system no longer seems to function, leaving the northern provinces with an acute food deficit. Moreover, urban residents in Korea are much more affected by the shortages than rural dwellers. Factory workers are without doubt the hardest hit, owing to the unemployment that has resulted from factory closings. City dwellers are attempting to make do as best they can. Many families have built hen houses on their balconies or have begun to raise pigs in their apartments.

What is more, as we will see later, the government's food distribution program is based on criteria that clearly exclude a sector of the population.

This serious food crisis obviously raises the question of whether famine exists in North Korea and to what extent. This is a sensitive and controversial subject. One of the characteristics of a totalitarian regime is the lack of transparency, its opaqueness. No one is in a position to confirm or deny the current figures of two to three million deaths since 1996.

In May 1999, for the first time, Korean officials verbally acknowledged a significant increase in the mortality rate (from 6.8 per 1,000 in 1993 to 9.3 per 1,000 in 1998), which would mean some 55,000 additional deaths per year, or 220,000 over a four-year period. Still, these figures appear to be conservative. At the end of 1998, a nutritional survey conducted by the United Nations Children's Fund (UNICEF), the World Food Program (WFP), and the European Union revealed rates of moderate malnutrition of 14 percent and severe malnutrition of 2 percent among children aged between six months and seven years old.

North Korean refugees accounts paint an even more tragic picture of the situation, of entire families decimated by illness, and of the lack of food. A recent study[2] of these refugees has shown that the mortality rate was very high (42.8 per 1,000) in 1995, 1996, and 1997 and that it was continuing to rise. The study also revealed that government rations were the main source of food for only 5 percent of the people surveyed and that, for nearly half of the respondents, picking fruits and gathering herbs and roots was their primary source of food.

Beyond the debate over numbers, the humanitarian situation in North Korea is undeniably critical, and people are dying of hunger and diseases associated with malnutrition. The complete collapse of the public health system (poorly heated hospitals lacking medicine) renders the country's inhabitants all the more vulnerable.

A Regime That Manipulates
Humanitarian Aid with International Complicity

Even though the North Korean system constitutes an impediment to efficient humanitarian aid, the use of the term *humanitarian* as a bargaining tool by certain governments has undercut demands by genuine humanitarian actors for control and freedom of access.

The humanitarian programs operating in Korea face numerous obstacles. The implementation and success of a program are hampered by the deliberate efforts of the authorities to limit the scope of humanitarian activities by placing restrictions on freedom to evaluate a situation, direct supervision of invested materials, freedom to evaluate the impact of programs, and direct access to beneficiaries.

For Koreans, national security and sovereignty are more important than humanitarian assistance. The humanitarian characteristics, even if recognized, are not acknowledged as arguments during negotiations.

In the minds of Korean officials, operational principles and humanitarian ethics conflict with the notion of national interest. The criteria for intervention and for providing aid to the population are viewed as affairs of state, and the system in place must, in principle, provide complete support to the population. It is also a means of controlling and monitoring the population. Organizations are allowed, or rather tolerated, in the country with suspicion and distrust because they are presumed to be hostile to the regime in place. These organizations have the potential to uncover and reveal the regime's weaknesses and also have the means of reporting the internal situation to the outside world by circumventing the country's strict, voluntary isolation. North Korean officials have clearly perceived the risk that Action Against Hunger may report to the outside world what we observe daily on the inside. The authorities view this potential as an essentially political capability.

Korean discourse has not changed. The government accepts only aid that it deems to be humanitarian, but only if it is not subject to conditions, which are always considered to be political. Moreover, the testimonials that Action Against Hunger is in a position to provide must take Korea's situation into account and moderate the criticisms that may be contained in the testimonials in light of their possible consequences, in order to retain our organization's capacity to bear witness to the situation.

One of the major constraints is that all humanitarian aid must be channeled through Korea's state distribution system. The regime thus controls the aid and provides aid only to those people whom it wishes to help. These people are not necessarily the same ones that the humanitarian organizations would like to benefit.

This situation presents a cruel dilemma and a vicious circle for the humanitarian organizations in Korea. Access to the most vulnerable sectors of the population is a major objective, but one of the reasons for their vulnerability is precisely their exclusion from the system under which humanitarian aid is distributed.

This may explain the coexistence in North Korea of two realities: the world to which humanitarian organizations have access and the world of those who are excluded, a world Action Against Hunger sees without being able to help. According to North Korean refugees accounts, the province of North Hamgyong, in the northern part of the country, is one of the areas most affected by famine, and people there are dying of hunger. There is no doubt that humanitarian organizations could save these people if they had access to them.

Even though statistics concerning North Korea must be treated with caution, the food deficit in 1999 was estimated at 1.3 million tons, as stated earlier. Food aid to North Korea in 1999, however, was just over one million tons! If the food crisis were merely a question of the quantity of food, one could say that the massive amounts of aid received by the country have resolved the problem. Yet famine has continued throughout the year, at least in certain parts of the country. This situation suggests that the problem is more complex than mere availability of food and that aid is probably not reaching those who are most in need.

In any case, Action Against Hunger's operational principles are under daily pressure. Because of their extreme suspiciousness, Korean officials are constantly seeking ways of preventing the organization from getting an accurate assessment of the humanitarian situation in the country and from understanding the way certain state structures, such as the public distribution system (PDS) and collective farms, operate.

The key to greater efficiency for the programs of Action Against Hunger lies in understanding how these structures function. But, in Korea, answers to these questions never come easily, if at all. Nevertheless, our organization's fundamental principles of intervention must be tirelessly maintained, explained, and defended to Korean officials; Action Against Hunger should know who the beneficiaries of its aid are, and distribution must take place under our organization's own supervision even within the overall system in place.

Too often, international political agendas are cloaked in humanitarian vocabulary and ensnare certain humanitarian organizations that are unaware or unable to avoid them.

The initial historical polarity between two blocs (the USSR and the United States) that started the conflict has given way to another polarity between the People's Republic of China, on the one hand, and the United States and its allies in the region, on the other hand. In this area where tensions between neighboring countries are high and well known and where U.S. and Chinese interests always lurk in the background, satisfactory diplomatic and military solutions are rare and complicated.

A peninsular perspective no longer suffices as an approach to a solution to the Korean conflict; its implications and ramifications are regional and directly affect all neighboring countries: South Korea,

Japan, and China. Russia today is no longer an integral part of the search for a diplomatic solution. Given the privileged ties and defense agreements between the United States and its allies in the region and concerns about strategic interests and the security of U.S. troops in the region, a purely Korean solution to the conflict seems unlikely. North Korea, however, has a multifaceted diplomatic approach. It wants to first try to negotiate its best deal with the United States alone, since North Korea would no longer be at war with the United States and only with South Korea. Then it envisages a resumption of diplomatic relations with the South.

Koreans would like to see an exclusively Korean solution, which would satisfy peninsular nationalism by excluding any other parties. This is true not only because the United States still represents the hereditary enemy, but also because North Koreans do not hide their deep suspicion of their Chinese neighbors.

The nuclear argument, however, so well employed by North Korea and the United States as an international bargaining chip and means of entry into the country, eliminates all possibility of a pan-Korean solution. Recent developments, following the discovery by a U.S. satellite of a large construction site suspected of being a future underground nuclear site, have demonstrated the use of the nuclear argument by the United States and North Korea. The Koreans have put a price on the authorization of U.S. inspection visits to the site, estimated at $300 million. The United States cannot agree to pay for this right; according to the agreement on nuclear assistance signed in 1994 by North and South Korea, Japan, and the United States, inspectors should have the right to visit the site in order to verify that the agreement has been respected. Nevertheless, the United States does not wish to pass up an opportunity to be able to enter the country and has succeeded in modifying the original terms of the bargain by having the Koreans accept payment for their authorization in the form of food aid (300,000 tons of food aid and agricultural assistance). It is now known that this aid will be channeled through the United Nations and U.S. international aid organizations. These humanitarian organizations will therefore transform what is really bilateral aid into "humanitarian assistance" in response to military and political objectives that are in no way humanitarian. This blurring of the distinction between the two types of assistance is extremely harmful to the humanitarian ethic.

Viewed in this light, humanitarian assistance to North Korea takes on a different perspective:

- The North Korean regime's extortionist policies and its capacity for mischief are being used as leverage to secure more aid that, in fact, helps to reinforce the regime and has little impact on the most vulnerable sectors of the population.
- U.S. support seeks to make the North Korean regime heavily dependent on U.S. aid while allowing the United States to increase its leverage with North Korea.

The abandonment of all requirements for control by certain United Nations agencies or nongovernmental organizations (NGOs), whose practical approach is to make gifts without any effective control over them, merely encourages Korean officials to reject humanitarian principles of operation. This practice is most certainly detrimental to humanitarian aid as a whole.

Large quantities of food are in fact delivered to Korea in the form of gifts. This aid has been integrated into the national distribution system, to be divided up and sent to designated zones and recipients. The permanent presence of expatriate personnel is an essential element in the supervision of this distribution, since it is always very difficult to follow the paths taken by the aid and to ascertain who the beneficiaries will be.

During 1998, the organizations working in Korea were split into two groups, one from the European Union that insisted on strict respect for the humanitarian principles of aid distribution and another, from the United States, that favored "no conditionality," or aid without any conditions attached. It is easy to see behind these two stances the political positions that differentiate the two principal aid donors involved in the Korean crisis.

Questions can be raised about the genuineness and bases of the U.S. "no conditions policy" when U.S. aid representatives announce at an international conference that malnourished children are not involved in politics and that U.S. aid will therefore be provided without conditions. Questions can also be raised when it is revealed, moreover, that in return for the authorization for U.S. inspectors to visit a suspected nuclear site, North Korea will receive agricultural assistance for potato farming along with thousands of tons of food aid.

The U.S. approach to North Korea is relatively straightforward: zero risk for U.S. soldiers in South Korea, control of nuclear armaments, and ongoing efforts to defuse the crisis in a soft landing approach by adapting or transforming the current political and economic system. In order to achieve these objectives, a U.S. presence in North Korea is a valuable asset; a link must be established, a sort of indirect diplomacy that could be put in place before a more direct relationship is developed if circumstances so permit. Certain U.S. NGOs could fill this role.

The sums invested by the United States in the process of stabilizing the peninsula over the past years, especially its investments in food aid, represent a significant bargaining chip for the application of U.S. policy, either through the United Nations or through NGOs. Will the large scale of the aid provided create a North Korean dependence on U.S. aid? NGOs will have to find a way to develop programs in North Korea while respecting and ensuring respect for the general principles of intervention that were accepted in 1998 by all of the humanitarian organizations and agencies present in North Korea and that comprise the only document that is common to the entire humanitarian community, with the exception of aid donors.

More specifically, today certain organizations distribute hundreds of thousands of tons of aid (medical, foodstuffs, agricultural, and so on) with very limited means of supervising the distribution. This method of operation and the leeway it allows Korean officials feed fears that the most vulnerable sectors of the Korean population have little hope of benefiting from the manna. Action Against Hunger, despite the introduction in Korea of the most rigorous logistical protocols possible and with nine expatriates permanently in the field, has great difficulty in ensuring that there is no diversion of the hundreds of tons of aid that it ships to the country and has doubts about the possibility at the present time of gaining access to the most vulnerable sectors of the population. One can only admire the United Nations agencies that claim that they are certain that the hundreds of thousands of tons of aid distributed in North Korea reach those sectors of the population most in need. Admirable but doubtful.

The fundamental difference between the U.S. and European approaches could lead to a risk that the Korean authorities will begin to compare different organizations, their conditions for distribution of aid, and their programs and then make them compete against each other. Only those conditions that are most advantageous to the Korean system would be accepted as the conditions for the distribution of aid in Korea, all with international support (mainly U.S., given the amount of aid and the weight of the organizations waiting to enter the country), and it would then become difficult to maintain a strict respect for humanitarian principles.

There can be no ethically acceptable and operationally efficient humanitarian interventions in North Korea until such time as the international community adapts a common and agreed-upon position.

Notes

Christophe Reltien is former Action Against Hunger chief of mission in Korea.

1. FAO [Food and Agriculture Organization]/WFP [World Food Program], *Crop and Food Supply Assessment,* 1998.

2. Rising mortality in North Korean households reported by migrants in China, Johns Hopkins School of Hygiene and Public Health, 1999.

16

Lessons from
the Kosovo Tragedy

Sylvie Brunel

Nongovernmental organizations (NGOs) have complained loudly, and to no avail, that the North Atlantic Treaty Organization (NATO) did not acknowledge their true contributions in Kosovo. We must therefore draw lessons from the recent events in the Balkans.

Lack of Appreciation for
NGOs' Experience with Crises

NATO's failure to achieve the initial goal of its operation, namely, for Slobodan Milosevic to immediately cease his criminal actions against the Albanian "minority" (a minority in political but not in population terms) in Kosovo, should lead us to question the tactic employed. Humanitarians know from their experiences in Sudan, Kurdistan, and Bosnia that aerial bombardments have never forced the quick surrender of a dictator if they are not followed up by the deployment of an intervention force on the ground that has a genuine mandate to put an end to the fighting. The aerial bombing gave Milosevic, who expected nothing less, a ready excuse to complete his ethnic cleansing operation undisturbed and without witnesses, since the Organization for Security and Cooperation in Europe (OSCE) observers and NGO members had been forced out of the territory.

Would NATO intervention on the ground have prevented the "cleansing" of villages and regions suspected of complicity with the Kosovo Liberation Army (KLA), or would such intervention on the contrary have led to widespread carnage? It is a question difficult to answer because Milosevic's behavior has been so unpredictable since the early 1990s. One cannot help wondering, however, whether the Western democracies, by limiting themselves to high-altitude bombing, unintentionally initially facilitated the task of a dictator whose aim was to "cleanse" Kosovo. That was obviously the opposite of what they intended. In dealing with NATO, which operated with an almost total lack of transparency, the humanitarians, who were divided and unclear as to their exact role in such circumstances (should they enter the political fray or preserve their sacrosanct "neutrality"?), stood by, powerless, as the chronicle of a tragedy foretold unfolded. While a review of the situation in Somalia and Rwanda confirmed that preliminary consultations had taken place with the military, this time humanitarians have been kept in the dark about decisions taken by NATO states' governments. The effect of this was to reduce the effectiveness of the advocacy role that humanitarian organizations have decided to assume in situations where crimes are being committed and only their action in the field can bring a measure of relief to the suffering, though without putting an end to it. In Kosovo, NGOs have certainly played a decisive role in sounding the alarm, but above all they gave NATO a humanitarian justification for prosecuting the war. That led French writer Jean-Christophe Rufin to say that NGOs in Kosovo unwittingly served as the "trigger" for the warmongers.

Weapon of Hunger Used to Eliminate an Unwanted Population

Once again the weapon of hunger, which we now see being used almost systematically in the new conflicts in the South, has been deliberately used against a political and ethnic "minority." Victims for years of discriminatory practices in access to food, the Albanian Kosovars have seen their crops and stocks of food destroyed or pillaged since the NATO bombardments began, and they themselves have been forced into exile. Throughout their deportation they were denied any food assistance, which led to the deaths of the most vulnerable among them—the elderly, young children, and the sick. The survivors arrived at the frontiers exhausted, humiliated, their identity papers and their belongings confiscated. Above all they were psychologically destroyed.

The destruction of villages and killing of men of fighting age, who were suspected by Serb forces of belonging to the KLA, are proof that for Milosevic the process of getting rid of Kosovo's Albanian population is part of a long-term strategy aimed at preventing their subsequent return and at settling the problem of Kosovo once and for all by eliminating all non-Serb minorities. While the return of the Kosovar refugees after eleven weeks of NATO pounding of Serbia shows that this strategy ultimately failed, it has taken a frightful toll in human lives, as proven by the discovery by the Kosovo Force (KFOR) of mass graves in Albanian villages that had been reduced to piles of rubble.

The Militarization of Humanitarian Operations

The confusion between military and humanitarian operations, already condemned in Somalia and Bosnia for its perverse effects, reached its height in the Balkans, with NATO providing the after-sales service, that is, the reception of refugees after the bombardments. Not only has the military reinvented or rather reimprovised the techniques of humanitarian assistance to deal with a much larger influx of people than it had expected, it has also refused to draw upon the know-how and experience of the "real" humanitarian agencies, even though this might have spared NATO many difficulties. For example, the military and the authorities of the "host" countries (a term hardly suited to the case of Macedonia) considered NGOs to be undesirables and nuisances who should be kept at a distance, whereas NATO favored any means that increased the "visibility" of its own humanitarian actions. Each member country's army set up at great cost its own model camp (in reality often erected on unsuitable or unhealthy sites). In fact, these camps housed few people, since the Albanian community in Macedonia, Montenegro, and Albania sheltered the bulk of the refugees in their homes, even though they received only a tiny portion of the humanitarian aid.

This confusion between military and humanitarian operations continues to reveal both the limits and the dangers of the technique, exposing humanitarian teams to the risk of marginalization or even reprisals and thereby undermining their effectiveness and calling into question the very concept of operational neutrality that had, until now, protected NGOs from suspicions of partiality. The confusion also demonstrates that the army, as in the past, still considers itself much better equipped than civilians to carry out such operations as the building of camps and tents that require prompt and large-scale logistical intervention. Yet, twenty years of a "borderless world" have permitted NGOs to pass from the stage where they warn about tragedies to the stage where they are also capable of dealing effectively with them.

Extensive Media Coverage
Leads to the Same Incorrect Responses

Once again, the media images of hordes of exhausted refugees walking along mountain roads, being driven toward the border both by armed soldiers and by their fear of antipersonnel mines, which obliged them to follow the paths marked out by their torturers, provoked a vast surge of generosity in a Western public that is anxious to provide aid and to demonstrate solidarity. Yet once again errors were committed or even encouraged: The appeal to individuals to make their contributions in kind in order to relieve the suffering of the refugees and the request for people to mail off their little packets of noodles and sugar from local post offices created great difficulties. Transporting the food thus collected to processing centers, unpacking and then repacking it in an easy-to-use form, then transporting the pallets in cargo vessels and attempting to unload them in clogged ports all create a real logistical nightmare in every sense. It might also be mentioned that the economies of the host countries are collapsing from the massive influx of goods that could have been procured right there much more easily, cheaply, and conveniently. In June 1999, thousands of tons of humanitarian aid, which had not been cleared through customs, were still rotting in the port of Durès in Albania, the object of the covetousness of the Italian-Albanian mafia.

Once again, and in spite of repeated warnings by NGOs that have experience in disaster relief and that are constantly suspected of *pro domo* advocacy, we have witnessed the use of the myth of "the truck to the rescue" that collects any kind of item willy nilly and ships it at great expense in order to distribute it to anybody. How can we be surprised, after such errors, when all kinds of illicit trafficking proliferate on the fertile ground of humanitarian aid? As for the content of what is actually delivered, we must also question the selection: The garbage cans of the camps very quickly overflow with the leftovers of our generosity, which is certainly very great, but also unselective. Kukès thus very quickly became a gigantic public garbage dump. We have also witnessed the scandalous spectacle of convoys of trucks opening wide their rear doors to disgorge in disorder and in a general free-for-all a few miserable parcels to crowds that have stood patiently waiting for hours, only to close their doors again and flee like criminals as soon as the cargo is discharged, for fear of being lynched by those who waited in vain. Unfortunately, this lowest form of humanitarianism continues to bring in contributions in major disasters that become media events, and some journalists themselves do not hesitate to encourage it.

The Limits of Emergency
Disaster Relief in the Balkans

After a shaky beginning marked by amateurism and guesswork, the NGOs like to present themselves now as increasingly effective and professional. Yet, what is the lesson of the impotence of the NGOs not only in Kosovo itself, but also in the neighboring countries where they have been restrained as much by NATO forces as by national armies anxious to stop the floods of undesirable refugees that threaten to disrupt the local ethnic and political balance? The question of access to victims has taken on added urgency. This time, not only was access to the disaster area itself, Kosovo, denied by the criminal regime that is the cause of the tragedy, but it was also considerably restricted in Montenegro, Albania, and Macedonia. Even though humanitarian law exists on paper, it still needs to be enforced in practice.

As for humanitarian workers themselves, the time is long past since they crossed the most tightly sealed borders clandestinely and illegally: Kosovo at the end of the 1990s is no longer Afghanistan in the early 1980s. Did anyone then imagine NGOs at the frontiers of the martyred country patiently awaiting the arrival of refugees, as happened from March to June 1999 during the NATO bombing? Humanitarians today have paid too high a price for their freedom to operate in the new conflicts of the South and East to be willing to thoughtlessly place in danger the lives of their volunteers, who are now more vulnerable than ever. NGOs have suffered twice as many fatalities in the past five years as in the first twenty years of our borderless world. Today they are no longer behind the front lines but on the front line, actively involved in spite of themselves in conflicts where their involvement is much more important than in the past: Their arrival on the scene is now one of the objectives of modern conflicts, because of the financial bonanza and media coverage that they attract. Never have security concerns been so high on the agenda. It is true that NGOs have compensated for their lost audacity with increased efficiency and even greater professionalism. Yet there is still room for improvement.

Problems in the Very
Nature of the Assistance Rendered

For all that humanitarian agencies are efficient when treating "physical suffering" by supplying survival kits—food, drinking water, vaccines and medical care, shelter, and blankets—they are still deficient as far as the other needs and demands of victims are concerned. In Goma, in Somalia, or after the passage of Hurricane Mitch, the NGOs worked wonders because they were providing relief to populations that lacked the bare necessities and were used to living in the most precarious conditions in their regions of origin. On the borders of Kosovo, as in Bosnia or in Kurdistan in 1991, "basic" humanitarian aid very quickly reaches its limits. The similarities in culture and in living standards between victims and their rescuers makes the latter suddenly aware of an underlying need for psychological assistance, which they could afford to ignore elsewhere because it was masked in part by the need to respond to urgent physical needs. In Rwanda, Somalia, or Burundi, the psychological distress of the populations, in a state of shock after what they had just lived through, was just as strong as in Kosovo, but humanitarian workers were often less conscious of it because the means of communication were often more limited.

In Kosovo, the people we dealt with were people "like us," with the same level of development and culture. The difference was that they had just lived through a terrible physical and moral trauma. Delivering enriched flour and plastic sheeting may be a response to real needs in the early stages, since refugees cross the border exhausted and starving. But very quickly the victims' demands and the variety of their needs begin to pose serious challenges for their rescuers. The challenges come first of all in the area of food and hygiene; millet, corn, sugar, oil, and salt may be sufficient for food rations in Africa, but the refugees in Kosovo demanded rather more varied meals, such as breakfasts consisting of prepared dishes, coffee, and so on. Then come the challenges at the moral level; like the Kurds, the Kosovo refugees felt humiliated that their expectations were reduced to simple physiological needs when they had just lost their homeland. Everything happened as if, once again, their rights as citizens were being denied.

Few humanitarian organizations try to relieve the trauma experienced by providing genuine psychological support, a listening ear, or legal and administrative assistance. The rare telephones put at the disposal of the Kosovars to enable them to contact their loved ones were more precious to them than the thousands of jars of jam and sundry items sent by the outside world, most of which ended up in the garbage (in a mismatch of food aid that is regrettably common, we even saw salami being delivered to Muslims!). There was a profoundly shocking contrast between "humanitarian workers" bedecked with ultramodern communications gadgets (even though satellite phones, unlike cordless phones, did not work well in Albania) that enabled them to stay in touch with their headquarters, their families, and journalists, on the one hand, and the refugees waiting for hours to try to contact their loved ones just to tell them that they were alive, on the other hand. Should not humanitarian aid start there?

Civilians Are the Real Victims of Modern Wars

Two new concepts—that of "zero fatalities" introduced by Bill Clinton after the Somalia experience, which consists of not risking the lives of U.S. soldiers in foreign theaters of action, and that of the now widespread tactic of "human shields" used in Iraq—have once again placed civilian populations at the front line, particularly its most vulnerable sectors. The return home of three U.S. soldiers whose F-17 warplane had been shot down during the Kosovo war seemed to carry an emotional charge more intense than the harrowing ordeal of thousands of unknown families. Everything these days suggests that the lives of a handful of career soldiers were infinitely more precious than those of thousands of women, children, and the elderly. This hierarchy merely signals a return to the rule in force in traditional civilizations, where priority was given to protecting the adult male because it was he who had the capacity to fight and to obtain food for the group. So-called surgical strikes, sophisticated technologies such as those that incapacitate electrical systems, and the imposition of embargoes are all part of the myth of the "clean war" that is, however, just as dirty as traditional war, since all the forces involved claim civilians as their first victims, while the armies themselves are ensconced in the rear with their legions of warriors intact. Will we know one day how many human lives the Yugoslav army did in fact lose? Without a doubt, the number of soldiers killed is derisory compared with the number of civilian victims.

This refusal to commit troops on the ground even leads to a preference for aerial drops of food, without any precision whatsoever, in the guise of assistance targeted to victims. The practice of "humanitarian drops" already begun in such places as Kurdistan and Sudan is becoming widespread. This is new proof, however unintentional, that part of the West would like to offer charity to those in need, provided that they do not come into contact at all with the victims, perceived as plague-infested, flea-ridden people who must be kept at a distance. Compassion yes, but from a distance; contact, certainly not.

On the other side, people rally around a dictator who is now seen as a martyr, and the resentment builds against the bombs descending from the sky and indiscriminately striking civilians. "Collateral damage," claims the Western righter of wrongs by way of excuse, a phrase so casual (to say the least) that it stirs up even more resentment. Intensified by clever propaganda, a feeling of profound injustice in the face of an intervention that is perceived as unjust galvanizes the Serbs—as it did the Iraqis, Sudanese, and Afghans—against a smug, self-assured, and domineering West that purports to give lessons to the rest of the world. It only remains for the Saddam Husseins or Milosevics of the world to cultivate hatred of the Other in order to prosper in full impunity in the fertile soil of nationalism, especially since the West has repeatedly shown that it prefers to negotiate with a strong dictator who is in charge of his country rather than risk chaos and the destabilization of entire regions by putting into power opposition groups that are often divided and weak.

For humanitarian organizations, there is a real dilemma. They want to relieve the very real suffering of populations subjected to an embargo or to sanctions, even if that suffering is not comparable to the suffering of minorities that are victims of their dictator, such as Kurds and Shiites in Iraq, Albanians in Kosovo, Nubians and the peoples of southern Sudan, and the non-Pushtun minorities of Afghanistan. The decision to bring aid to those populations, however, is to give the impression of taking sides, to make a choice that may be badly viewed (by donors, journalists, public opinion). The Serbs of Kosovo are in turn experiencing their own ordeal of exodus. Aside from some nations such as France, with its well-known Serb affinities, the world hesitates to come to the rescue of these "bad victims." It goes without saying that dictators are skilled at exploiting such aid in order to embellish their propaganda. Slobodan Milosevic's wife thus presides over the Yugoslavia Red Cross. Saddam Hussein, who cultivates Western opinion makers in order to publicize the ravages caused by the embargo to his country, prohibits NGOs (which wish to relieve the suffering of the Iraqi people) from intervening in the north of the country, among the Kurds, and in the south, among the Shiites.

Shortcomings of the United Nations

Even though the NGOs have done everything possible to remind NATO of their indispensable role in "humanitarian crises," they have not been firm enough in criticizing the United Nations High Commission for Refugees (UNHCR) for its shortcomings. The agency has been overwhelmed from all directions, as much by national authorities as by NATO forces. As usual, United Nations agencies were absent when the crisis broke out. As usual, they failed to become operational promptly enough to fulfill their mandate. On the borders of Kosovo, and particularly in Macedonia, families were arbitrarily separated and transferred (deported) to so-called reception areas without first having been registered, which was disastrous to subsequent efforts to reunite them. Given that the United Nations was not consulted before the start of the intervention and that NATO decided to forgo the Security Council's approval for fear of a Russian or Chinese veto, the United Nations once again discredited itself in the Balkans. Some years earlier in Bosnia, the UN's emissary had distinguished himself by the indulgence shown toward the Serbs who were guilty of a bloody campaign of ethnic purification.

What is the long-term plan today for the victims—the Albanian Kosovars returning to Kosovo? They are returning to their country where their homes have been reduced to rubble. The intervention force is likely to be in for a long stay in Kosovo, the new Palestine of Europe. Only a genuine Marshall Plan could rebuild this devastated region. It will indeed be launched to give impetus to a United Nations in search of a second wind and to galvanize for a little longer this Europe in search of itself that has found the soul it lacked in its coalition against a dictator. Nevertheless, there is reason to fear that the effort to rebuild a destroyed country, by mobilizing substantial financial investments, will be made once again to the detriment of development aid for the poorest countries, notably in sub-Saharan Africa, which has already been seriously affected by the threat of non-renewal of the Lomé Convention.

Once again, the tragedy of Kosovo shows us that the worst of disasters can happen at our gates, even in our backyards, without our being capable of anticipating or preventing such disasters, of stopping them, or of relieving suffering.

- We are not capable of anticipating or preventing the disasters. Bosnia, 1992; Rwanda, 1994: Kosovo, 1999—in this trilogy of the worst, tragedy unfolded live before our eyes while we, impotent, even involuntary accomplices, commented on the horror.
- We are not capable of stopping the disasters. It is only when the butchers have completed their job of cleansing that they finally lay down their weapons to take a breath and to negotiate a compromise—on a field of ruins on which they have been able to advance their pawns.
- We are not capable of relieving the suffering of those who

have been butchered and of bringing the perpetrators to justice. The ad hoc tribunals are overwhelmed by the scale of the task at hand, while the world very quickly opts for a convenient amnesia with the token conviction of a few expiatory perpetrators "to set an example."

The term *humanitarian disaster* has often been used loosely where *human disaster* would have been more correct. For once, however, the terminology was appropriate in the Balkans: Yes, there was definitely a humanitarian disaster in Kosovo. It should lead the NGOs to question the relevance of their action in a world where they are systematically used as tools—a new unarmed branch of the great powers in search of new theaters of action—instead of constantly relying on a mandate for relief that they have conferred upon themselves and that they are unable to effectively discharge, in the absence of joint and concerted action, in the so aptly named "humanitarian disasters."

Yes, there certainly has been a humanitarian disaster in Kosovo. And a second one may well occur in the months or years ahead.

Notes

Sylvie Brunel is strategy adviser, Action Against Hunger.

17

A Code of "Good" Conduct?

Daniel Puillet-Breton

Nongovernmental organizations (NGOs) should be held accountable for their actions to the public, to private and institutional donors, and to the governments of the countries in which they operate. This obvious fact is not a recent invention; NGOs, sometimes from their very inception, have charters with principles of action to ensure transparency. Since 1979, Action Against Hunger has had a charter based on the fundamental humanitarian principles of neutrality, impartiality, and independence. This charter has been adopted by all sister organizations in France, the United Kingdom, Spain, and the United States.

The Right to Provide Assistance or the Right to Receive Assistance?

In the 1990s, the number and activities of humanitarian organizations increased considerably, especially in countries suffering from armed conflicts and crises. The range of different organizations and the diversity of objectives often cloud the perception that they are conducting strictly humanitarian operations. Humanitarian organizations have sometimes unwittingly helped to further complicate situations.[1]

In addition, the public and donor governments have increasingly focused on what is sometimes termed the "humanitarian circus" (the media portrayal of victim/savior) that threatens to undermine public support for humanitarian efforts. Linking theory and practice, academics who have analyzed the most professional humanitarian organizations describe, and sometimes denounce, the advent of a "humanitarian bureaucracy" that creates its own self-sustaining cycle of demand.[2] Although these attacks are sometimes incomplete or off the mark, we must acknowledge that criticism of humanitarian efforts and critical self-examination are constructive and an encouraging sign of maturity. New perspectives integrating war economics provoke organizations to develop a more sophisticated understanding of the conflicts in which they are involved and the impact of their programs.[3]

This necessary critical analysis is linked to efforts for a better coordination of humanitarian organizations whose objective is to establish standards to which they would in theory be held accountable by the public and by the beneficiaries of their programs.

In 1994, eight of the oldest and largest humanitarian organizations worldwide met and established a Code of Conduct for disaster relief programs.[4] This action acknowledged that when the organizations should have been flexible and responsive to humanitarian "problems" in the 1980s, most of them were still more or less in the process of establishing themselves as institutions.[5] The Code of Conduct is a reflection of this phenomenon insofar as it has remained centered around these eight large organizations.

In 1996, over 103 international signatory organizations pledged to follow "principles of behavior" and "guidelines" (recommendations contained in three annexes to the code) for disaster relief operations.[6] The main principles are as follows:

1. The humanitarian imperative comes first.
2. Aid should be given regardless of the race, creed, or nationality of the recipients and without adverse distinction of any kind. Aid priorities should be determined on the basis of need alone.
3. Aid should not be used to further a particular political or religious viewpoint.
4. Humanitarian organizations must endeavor not to act as instruments of government foreign policy.
5. Local cultures and customs must be respected.
6. Disaster responses must be built on local capacities.
7. Ways must be found to involve program beneficiaries in the management of aid relief.
8. Relief assistance must seek both to reduce future vulnerabilities to disaster and to meet basic needs.
9. There must be accountability to beneficiaries and donors.

10. There must be recognition of the dignity of disaster victims in media activities.

These principles are "offered as guidance." According to the code, they are not "legally binding, ... nor do we expect Governments and inter-governmental organizations to indicate their acceptance of the guidelines ... although this may be a goal towards which to work in the future." Ultimately, the objective is to create "a spirit of openness and cooperation so that our partners will become aware of the ideal relationship that we seek with them."

The Code of Conduct reflects the main goal: the voluntary and unilateral effort (see the "Purpose" section in the preamble to the code) of international humanitarian organizations, above and beyond their diversity, to establish the basis for self-regulation in the operational practices of signatory organizations. These principles should guide coordination in the field and help to pressure traditional humanitarian partners: donor governments, host governments, and the United Nations. It is interesting to note that the principles intended to humanize warfare are defined in the Code of Conduct as principles of "conduct" without mentioning protection; they "will be interpreted and applied in conformity with international humanitarian law" in the case of armed conflict.

The code is now being supplemented by Minimum Standards in Disaster Response (the rules of the game in some respects) that are to be used to evaluate, define, and conduct humanitarian operations in accordance with internationally recognized professional criteria. The Ombudsman Project will allow the beneficiaries of humanitarian programs to collectively demand accountability of humanitarian organizations.[7]

In general, the "international aid industry" should have a system that is no longer based on the right to provide assistance but on the right to receive assistance. Although this international ethic is in the making, there are still a number of questions to resolve in the application, enforcement, and respect of the principles by humanitarian partners, since it is a unilateral and voluntary code.

Applying the Rules of Good Conduct to Nondisaster Situations

The definition of a "disaster," when examined closely, is either too restrictive or too universal: The authors of the code defined it as "a calamitous event resulting in loss of life, great human suffering and distress and large-scale material damage." In many cases it is difficult to determine the degree of "distress." And what is the threshold for "large-scale" material damage? Does a strict interpretation of "disaster" require all four factors, or can they be taken separately? By what standard should we judge "political" disasters, especially if they involve "distress" but not necessarily serious material damage or human suffering (assuming the authors intend to differentiate between moral and physical suffering)? "Calamitous event" is the most important word in the definition. But to qualify it as a "disaster" requires the subjective measurement of suffering and human distress, which is the essence of the problem in aid assistance.

Recent examples of disaster relief operations demonstrate that the Code of Conduct formalizes the spirit of cooperation and emphasizes the primacy of humanitarian principles. Liberia is an interesting case in this respect; cooperation between organizations led to a Joint Policy of Operations to limit the negative side effects of humanitarian aid in the country.[8] The policy disentangled the economic impact of assistance from the political interest of actors in the conflict (including ECOMOG, the Economic Community of West African States Monitoring Group) and created a united front in dealing with the United Nations system and donor governments.[9]

But why is the code only specifically applicable to disaster assistance? Do not the situations that exist prior to disasters (where do they begin and end?) contain their causes? Considering only natural disasters, one can identify such preexisting vulnerabilities as endemic poverty and the position of minorities in the social, economic, and political spheres. These vulnerabilities are such that they exceed the capacity of potential victims to defend against the impact of disaster (or to prevent disaster).

Both a priori and a fortiori, the rules of good conduct are also useful in "development" situations.[10] Too often, emergency aid organizations appear to be responsible for the "perverse" and often surreal character of disaster situations. International organizations, including the United Nations and local development groups, do not exist in a political void created by the magic of development. Far from it, the development and aid policies of donor governments have been frequently castigated for their partiality. How many times have we seen development programs—in fact, "white elephants"—greedily consume public funds and money from the international community without developing the capacity of communities to effectively defend themselves in the future? Disaster situations often reflect both the failure of development policies and an absence of preparation. The sustainability of development programs should also be measured in term of capacity to prevent disasters.

As for disasters, why does the code not apply to private companies operating in the country, since these are often used by the parties to the conflict as a means of support or to legitimize their dubious sovereignty. There is no lack of examples: the Taliban and the pipeline business in Afghanistan; Laurent Kabila's new Democratic Republic of Congo and Canadian mining companies; the factions and government of Sierra Leone and De Beers diamond company; the Liberia of Charles Taylor and timber companies; the Khmer Rouge and Thai companies; and so on.

Moreover, are the principles of conduct not contradictory when they affirm that "we shall attempt to build disaster response on local capacities" without providing for the dissemination and approval of the code by local organizations?[11] Do they have access to the same information as international organizations? Were they consulted in the formulation of these principles, or of any others? Some organizations frequently point out that the code is aimed at the most powerful humanitarian organizations without really taking into account the quality of the work of local organizations.

The authors of the code therefore need to devote more attention to this problem in order to clarify the exact scope of its application. It seems to us that the rules elaborated for disaster situations are just as valid for nondisaster situations.

Enforcement Mechanisms

Organizations that have subscribed to the Code of Conduct have not yet clearly defined the criteria for its application and enforcement. At present, implementation of the code relies on the good will and self-regulation of participating organizations. A signatory organization that does not respect the code's principles could find its operations rapidly and temporarily marginalized. Operational standards should in theory give more objective substance to the principles that have been established, and where problems arise, a mediator would intervene to establish a fair solution.

A number of potential disaster situations, because they were not recognized as disasters, have demonstrated the limitations of the Code of Conduct as regards external or internal mechanisms to monitor compliance and respect for its principles. A case in point was the famine in the Democratic People's Republic of Korea (North Korea) in November 1997.

Meetings about that situation were held in several countries in Western Europe and in the United States. In some instances, only humanitarian organizations attended the meetings, while others were attended by the United Nations (including the United Nations Children's Fund [UNICEF]), humanitarian organizations, pressure groups, and donor governments.[12] On a number of occasions during these formal meetings, some organizations presented "excuses" for their lack of data or elaborated upon press releases prepared by their public relations departments that were published in the press and aired on television.

The problem of famine in North Korea urgently raises the question of professionalism in the evaluation of disaster situations. In September-October 1997, for example, UNICEF announced, without any scientific basis, that eighty thousand Korean children under the age of five were severely malnourished (UNICEF had at that time only two vehicles in North Korea). A month later, during an informal workshop about Korea in Geneva, a UNICEF representative declared that there was no famine in the country. In Rome, a World Food Program (WFP) representative acknowledged in September 1997 that the way in which the data collected were processed probably greatly overestimated the food deficit. Regardless of which report was ultimately correct, this example demonstrates how the timing of appeals for fund by the United Nations system, rather than professional judgment, can result in statements that contradict each other from one month to the next. The stakes in the numbers war are high for all humanitarian organizations, since they influence the level of support that will be forthcoming from the public and from donors.

If a mediator and operational standards had existed, could these hasty and unfounded declarations have been corrected?[13] Given the overpoliticization of the debate and operations in North Korea, data and information could have been more effectively monitored and rejected or merely corrected in the light of the operational standards and principles. Even so, this would not prevent an organization from crossing the line by citing figures without any evidence and without fear of general opprobrium or censure.

Thus, while the code and its operational standards can be effectively monitored, they do not a priori guarantee proper conduct or a high level of professionalism. Monitoring is thus largely reactive, a posteriori, and dependent on an organization's being able to admit to its peers that it might have committed errors or violated the code. And what about transparency vis-à-vis the public? Would it not be more forthright to explain to donors that there is a need for humanitarian work in North Korea, not because a given organization has an expert knowledge of the situation and is certain of the statistics but precisely because of the absence of reliable figures? All humanitarian organizations recognize that there are serious hunger and health problems, but there is no means at present of gauging the extent of the problem. It is precisely this lack of information that is worrying and that justifies, on professional grounds, a humanitarian presence in North Korea.[14]

However, this goal of transparency will probably never be fully respected: To date no organization has admitted its errors publicly, and many do not dare to state, in professional terms, the true motivation behind their operations and their presence.

Paradoxically, the Code of Conduct is relatively clear on this point: It is best to act according to the rules from the very start. In other words, the code should be observed even before the operation begins, even when it is unclear whether a genuine disaster has occurred.[15] Among the mechanisms of a posteriori monitoring, note should be taken of the efforts of one organization in particular that chose to support the United Nations system in order to work from within the structure of both the United Nations and other organizations or newcomers to the field wishing to monitor and correct the strategies adopted. The humanitarian objectives of the humanitarian organizations represented at this meeting were not all the same.

Monitoring mechanisms are still therefore relatively informal and unsatisfactory to the public, to which the code sought to offer an additional guarantee of transparency. In short, the code is relatively superficial because its only means of enforcement is the reputation of organizations among their peers. However, for the time being, the Code of Conduct, Operational Standards, and the Ombudsman Project are the only mechanisms in place to monitor compliance with the principles of good conduct.

Ensuring Respect for the Code

In theory, the code has no legal force, even though it sets out the "rules of the game" that, as we know, have customary value and tend to create a legal or juridical effect.[16] But the code itself states that "in the event of armed conflict, the present Code of Conduct shall be interpreted and applied in accordance with international humanitarian law." The code's scope is such that, in cases of armed conflict, it is necessary to interpret it in a manner consistent with international humanitarian law. The authors of the code might just as well have omitted the interpretation.

The absence from the code of any theoretical legal force reflects the authors' wish to preserve the most homogeneous corpus of law possible for situations of conflict and to recognize the primacy of international humanitarian law. This approach tends logically to favor the International Committee of the Red Cross (ICRC), even though the ICRC is now beginning to admit the possibility of closer collaboration with other humanitarian organizations, particularly "in the evaluation of situations in the field and advocacy in favor of greater respect for legal standards" of protection in time of conflict.[17] This collaboration should therefore be pursued in a concerted manner in the field. International humanitarian law provides the bases for this consultation, but the Code of Conduct will no doubt facilitate more flexible and certainly easier collaboration. The text of the Code of Conduct is in fact more accessible to NGOs as a group than the Geneva Conventions and its Additional Protocols, which, as the ICRC has quite rightly argued, require a staff of legal specialists.

However, one of the major problems envisaged in the text is that of the future, when considering that its signing could be "a future objective." The recent case of Sierra Leone seems to require an acceleration of the process. The British government, which has been very active on the case, has in fact recently demonstrated that a government could, on the one hand, promote or even demand that NGOs abide by the code and, on the other, conduct its humanitarian aid policy in a way that violates not only the principles of the code but also human rights and international humanitarian laws. When the newly elected government of Ahmed Tejan Kabbah fell, the British government relied on ECOMOG, whose operations were led by Nigeria, and on the United Nations to obtain the imposition of an embargo against Sierra Leone, excluding, in principle, humanitarian supplies. For six months beginning in March 1997, all goods intended for humanitarian programs should have first received an exemption from the United Nations and authorization from ECOMOG to cross the Sierra Leone–Guinea Conakry border. The junta that deposed Tejan Kabbah found itself in January and February 1998 in political and military difficulties and fled the capital, Freetown. After being a "refugee" under the protection of ECOMOG in neighboring Liberia, the deposed president returned to power on 10 March 1998 with strong support from the British government. Humanitarian aid policy, contrary to what was officially maintained, changed from one day to the next, and suddenly it was possible to support humanitarian organizations only in "secured" zones under the indirect control of the president through the intermediary of ECOMOG.

This policy was based on a white paper that argued that humanitarian aid should be based no longer on needs but on legality. In this sense, support for the embargo was equated with support for a foreign policy that advocated a return to democracy, specifically by punishing (as the U.S. government does from time to time[18]) forced takeovers, and coups d'état. It was striking to observe in this case how funds intended for humanitarian aid were completely cut off and restored only in January 1998, when the junta began to show signs of weakness in the field. The active collaboration with ECOMOG, especially under its Nigerian leadership, raised questions about the consistency of this foreign policy: How can one demand the restoration of democracy and at the same time rely on a force led by a country whose government is itself under sanctions for its human rights abuses? The defenders of the arms embargo against Sierra Leone were themselves later suspected of not observing the embargo. In May 1998, the British press revealed that Sandline International, a private company based in London that provided the services of mercenaries, might have been allowed to import weapons to support the president's return to power under the very nose of the British representative in Sierra Leone.

These recent events demonstrate that the rhetoric of governments has always had a strong tendency to manipulate humanitarian aid, whatever its foreign policy stance. This is nothing new, and it is not confined to one country.

Should governments and the United Nations be called upon to sign the Code of Conduct, especially if they are considering collaborating with or funding NGOs in the field, based on the latter's observance of the Code of Conduct? In theory, signature of the code promotes respect of its principles. And, above all, if NGOs themselves elaborate a code of conduct and call upon governments to respect its principles, why not go further and vigorously disseminate the code so that governments that are most active in foreign policy matters might be gradually persuaded to sign.

The authors of the code envisaged signature by governments as a real goal that could become a necessity. As long as governments wish to continue using humanitarian aid as an instrument of foreign policy, this should be done on the basis of a document respected both by NGOs and by the governments themselves, as long as governments contract out humanitarian aid to the NGOs. Otherwise, humanitarian organizations will have to be satisfied with a framework for action that, though ideal, will constrain their operations but not be binding on donor governments and on the United Nations.

One can draw four main conclusions from these observations:

1. Signature alone does not suffice to guarantee respect for the principles and thus their application.

2. Failure to sign the Code of Conduct does not mean that an NGO is not behaving in accordance with its principles.
3. Furthermore, the question of the scope of the code's application—that is, should the code be applied even if it is unclear whether a disaster has occurred—remains crucial. The answer is yes, since the best way to apply the principles is still to respect them whatever the situation. This is what the code means, when it declares under "object" that "implementation depends on the determination of each subscribing organization to respect the norms which it establishes."
4. Last, monitoring remains very weak. Nothing guarantees that the future existence of Operational Standards or of a mediator will correct this situation.

Above all, the code is a flexible, nonbinding, and voluntary reminder that humanitarianism in both foreign and domestic policy remains essential if we are to be consistent and relevant. In any event, humanitarian aid must always be accompanied by protection. Blocking aid often means that those who have the means of providing protection for those most in need are deprived of any possibility of doing so.

In the final analysis, we may say that the code is a necessary tool but not sufficient in itself. The tendency toward institutionalization that it represents does not guarantee respect for fundamental humanitarian principles and human rights by NGOs, governments, and the United Nations.

The monitoring of activities through the Ombudsman Project and the Operational Standards is no substitute for the special and additional effort needed to disseminate the code and to encourage donor governments, and in particular the United Nations, to sign it. Otherwise, humanitarian organizations could find themselves in an aid system burdened by onerous constraints, which would give governments and donors even more reason to withhold humanitarian aid while using as a pretext the principles enshrined in the Code of Conduct.

We may have to acknowledge in the end that humanitarian principles are not universally perceived in the same way and that, despite the respect they demand, they remain a matter of human passions—compassion and solidarity—that belong to no one or, quite on the contrary, to everyone. Humanitarian intervention in the field teaches us the enduring lesson that commitment is necessary but never sufficient. And that no government and no institution can claim to arrogate to itself.

Notes

Daniel Puillet-Breton was the executive director of Action Against Hunger in London until February 2000.

1. The military-humanitarian interventions in Somalia in 1992 are an example.

2. See Mark Duffield's study *The Symphony of the Damned* (University of Birmingham, 1996).

3. As we know, aid is susceptible to all kinds of evils. Humanitarian aid is often criticized for participating in the economic dynamics of conflicts (how can we deny it?); it can easily fail to protect those it was intended to benefit. It is increasingly politicized and compromised by the growth of military-humanitarian interventions (interventions for humanitarian reasons supported by the United Nations or by NATO).

4. The eight organizations were the Caritas International, Catholic Relief Services, International Federation of Red Cross and Red Crescent Societies, International Save the Children Alliance, Lutheran World Federation, Oxfam, and the World Council of Churches.

5. A representative from one of the founding NGOs recently remarked that the Code of Conduct should not negate the diverse mandates of the signatory organizations. He also stated that the code should not promote a vision of one single type of humanitarian organization, which he felt was a dangerous notion because it did not guarantee that humanitarian principles would be respected in any case (London, 12 March 1998, Overseas Development Institute conference).

6. Recommendations to the governments of disaster-affected countries (Annex I): 1. Governments should recognize and respect the independent, humanitarian, and impartial actions of humanitarian organizations; 2. Host governments should facilitate rapid access to disaster victims for humanitarian organizations; 3. Governments should facilitate the timely flow of relief goods and information during disasters; 4. Governments should seek to provide a coordinated disaster information and planning service; 5. Disaster relief in the event of armed conflict.

Recommendations to the donor governments (Annex II): 1. Recognize and respect the independent, humanitarian, and impartial actions of humanitarian organizations; 2. Provide funding with a guarantee of operational independence; 3. Use their offices to assist humanitarian organizations in obtaining access to disaster victims.

Recommendations to intergovernmental organizations (Annex III): 1. Recognize humanitarian organizations, local and foreign, as valuable partners; 2. Assist host governments in providing an overall coordinating framework for international and local disaster relief; 3. Extend security protection provided for UN organizations to humanitarian organizations; 4. Provide humanitarian organizations with the same access to relevant information as is granted to UN organizations.

7. The operational standards are also called the Sphere Project. The Ombudsman Project is Projet Médiateur in French and has been renamed the Humanitarian Accountability Project (HAC) 2000.

8. The Joint Policy of Operations is an international collective effort of NGOs, including Action Against Hunger, Medecins sans Frontieres (MSF),

Save the Children Fund (SCF), World Vision International (WVI), Cooperative for American Relief to Everywhere (CARE), and the Oxford Committee for Famine Relief (Oxfam), to name only a few.

9. This followed the looting of supplies and equipment of practically all the organizations. Action Against Hunger in 1997 luckily escaped warring factions attacks in Monrovia.

10. How should a country's level of development be evaluated? What is the capacity of social and political entities in the country to organize? Even countries that are considered "developed" by Western standards are not necessarily well equipped to manage humanitarian disaster relief.

11. The quotation is from the Principle of Conduct 6.

12. An informal workshop on the Democratic People's Republic of Korea was held by UNICEF in Geneva, October 20–21, 1997.

13. In March 1998, the logistical management of all humanitarian operations in North Korea was in the hands of the government, in particular, the Relief Committee for Flood Damage (RCFD). Only a small portion of aid was possibly considered as humanitarian, thereby preventing monitoring. Food security and nutrition surveys conducted under the aegis of the United Nations were unable to apply the standards necessary for publication that are currently used in the humanitarian profession.

14. The famines in northwest China in 1927 (sixty million victims) and in the Ukraine from 1932 to 1934 are evidence of this problem. Many Western visitors did not report these famines because they did not themselves observe them. See the excellent book by Jasper Becker, *Fantômes affamés* (London: John Murray Pub., 1997).

15. Many of the organizations at conferences and meetings on North Korea were not yet operational or had not been able to evaluate the country's needs in a free or reliable fashion in 1997. A number of them published baseless statistics on the number of famine victims without having set foot in North Korea at all; the reports were intended to promote campaigns to fund their future work in the field. The North Korean government was their exclusive source of information and currently continues in this role.

16. The Working Environment section of the code specifies that the guidelines are not "legally binding."

17. See Carlo Von Flue and Jean Philippe Lavoyer, *Revue du RRN, ODI, ICRC* in "*Comment les ONG peuvent-ils aider à promouvoir le Droit International Humanitaire?*" [How can NGOs help promote international humanitarian law?] November, 1997.

18. However, since 1989, U.S. law prohibits cutting humanitarian aid for political reasons.

18

Standards and Quality Assurance

Pierre Perrin

Quality assurance is a given in all spheres of activity, but the definition of *quality* will differ from one field to another. In the field of economics, quality is a combination of two elements: consumer satisfaction and the best economic return. The first should lead to the second, which is the ultimate goal. In the humanitarian field, success is always measured with respect to victims: best possible guarantees of protection and assistance. Striving for the most economical solution possible should be a concern, but the blind application of economic laws to humanitarian operations risks running counter to the fundamental humanitarian principles of compassion and impartiality. Today, humanitarian interventions seem to be based more on cost/efficiency criteria than on the needs of victims, and we must therefore remember this basic principle when referring to quality assurance that, in the humanitarian field, must be focused on victims.

Bases for an Effective Humanitarian Operation

Two elements are fundamental for a successful humanitarian operation: focusing action on the victims and following a logical approach.

This article is based on a seminar organized by the International Committee of the Red Cross (ICRC) in Geneva on 14 December 1998 and published with the kind permission of the ICRC.

The goal of humanitarian intervention should always be to assist those who have the right to humanitarian aid, that is, the victims. The use of a logical approach has long been applied in humanitarian operations in which certain planning and operation elements are present.

Planning should include:

- An accurate study of the situation, including an analysis of victims' needs; the economic, cultural, and political context; and potential obstacles. The choice of a strategy that is most appropriate to a specific situation at any given time depends upon the depth of the study.
- An overall analysis of the needs of victims in order to avoid partial measures that neglect entire aspects of victims' needs.
- Definition of overall goals according to the needs of victims. Operations in which the mobilization of resources becomes an end in itself should be avoided.

The search for effectiveness during the operational phase is based upon:

- Consistency with stated goals;
- Observance of the implementation procedures decided upon in the planning stage;
- Mobilization of adequate resources, ensuring, for example, that the skills of operational personnel match the activities that are to be undertaken;
- Refinement of the operation based on regular review of the overall situation, of the data collected during monitoring, and of the results of evaluation exercises.

The search for quality must be pursued at all levels. Activities of a very high standard will be irrelevant if the supporting analysis is of poor quality.

Components of a
System of Quality Assurance

The basic elements for ensuring the quality of an operation are analysis and planning, program implementation, monitoring, and evaluation. A system of quality assurance should go even further, however. Planning goals and implementation procedures should take into account norms that may be international, local, or specific to a particular organization. These will be essential for evaluating outcomes in order to permit useful comparisons to be made. An expert knowledge of these references is a necessary component of quality assurance.

Evaluations are not only a management tool but also an indispensable element for developing institutional memory. That memory should not be a passive database but an instrument for the development of institutional policies that combine the necessary evolution of strategies and procedures with the lessons learned in the field.

The next step will be to ensure that those responsible for the implementation of policies and procedures thoroughly understand them. Training is therefore another key element of any system of quality assurance.

Each element of this "quality assurance system" should have its criteria for ensuring quality and the necessary monitoring mechanisms. For example:

- Situational analyses should be conducted with rigor using available tools of analysis.
- Services provided should match the quality criteria identified for this type of service.
- Mechanisms for the ongoing follow-up of activities should be in place and functioning.
- Evaluations should be planned.
- References appropriate to the context should be used.
- Intervention policies should be regularly reviewed and updated.
- Training programs should effectively prepare personnel for future responsibilities.

A system of quality assurance will not be effective unless there is coordination among the various components of a program. Mechanisms must be in place so that:

- The results of evaluations are systematically used to reorient activities, feed the institutional memory, develop action policies, and provide a practical basis for training.
- Evaluation standards are used at three stages of intervention: planning, implementation, and evaluation.
- Training equips staff with the skills needed to implement

planned activities, which requires a constant exchange between management and staff in order to ensure the best possible match between tasks and skills.

One can imagine an infinite number of possible connections among the various elements of a quality assurance system. Each organization is responsible for identifying the linkages that it wishes to institutionalize in order to develop its own system of quality assurance.

Establishment of a System of Quality Assurance at the ICRC

By applying this concept, the ICRC is able to monitor the progress made in the search for quality within the institution. The following are examples of how this takes place:

- Planning for Results is a new planning tool introduced in September 1998. It emphasizes rigorous analysis of humanitarian situations and the establishment of goals as a function of the needs of victims.
- For monitoring purposes, an analytic accounting system will link each activity to its real cost, thus enabling organizations to accurately respond to donors.
- The intention to carry out impact assessments was stated in the ICRC "Future" plan. An assessment policy has been defined and the structures for its implementation established.
- ICRC action policies are regularly revised and developed. The policy of assistance to war wounded was one such program.
- Training remains a priority and offers a range of opportunities from loyalty to ICRC to specialized courses in international humanitarian law, public health, and so on.
- Operations at the management level permit closer links to be established among operational activities, resource management, evaluations, studies, and policy development.

By using this approach it is possible to pinpoint the role of benchmarks within quality assurance systems. Such benchmarks are vital to the success of operations, provided that they are interpreted in a way that takes account of the specific characteristics of each situation, including constraints, the socioeconomic environment, and cultural criteria. Lastly, one must not forget that, in the humanitarian field, a system of quality assurance seeks above all to ensure that interventions provide an effective response to the needs of victims.

Notes

Pierre Perrin is medical director at the International Committee of the Red Cross, Geneva.

19

Humanitarianism—
A Changing Concept?

Jean-Luc Bodin

Under the auspices of the Steering Committee for Humanitarian Response (SCHR), a number of major humanitarian agencies in 1992 established a Code of Conduct for Disaster Relief Operations. The code was signed by over 150 organizations. Later it was supplemented by a number of initiatives, including:

- The Sphere Project, a Humanitarian Charter and Minimum Standards for Disaster Response for humanitarian activities in the field;
- People in Aid, a code of best practices to improve the quality and efficiency of aid workers' management;
- The Active Learning Network for Accountability and Performance, a network of research and information for humanitarian organizations;
- The Ombudsman Project, a vehicle for managing and monitoring the implementation of all humanitarian projects through the intervention of a mediator.

The idea of a universal ethic and a mode of action common to all humanitarian organizations is seductive. Most of the principles posited in the Code of Conduct and the humanitarian charter of the Sphere Project are incontestable: the right to live in dignity and nondiscrimination. No serious humanitarian agency would dispute these basic rights. Action Against Hunger, from its inception, has had a Charter of Principles based on fundamental humanitarian rights, which it strives to respect in all of its operations. Even so, a universal charter is not valid. Each nongovernmental organization (NGO) represents a commitment by a group of people with their own specific mandate and their own version of a charter and ethical principles that one should respect. Impartiality may be interpreted as the principle of nondiscrimination in implementing actions, while neutrality comes into play at the operational level and obliges (as far as possible) an agency to intervene regardless of the "side." But as we consider the notions of impartiality/neutrality, it is clear that no one will have the same definition. This would play into the hands of some organizations that would refuse to accept strict adherence to such principles, thereby proving that a common code of ethics would not be practical. A strict universal ethic will not work.

Defining operational standards in the areas of nutrition, food security, water, sanitation, health, and victim services led to productive discussions in working groups. No one will contest that this effort resulted in substantial improvements in the coherence and coordination of technical operations in the field.

The question that remains is how to apply these principles and standards. There is an obvious risk of imposing excessive uniformity on humanitarian activities. While such an approach could definitely facilitate exchanges between the different agencies, thus making them more efficient, it can never replace the goals, ethics, or methods of operation that are unique to each humanitarian actor.

Another risk resides in the ambiguity of terms used for the implementation of these principles and standards. Political and economic conditions are not mentioned, since the situation is described in ideal, even utopian terms, yet they constitute one of the primary obstacles to intervention. What will happen when the lack of security and lack of access to victims make it impossible to achieve the stipulated goals of these projects? Should we refuse to act on the grounds that one cannot do enough, or should we continue anyway because our primary mission as humanitarians is to be there, even though what we do may never be sufficient? If the objectives of these projects remain as points of reference, that in itself could be a positive thing if the project remains incomplete; but if we adopt a legalistic approach, the danger becomes great. Expressions such as "what the populations have the right to expect from humanitarian assistance" or "develop standards of performance that can be measured" should be quite rightly questioned. Donors would then be authorized to condition their support for a particular mission on its "results," if they do not already do so. This could be an additional argument to reduce the scale of projects.

As Daniel Puillet-Breton explains in Chapter 17, the legal framework for humanitarian operations is still weak. There is no real monitoring of the observance of these standards, only a vague and unclear reference to a mediator. Neither is there any real obligation on the part of states whose first obligation, nevertheless, is to provide assistance to their populations. Before devising a new set of laws for beneficiaries, let us do everything possible to ensure compliance with existing laws, in particular the Geneva Conventions and the Universal Declaration of Human Rights. It would be dangerous for humanitarian organizations to abandon these norms, when mechanisms for monitoring respect for fundamental rights do not function.

Everything depends then upon the application of these universal standards. Faulty interpretation would leave the door open for actors whose objectives are not exclusively humanitarian. Obviously, NGOs cannot achieve everything based only on their good will. The largest possible number of organizations should accept these principles and standards, as Pierre Perrin argues in Chapter 18. They should be guidelines but not become a new international norm that structures or even regulates a humanitarian world that has lost its independence. Let us not misunderstand our goals, which are based first and foremost upon humanitarian principles. In Burundi, for example, a study has demonstrated how technically oriented objectives could become a trap. In fact, correctly applying technical standards does not necessarily mean achieving humanitarian goals—taking care of 500 children is not an end it itself, when several thousand other children continue to suffer from hunger a few kilometers away.

The stakes in this question are high: What constitutes humanitarian intervention? Does an organization become humanitarian the moment it respects the norms? Is it the operation or the organization that is deemed humanitarian? The danger, aside from political exploitation, is that new actors in the field may be humanitarian in name only. Confusion already reigns. During the Balkan crisis, we witnessed a perverse form of globalization: NGOs, United Nations agencies, the Red Cross, the military, religious organizations, civil society, and States were all "humanitarian," everything was "humanitarian," and the general perception of others, donors, victimizers, and victims was summarized in one acronym: NATO (the North Atlantic Treaty Organization). When impartiality and neutrality are not respected, one should not be surprised if Serbs, but also all the other forgotten populations in Sudan, North Korea, or elsewhere, are critical of "humanitarian operations."

This is why ethical and technical aspects of the question must be appreciated for what they are, namely, points of reference. The priority must continue to be quality and not be obscured by quantitative aspects that draw attention away from the spirit of initiative and solidarity that lies at the heart of humanitarian action.

Notes

Jean-Luc Bodin is executive director of Action Against Hunger–France.

20

Security: A Key Component of Humanitarian Action

Pierre Gallien

Over the last decade or so, humanitarian assistance operations have had to face increasing difficulties. The situations in which aid organizations are required to intervene are becoming more and more complex. Logistical and administrative constraints have been compounded by political and media-related issues and security problems. Ensuring the security of humanitarian personnel today presents major challenges.

The dangers faced by relief teams are not only greater but are now directly targeted at their personnel. Violence has become commonplace and is being increasingly used against humanitarian workers to influence their work. In some places, those using violence do not want embarrassing witnesses; in others, control is sought over the distribution of foodstuffs. In yet other places, attempts are made to influence international decisions through, inter alia, death threats, kidnappings, and attacks. No method is excluded, especially since in most cases no serious investigation is undertaken to find and punish the guilty parties.

Unfortunately, this violence against humanitarian relief personnel is but a small part of the problem. In many situations, the civilian population is used, manipulated, or oppressed by the parties to the conflict, in violation of the fundamental principles of international humanitarian law. Humanitarian teams are then faced with security problems in trying to maintain direct access to victims when the parties to the conflict knowingly and willfully fail to ensure their safety.

Action Against Hunger
and Security-Related Incidents

Information compiled by Action Against Hunger shows that during the late 1990s the organization faced major security crises each
year:

- In 1995, Rudy Mark was kidnapped in Mogadishu, Somalia,
  while on his way to the airport in a vehicle that was clearly
  identified as belonging to Action Against Hunger. Two Somali
  staff members were wounded in this attack, which was really
  aimed at the work of the organization. Thirty-seven days of
  negotiations and the support of the entire humanitarian relief
  community were necessary before Rudy was released. Today,
  only five organizations are still working in Mogadishu.
- In 1995, in Gitega, Burundi, grenades exploded simultaneous-
  ly in the offices and homes of four of the five humanitarian
  organizations present in the town. Sylvie Fehlbaum and Pierre
  Gallien were injured in the explosions (fortunately not seriously). In the weeks prior to the attack, government and rebel
  troop movements had forced some of the population to abandon the urban area in order to escape the atrocities of the
  armed groups. Following this attack, the organizations present
  in Gitega were forced to suspend their operations for several
  weeks.
- In 1996, Michael Penrose and Frédéric Malardeau were kidnapped in Grozny, Chechnya, and held for twenty-six days
  while the city was subjected to heavy bombardment by the
  Russian forces. In the months that followed, the proliferation
  of kidnappings forced most organizations to withdraw from
  the country.
- In 1997, Frédéric Michel, Daniel Llorente, and five members
  of our Afghan staff were arrested by the Taliban militia and
  accused of having been present at the party held to bid
  farewell to the team's medical officer, at which a few women
  were also present. Despite intense pressure from the international community, they were condemned to several weeks of
  imprisonment. While Frédéric and Daniel were especially well
  treated, the Afghan staff were subjected to physical abuse. A
  few months later, all of the nongovernmental organizations
  (NGOs) present in Kabul were forced to withdraw in the face
  of the intransigence of the Taliban, who wished to impose

rules of operation that were contrary to the core principles of humanitarianism.

- 1998: In Sierra Leone, the forces of ECOMOG (the Monitoring Group of the member countries of ECOWAS, the Economic Community of West African states) launched a surprise attack on Freetown to restore to power the democratically elected president Ahmed Tejan Kabbah. The military junta and the Rebel United Front (RUF), the main rebel movement in Sierra Leone, were then beaten back and retreated in disorder, looting and committing atrocities. All the relief organizations present in the country were surprised by this movement and, in light of the risks they faced and the widespread looting of their operations, were forced to evacuate their workers under difficult conditions.
- In 1999, Eric Courly was kidnapped in Ethiopia while traveling in the south of the country for work-related purposes. Five weeks of negotiations were needed to secure his release.

For nearly two years now, the Humanitarian Safety and Protection Network, a comprehensive program undertaken in close collaboration with other European NGOs, has sought to develop the institutional memory of organizations in order to gain greater familiarity with the scope and nature of the dangers faced by their personnel in the field.[1] This initiative begun by the Paris Office of Action Against Hunger in 1998 was extended to the other members of the Network (Madrid, London, and New York). During these two years, it has highlighted a number of important elements. The proposed classification draws a distinction among three groups of incidents, based on their nature and inherent objectives:

- Acts of banditry, characterized by the search for short-term economic gain;
- Acts of terrorism, attacking the very values of the organization;
- Acts of war and police actions, in which the actors identified with the conflict are directly involved.

In 1998, three-quarters of the missions of Action Against Hunger that were monitored by the Paris office faced security problems of varying degrees of seriousness.[2] In all, fifty-six situations of insecurity had to be dealt with. Of these, sixteen involved the evacuation of personnel. The security-related incidents are detailed in Table 20.1.

Table 20.1   Security-Related Incidents, 1998

	Number	Percentage
Acts of banditry	15	37.5
Acts of terrorism	9	22.5
Acts of war and police actions	16	40

During the first five months of 1999, half of the teams in the field had to face at least one security problem, or thirty-six altogether. Today, 40 percent of heads of mission consider security as a priority element of their work. In the most sensitive situations, this element may account for more than half of their working time.

Table 20.2 offers a more detailed analysis of the nature of these problems.

Table 20.2   Security-Related Incidents, 1999

	Acts of Banditry	Acts of Terrorism	Acts of War and Police Action	Total
Specific death threats	2	3	5	10
Theft of material	7			7
Requisition of material			2	2
Arbitrary detention			4	4
Verbal aggression		1	4	5
Threat of physical aggression		2	2	4
Intrusion by military			1	1
Murder		1		1
Kidnapping		1		1
Bombardment			1	1
Total	9	8	19	36

It has become evident that the violence is aimed directly at the organization. Of the thirty-six incidents reported, only one was due to a nondiscriminating danger resulting from a military action (bombardment). The other thirty-five were all directed against the organization, either to seize its property (ten thefts and requisitions of equipment) or to prevent it from carrying out its activities.

The number of incidents related to banditry and terrorism (nearly half of the incidents) is also notable. This type of incident is now becoming more and more violent. Another obvious conclusion is that most incidents reflect a lack of respect for humanitarian action by the parties to the conflict themselves.

Unfortunately, this type of situation is true not only for Action Against Hunger. All humanitarian organizations, including the United Nations and members of the Red Cross, now face similar problems.

Humanitarian Operations in Increasingly Complex Situations

These dangers are of course not new and are inherent in the type of humanitarian relief activity to which we are committed: we are as close as possible to the victims of hunger. However, there have been significant changes in certain aspects of our work. It is essential that humanitarian organizations take these changes into account in their operations in order to address them effectively without losing sight of the core principles that govern their actions.

It is clear that the nature of conflict has changed since the end of the Cold War. A review of these structural changes and their effect on the way in which violence is expressed is a necessary but not sufficient phase for understanding the phenomenon as a whole. Humanitarian relief organizations for their part have also changed in terms of the way they operate and of their relations with political and media figures. Their challenge now is to take stock of the situation and come up with new approaches to their work that are perhaps less standardized, more creative, and better adapted to local conditions and constraints.

The collapse of the Soviet empire brought about a radical change in the order of international relations. The East-West divide and the fear of recourse to nuclear weapons had made it possible to normalize certain types of situations. The ideology of these two large blocs clashed within zones of influence, with each party relying on its political and economic support for friendly regimes or certain rebel groups, as circumstances dictated. In a certain sense, this situation made it possible to control and contain confrontations. It was therefore assumed that, after the fall of the Berlin Wall, the different rebel movements would gradually fade from lack of financial and technical support.

The bitter reality, however, has been that the opposite happened. Over the past ten years, the number of conflicts in the world has increased dramatically, often exceeding in horror the limits of our understanding. From Liberian child-soldiers to the bombardment of Grozny, including armed bands in Somalia and the genocide of more than 500,000 Tutsis and moderate Hutus in Rwanda, these new conflicts seem to be characterized above all by an indescribable chaos in which only the strongest survive and where there are no rules.

The collapse of communism has indirectly resulted in the emergence of two related phenomena. On the one hand, it has contributed to the weakening of a large number of states. On the other, it has promoted globalization and the development of the market economy.

The decline in aid-flows from most countries in the North has caused difficulties in many developing countries burdened by heavy administrative structures. Many of them have been forced to comply with the recommendations of the International Monetary Fund and undertake structural reforms for which there have been varying degrees of political acceptance. For Béatrice Hibou, these liberalization reforms have also had "unexpected and often undesired lateral effects: reduction in budgetary expenditure that place administrations in difficulty, delegitimization of government bodies, decentralization of decision-making authority, emphasis on external over internal legitimacy, quickness of action over modalities and results over means."[3] In keeping with this new trend toward liberalization, a number of state functions have been privatized. The increase in the number of NGOs has been a characteristic of this phenomenon.

In the face of this weakening of the state, demands for the recognition of group identities, which had been throttled in the past, have found fertile ground for expression. In many countries, moreover, the phenomenon of rural exodus has led to the collapse of the family unit and to the loss of the values and references of the rural world. This new urban population, relegated to the poor neighborhoods of the cities, thus finds itself in contact with the values of modernity (especially through television) yet unable to enjoy its benefits. Faced with poverty and unemployment, this population provides fertile ground for increased crime and the emergence of new forms of social protest. According to Jean-Christophe Rufin, far from a loss of the ideological values of rebel movements, we have witnessed the emergence of new forms of doctrine based on the appropriation of local ideological values that have been integrated into more modern political constructs. For example, the doctrine of the RUF combines the values of a return to sources and a base of Marxist organization.

The survival of old movements and the emergence of new ones

have been possible only to the extent that the economic environment has permitted them to exploit independent resources. The globalization of economic exchanges has seen the rapid development of new operators without any real oversight by state entities. Client networks have been privatized and more specifically internationalized, thanks to unprecedented developments in the communications sector. The mafia and major international organized crime have expanded to the point where their economic weight is greater than the budget of certain countries. Globally, between $750 and 1,000 billion per annum are controlled by the mafia. By way of comparison, the gross domestic product of a country such as Mali, which is among the poorest in the world, is approximately $6 billion.

The different rebel movements have rapidly adapted to this new environment and have developed new strategies. They have compensated for the fall-off in international support from states by developing new economic links. In Mogadishu, Somalia, as the country was just emerging from one of the worst famines in its history and the city was controlled by armed bands, it was easy to telephone to the other end of the world using the satellite services of a private company operating in the city. Similar examples have prompted Roland Marchal to write that "Mogadishu is today more closely linked to the world outside than it has ever been for the thirty years of its existence as a State."[4] This situation is not specific to Somalia. In Angola, exports of diamonds have increased sharply over the past five years, providing annual income estimated at more than $500 million for the National Union for the Total Independence of Angola (UNITA), the main armed movement opposed to the government. In Liberia, exports of exotic woods have never ceased and have even increased during the conflict, thus permitting Charles Taylor to finance his war effort.

This new situation has led a number of guerrillas to redefine their strategies by incorporating an economic dimension into their ideological objectives. There should be no mistake about this. In most cases, theirs are not genuine economic activities that seek to redistribute a part of the benefits to the populations; they are predatory activities based on the reckless exploitation of the country's natural resources. The fields of activity are generally limited and involve mainly the uncontrolled exploitation of mineral resources or control over certain agricultural products. Processing industries that require major investments and stability in order to ensure a return on investment are few and are to be found mainly in particular sectors of activities, such as petroleum resources (Angola, Congo) or drug refining (Colombia, Burma, Afghanistan).

In this situation, two elements thus assume importance: the geographical and the human. The fight is over a territory and access to and control over resources or their marketing routes. What is worse, the civilian population needed to produce these revenues is also at risk. The use of violence as a means to acquire and control has become widespread, particularly given the popular view that the international community is powerless to punish such acts.

Lastly, alliances and fault lines between states have steadily been redrawn around new actors and around political and economic stakes, which have become more regional in character. In Congo-Brazzaville, in 1997, the committing of Angolan troops alongside the militia of Denis Sassou N'Guesso was the decisive factor in assuring his accession to power. In the new Democratic Republic of Congo, the involvement of countries such as Angola, Rwanda, Uganda, or Zimbabwe is an essential element for understanding the dynamic of the conflict. Also noteworthy is the role of Nigeria in the conflicts in Liberia and Sierra Leone or that of Ethiopia in the anarchy that prevails in Somalia. Although predominantly in Africa, these new power plays are also to be found in other continents. There are situations in Afghanistan and in Iraq; closer to us is the intervention of the North Atlantic Treaty Organization (NATO) in the crisis in the Balkans. These situations encourage the development of microzones that are organized around local potentates whose conflicts and violence bear only limited connection to national frameworks.

The chaotic forms of current conflicts can therefore be understood only through a multifaceted framework of analysis that takes full account of the following:

- ideological and identity-based claims;
- economic assets, means of exploitation, and marketing channels;
- interstate dynamics.

Since each of these elements has its own dynamic and its own geographical parameters, it is possible to find coexisting within a single country parts of the territory that are perfectly peaceful and others that are humanitarian crisis areas.

Similarly, it is clear that the dynamic of these conflicts can no longer be analyzed within a linear framework of the type of crisis in which emergency leads to rehabilitation that leads to development. What is now needed is a new cyclical approach in which periods of violence are followed by periods of calm.

Today's Current Humanitarian Responses

Faced with these changes in the environment in which they operate, humanitarian organizations have had to adapt to the new situation. Some of these changes have been the direct results of the new constraints that have been identified, while others are associated more with the broader changes taking place in the sector. To some extent, these changes have also influenced the forms of violence with which humanitarian personnel are confronted.

Humanitarian assistance provided through NGOs has increased largely at the expense of bilateral aid. The number of organizations involved in current areas of crisis, such as the Balkans, far exceeds the number that intervened in Ethiopia in 1985. More than two hundred organizations provide assistance to Albanian refugees as compared with only a handful fifteen years ago. This proliferation of organizations in crisis situations is accompanied by a certain form of competition—for new funds but also to secure sufficient media coverage or to burnish the reputation of the organization. It follows therefore that organizations are implicitly pushed into operating closer and closer to areas of conflict.

On the other hand, the term *humanitarian* has been much overused during the past few years. Humanitarian assistance is presented to the public as a coherent whole, with values, principles of action, and modes of operation that are shared and recognized by all actors. Donors, United Nations agencies, Red Cross movements, and nongovernmental organizations are cited indiscriminately. While this image may be attractive, it does not reflect the reality on the ground. The humanitarian family embraces a very diverse range of actors who no doubt share the same aim but who are not always in agreement on how to achieve it.

The attitude of the political authorities in recent years has only worsened this confusion. More and more, they give the impression of wishing to use humanitarian assistance as an instrument of foreign policy. The U.S. position on the food aid provided to North Korea is perhaps the most glaring example. In each major crisis of the past few years, we have seen in the same theater of operation humanitarian and military operators working in complete synergy. This was the case in Somalia and Rwanda, and we have just entered into a new phase with the crisis in Kosovo, where the same actors both wage war and conduct humanitarian operations.

More and more, humanitarian organizations are endeavoring to go beyond their roles of merely delivering aid. Recognizing that humanitarian assistance is nothing but a placebo if unaccompanied by political action to help the conflicting parties reach an agreement, these organizations seek to grab the attention of the political authorities and the public at large by relaying the suffering of the population. Present in the field, they are firsthand witnesses of the reality on the ground. The development of the media has amplified to the extreme this activity of witnessing. Pursuing this logic even further, some NGOs have become directly involved in diplomatic peace-building initiatives.

The image that results from this situation is particularly confused. The perception of a neutral and impartial humanitarian relief movement is increasingly open to question. In the Balkans crisis, hundreds of organizations were active in Albania and Macedonia, fewer than a dozen were present in Montenegro, and those that were allowed to enter Kosovo could be counted on the fingers of one hand. Did the civil population remaining in Kosovo have so few needs? No, but neither NATO nor the Serbian army could guarantee an adequate level of security, while permitting the organizations to operate independently.

The work of humanitarian organizations and their approach to problems have also evolved. The programs and budgets that they manage sometimes amount to several million dollars. In recent years, humanitarian relief organizations have markedly developed their capacity for intervention and rapid deployment. Logistical constraints have been removed. Prepositioned stocks of supplies can be mobilized and used from one day to the next in the event of a major crisis. Supplies themselves have become specialized to fit the specific needs of humanitarian emergency situations. New well-drilling equipment, specific re-nutrition products, and water supply kits are all positioned in such a way as to respond rapidly and effectively to emergency problems. The logistics list of Doctors Without Borders is illustrative in this regard: cholera kit, car maintenance kit, and a kit for the restoration of hospital services are all available to provide an immediate humanitarian response.

This technical choice of relief organizations also relies on a more professional international staff. Their work in the field is focused on technical expertise and on the supervision and training of national teams. To some extent, this tendency has unfortunately developed at the expense of the quality of the relationship between volunteers and aid beneficiaries. It is not that volunteers no longer have the desire, but rather that they no longer have the time to listen to beneficiaries and to try to better understand the background to the crisis. The volunteers are caught between administrative constraints on the one hand and the need for immediate operational responses on the other. This situation is made worse by the fact that the average time spent by a volunteer on a difficult mission rarely exceeds one year.

Rapid rotation of personnel in the field is thus accompanied by a significant loss of mission memory. Serious incidents naturally remain in the collective consciousness of countries, while nearly all "secondary" incidents are forgotten once they have no major consequences. In terms of analysis and of individual behavior, these episodes are particularly important and significant. The perception of insecurity is not always evident. Often problems arise suddenly and surprise relief teams. Knowing that death threats are a common practice in Burundi can no doubt influence the manner in which problems in that country are approached and resolved. This phenomenon of amnesia is reinforced by a certain taboo observed by organizations against investigating the causes of each incident and discussing their conclusions with other partners.

Last, humanitarian organizations have also had to adapt to the increase in the risks that they face. They have sought to limit the risk of incidents by taking protective measures. The increasing sophistication of their communications systems is illustrative of this trend. The use of radios, walkie-talkies, and satellite telephones is today widespread in sensitive missions. Radio contacts between the different operational centers are often a daily measure that has frequently permitted dangerous situations to be avoided. Travel by convoy has become common, and if access by road is too dangerous, helicopters or small airplanes are used. The use of four-wheel-drive vehicles is today so widespread in the world of humanitarian relief organizations that these vehicles have become their distinguishing characteristic. In most situations, these measures have been required to be able to conduct relief operations, but the almost automatic recourse to them has also created a number of paradoxes. Indeed, in certain situations, it is these same measures that can give rise to situations of risk. The excessive use of high-technology equipment or of four-wheel-drive vehicles in environments without structures is never without consequences: Either it provokes greed, or it creates a certain distance between the population and humanitarian relief workers.

Some organizations are now seeking to promote a centralized and collective system of security management in each country by institutionalizing the function of security officer. Others have tried recourse to private organizations to manage all of these problems for them. However seductive these approaches may appear, they can lead only to impasse.

By developing security procedures without weighing any other factors, humanitarian organizations run the risk of cutting themselves off from their environment and their raison d'être, which is to provide relief and protection to populations in need.

More than ever, the management of security must rely on a careful review of the operational context at the local level. It is only at this level that humanitarian organizations can hope to understand the nature and dynamics of the situations in which they are involved and thus to identify the risks to which they are exposed. Security management can no longer be conceived of as the mere application of rules and procedures that a nurse is required to follow without understanding their real purpose. Each rule, each decision must involve the individuals and organizations taking them. Moreover, each worker must be able to appreciate the collective aspect of the decision. According to most heads of mission of Action Against Hunger, the difficulty lies not so much in defining procedures as in ensuring their acceptance and implementation by the team as a whole. The notion of security must be integrated at all levels of operation. The definition of programs and communication policies, greater awareness of individual conduct, and assurance that operations are conducted with respect for the local culture are elements that should underpin a comprehensive security strategy.

This approach must be promoted and encouraged by working within each organization but also by inter–NGO projects designed to approach these problems in a rational way.

Today, only a few initiatives seek to promote the integrated management of security within NGOs. The training programs proposed by InterAction, Bioforce, or RedR must be viewed in this light, and the applied research undertaken by the group Emergency Rehabilitation and Development must seek to highlight this new approach that involves analysis of particular situations. The project Humanitarian Safety and Protection Network is for the moment the only program that is directly aimed at NGOs to try to develop a comprehensive analysis of the problem based on concrete elements, the idea being to compile reports of security incidents in a computerized database and standardize them as much as possible. The data can be easily stored at the respective headquarters, which will thus retain an institutional memory. The participation of a large number of organizations in this project will make these analyses more meaningful, thanks to a relatively standardized exchange of data and agreement on the conclusions thus elaborated.

All of these projects are aimed at assisting organizations to better plan their security management arrangements. They do not propose rigid and theoretical frameworks but try rather to promote a collective dynamic. These initiatives are substitutes neither for familiarity with the situation on the ground nor for the observance of procedures. Rather, they form part of a broader and more interactive security management system.

The security of humanitarian relief personnel today is a collective challenge, which is causing humanitarian organizations to question their very principles of operation. This challenge can be met only if each organization and each individual assumes full and complete responsibility.

Notes

Pierre Gallien is director of the Humanitarian Safety and Protection Network project.

1. Action Against Hunger participates in the Humanitarian Safety and Protection Network. It seeks to improve and standardize the compilation and storage of information related to security incidents with a view to more effective analysis.

2. Missions that are managed by the Paris office account for nearly two-thirds of all the organization's activities.

3. Béatrice Hibou, *Retreat or Re-Deployment of the State?* (n.p., 1999).

4. Roland Marchal, *Mogadiscio entre ruine et globalisation* (n.p., 1999).

21

Humanitarianism and the International Criminal Justice System: Abandoning Neutrality and Impartiality?

Carole Dubrulle

Over the past year, states have made considerable progress in advancing the notion of international criminal justice. The driving force behind these advances has often been pressure from nongovernmental organizations (NGOs) and civic movements. NGOs have also become involved in the functioning of international judicial bodies, following the example of recent experiences during the Kosovo crisis, when NGOs compiled testimony for forwarding to the International Criminal Court on the former Yugoslavia. Are such activities relevant and desirable for humanitarian organizations?

Historic Indictments for an Emerging System of Justice

The 1949 Geneva Conventions, whose fiftieth anniversary was commemorated in 1999, offered considerable hope that the words "never again!" would be given true meaning. Indeed, they established what is known as the principle of universal jurisdiction, by requiring states to seek out, arrest, and try the authors of serious violations of the conventions, wherever they may be and whatever their nationality. "To respect and to ensure respect for the present Convention in all circumstances" is the provision common to article 1 of all four conventions, which have been ratified by 188 states (in other words, by nearly all members of the international community).

However, states have always shown a marked disinclination to implement that provision, as they have been inclined to ignore all the coercive or simply investigatory mechanisms, which have sometimes accompanied later and more specific international legal instruments. By way of example, so far no action has ever been started before the International Fact-Finding Commission established in 1977 under Additional Protocol I to the Geneva Agreements.

In July 1998 the principle of a permanent International Criminal Court (ICC) to try the authors of crimes of war, crimes against humanity, and crimes of genocide was adopted in Rome, by 120 states. Numerous political obstacles have severely reduced the truly universal and independent competence that many, including NGOs, would like to see attributed to the court. Nevertheless, the establishment of this court marks a step forward in the campaign to establish an international criminal justice system, following the precedents of the Nürnberg and Tokyo military tribunals and the two ad hoc international criminal courts for Rwanda and the former Yugoslavia, which have recently handed down their first convictions.

As if the early prospect of an effective international criminal court had given the starting signal, extraordinary initiatives in the field of international justice have become the focus of media attention.

The first such case was that of the proceedings initiated by Judge Baltasar Garzon in Spain against General Augusto Pinochet of Chile, who was arrested in London on 16 October 1998 while on a private visit to England.[1] The Spanish magistrates claimed the right to try Pinochet in Spain for the torture inflicted on his opponents and requested his extradition on those grounds. After a series of rulings and reversals, including the historic ruling on 25 November 1998 not to recognize Pinochet's diplomatic immunity, the seven judges of the Chamber of Lords of the United Kingdom confirmed that ruling on 24 March 1999. Pinochet had enjoyed that immunity for over twenty years under an amnesty law voted upon at his initiative in Chile in 1978 and as a result of his obtaining in March 1998 the status of senator for life.

This ruling against a retired head of state could not but encourage other similar demands, such as for the arrest of Suharto, who had ruled Indonesia for more than thirty years.

Of even greater significance, however, was the indictment on 26 May 1999 for the first time of a sitting head of state. On that day, Louise Arbour, the prosecutor of the International Criminal Court for the former Yugoslavia, issued a warrant for the arrest of Slobodan Milosevic, president of the Federal Republic of Yugoslavia. The "recidivist of the Balkans" can no longer leave the territory of

Yugoslavia without risking arrest. It has taken ten years for the promoter of one of the most repugnant ideologies, which has several times been translated into deeds, to at last be officially designated as what he is alleged to be, namely, a criminal.

The rapid progress toward the establishment of an international criminal justice system has produced a sort of euphoria, with numerous scenarios that not long ago appeared improbable or even impossible now becoming achievable: Castro? Kabila? The Kurds? Tibet? And why not an international criminal court for Sierra Leone? And for Cambodia, to try the leaders of the Khmer Rouge, who were responsible for the mass killings that took place in that country between 1975 and 1979? The latter scenario is closest to being realized but is currently the subject of complicated negotiations between Hun Sen, the present prime minister of Cambodia, and Kofi Annan, secretary general of the UN. Halfway between "international" and "national" is the alternative concept of a criminal court "of an international character" for Cambodia, which would consist of foreign judges and prosecutors operating within a Cambodian court.

The purpose of an international criminal justice system is to compensate for the absence of a national response: When a state cannot or will not prosecute human rights violations committed on its territory, it is for the international justice system (this is the meaning of the principle of subsidiarity in the future international criminal court) or for a foreign court (in the Pinochet case) to take over. Fortunately, however, there are examples in which victim states dare to take direct charge of the confrontation with their history, and these amount to victories in the fight against impunity. South Africa established a Truth and Reconciliation Commission in December 1995 to shed light on the crimes of the apartheid regime that held power from 1948 to 1994. The commission, chaired by Archbishop Desmond Tutu, published its report on 30 October 1998. After ruling on whether or not a number of cases were deserving of amnesty, it handed over its cases to the South African justice system, which is now responsible for follow-up action. In Argentina, magistrates are prosecuting the former heads of the military juntas during the period of dictatorship (1976–1983), including former president Jorge Videla, who have been accused of the kidnapping of children. This is one of the few crimes, together with economic crimes, not covered by the amnesty laws. The indictments in Argentina would have been impossible without the tenacity of the Association of Grandmothers, the grandmothers of the Plaza de Mayo, who are today internationally recognized and who in 1996 filed a complaint for the illegal appropriation of the babies of their own detained and "disappeared" children. This tenacity illustrates the involvement and key role often played by civil society in influencing governments, which alone decide on the policies of national institutions.

Citizens' Groups

In France, Action Against Hunger joined the French Coalition for the International Criminal Court (ICC) and the group Article Premier. Article Premier is a group of organizations engaged in humanitarian activities, the defense of human rights, and the fight against social exclusion in France. It came together on the occasion of the fiftieth anniversary of the Universal Declaration of Human Rights in order to more effectively mobilize French public opinion and government authorities to ensure genuine respect for human rights in both foreign and domestic policy. In 1998, Article Premier was awarded the order of the Grand National Cause.

Accession to membership of the French Coalition for the ICC was justified by the pressing need to combat the impunity that still prevails in international relations. The emergence of an international criminal justice system as a new element in the sphere of international public relations is to the credit of states but also of citizens in a sometimes common effort to strengthen democracy. At the crossroads between human rights, human dignity, therapy, security, and the maintenance of peace, making everyone subject to the law is consistent with a certain line of political morality, and it is hoped that the treaty establishing that morality will not become yet another piece of paper. For that is precisely the weakness of international legal instruments: They proliferate but are rarely implemented.

Together with the victims, humanitarian organizations are the first witnesses of this dysfunction. It is true that civil society has succeeded over the years in organizing itself, campaigning, and gaining acceptance for its viewpoint on a number of key issues. It has done so by being on the cutting edge of international law through the establishment of new international conventions (Ottawa Convention on landmines, the Statute of the International Criminal Court). It has also used vigorous campaigns aimed either at combating processes that are underway (stopping the Multilateral Agreement on Investment [MAI]) or at the creation of new mechanisms (the introduction of the so-called Tobin tax of 0.5 or 1 percent on all capital movements to put into an international solidarity fund, which is the aim of the Association pour une Taxation des Transactions Financieres pour L'Aide aux Citoyens [ATTAC], an organization established in 1998 that has been gaining increasing international recognition). Nevertheless civil society still remains unsure as to the methods of action that should be employed downstream of international law: how to demand and monitor the full implementation of this law.

The experience of recent years shows that in order to be effective it is necessary to pool resources at both the national and international levels using the Internet, a tool that makes it possible to link and coordinate different initiatives at amazing speeds. Cooperation at certain times is also essential, however, between the public and private spheres. In order to move beyond the stage of protest and to achieve the desired goal of codification, coalitions must establish a permanent presence within international organizations and states. In the two recent examples of the Ottawa Convention and the Statute of the International Criminal Court, a parallel coalition of states referred to as "pioneers," supported in the rightness of their cause by the vigorous international campaigns conducted by NGOs, finally took up the cause and led it to a successful conclusion. These pioneer states included not only traditionally neutral states, such as Austria and Sweden, but also pillars of the North Atlantic Treaty Organization (NATO), such as Canada and Norway. It should also be noted that the Canadian Federal Parliament, together with the Finnish government, has already voted for the principle of a Tobin tax to put a brake on speculation in exchange markets.

This diverse coalition of states and NGOs has been consecrated in black and white in the text itself of the Ottawa Convention, while NGOs are involved in the regulatory functions of the state (armaments, criminal justice) and will have an active role to play in the universalization of the convention. Similarly, the statute of the ICC enjoins NGOs to participate in the functioning of the court.

Humanitarian Organizations Associated with the Proper Functioning of the International Criminal Justice System

NGOs will be one of the elements that will guarantee the relative independence of the court: The power of the prosecutor, who will have the power to initiate criminal proceedings, will in fact rely on information provided by NGOs, among others. This type of connection already exists for the two ad hoc criminal tribunals for Rwanda and the former Yugoslavia, which were established by resolutions of the United Nations Security Council.

Humanitarian organizations, because they are present in the field alongside the victims, have the capacity to sound the alarm and often assert in their statutes this role of bearing witness. But beyond the task of establishing the facts, they do not necessarily intervene in the process of identifying the authors of crimes against humanity. "Justice is rendered in the name of universal values that are non-negotiable," writes Patrick Baudouin, president of the International Federation of Human Rights Leagues, and some organizations have already established the connection between humanitarian action and justice. The fight against impunity is none other than a form of relief for victims, and the need for justice is as urgent as the need to eat or to receive medical care. Does not a human being who is hungry, beaten, or mutilated suffer both psychically and physically? And does not the therapy that seeks to repair the damage both individual and collective first require that justice be done? The notion of human dignity takes into consideration these two elements: Can one then claim to be seeking restoration while omitting to restore humankind to its full integrity?

The denial of justice is a serious affront, which can only lead to further injustices. The worsening lot of civilian populations in conflicts and the great frustration of humanitarian relief volunteers due to a feeling of powerlessness in the face of the absence or rather the nonactivation of juridical and political mechanisms to stop the spiral of violence should surely push such volunteers to ensure that legal proceedings are finally initiated against the authors of the most serious and massive crimes. Humanitarian work has but one objective: humankind. Merely by engaging in the fight for more effective justice, one finds oneself sliding into the political arena: Human rights? Rule of law? Justice? Democracy? Does not the Universal Declaration of Human Rights proclaim the freedom of mankind from "fear and want?"

Do the volunteers working on behalf of a humanitarian organization have to forget, in the name of humanitarian action, that they are also citizens and committed individuals? Will they themselves not lose a part of their own dignity by turning their backs on the need to see justice done, if their assistance is required for it to be done? Should they allow reasons of state to prevent them from denouncing obscenities, while international humanitarian law, to which they so often make reference, and more particularly the 1977 Additional Protocols to the Geneva Conventions have made states accept the notion that the offer of humanitarian and impartial aid cannot be construed as interference in an armed conflict or as a hostile act? In other words, as soon as humanitarian workers use testimony gathered from victims of discrimination for judicial purposes in a process initiated by the entities that are to establish responsibilities, as has been done during the crisis in Kosovo, do they then become the new righters of our planet's wrongs?

Consequences of the
Visibility of Humanitarian Organizations in Kosovo

Even though the war in Kosovo may have influenced the course of history, it still cannot change the meaning of words. Nevertheless, one of the consequences of this war is that it has cemented the abusive use of the term *humanitarian,* which has become fixed in people's minds as describing operations that have nothing to do with the word. The term now reinforces a customary use against which some humanitarian organizations, including Action Against Hunger, have fought. Indeed, a word used as a label seems to automatically confer respect and moral authority on anyone who places himself or herself under its banner.

Humanitarian, a term that has been truly consecrated at this end of the century, is now used to describe any event that involves a civilian population. Its highly positive connotation, associated with the idea of preserving human dignity in all circumstances, eclipses at the same time what previously was the accepted province of diplomacy, the military, development, and justice. In the wake of the "humanitarian disaster" of Kosovo, the commonplace occurrence of militarized humanitarian action or armed intervention for humanitarian ends has reached extremes. The confusion is total, the usurpation complete, while public opinion is misled about the ultimate objectives. Must we resign ourselves to this situation? "Humanitarian action has become the diplomatic form of mystification. Once private, it has become public and the unquestionable alibi of injustice," wrote Jacques Julliard in 1994, in an essay on the war in Bosnia that in a sense predicted the current crisis in Kosovo.[2]

Now this confusion is precisely the kind of juxtaposition that does not sit well with humanitarian organizations. Humanitarianism and justice must necessarily go together, and the link between the two bears testimony to this. There is no infringement of the principles here: Action and testimony are both part of the humanitarian vocation. Unfortunately, however, the Kosovo crisis and its intense media coverage have led to a kind of opportunistic shortcut that takes humanitarian organizations down a slippery slope and will lead perhaps to further confusion: Humanitarian organizations are becoming in charge of the proceedings! Because they cannot be direct witnesses to what is taking place inside Kosovo, humanitarian organizations have resorted almost avidly to gathering eyewitness accounts from refugees. Humanitarian organizations that are now unable to play their traditional roles are spurred on by encouraging pressures, notably from donors, some of whom would like to include the management of human rights within the scope of humanitarian activities; encouraged by their recent successes obtained from states in the normative field; and frustrated also after so many years of accumulation of injustice in this part of Europe. As a result they have demanded (perhaps too publicly) this new legitimacy, which is salutary in that it resembles a lifebuoy, providing for some organizations the only way to survive.

We are no longer sure whether these testimonies from refugees should serve the cause of justice—in this case the ICC for the former Yugoslavia (but if so, in order that the testimonies compiled can be used in the proceedings, there should be no publicity over them)—or serve to mobilize Western public opinion at the risk of justifying at the same time the NATO operation as a whole. Mobilizing public opinion could also mean that observers would draw and disseminate hasty conclusions, only to have those conclusions bitterly called into question, as we have seen in other crises.

Justice does not come as the automatic consequence of the sum of the injustices that are exposed. This kind of ostentatious determination to prove that the action of these new righters of wrongs, which humanitarian agencies appear to have become, is "protective" does not necessarily further the cause of justice: justice here today maybe, but what about justice elsewhere tomorrow?

Let there be no mistake about it: Action Against Hunger has also engaged in collecting testimony to try to understand what has happened inside Kosovo, to listen to what some, including Kosovar staff members of Action Against Hunger in Macedonia and Albania, had enough trust to share with us. "Charity without justice is fraudulent," Jacques Julliard further noted in *Ce fascisme qui vient*. Yes, and NGOs are the first to proclaim this quasi-political form of commitment. But we must be careful lest this role of bearing witness (quite imprudent in its visibility) produces a boomerang effect in the long term and in situations in which we will no longer be on the same side as the party with the most firepower. This boomerang effect might be the opposite of what we seek to achieve; in other words, it might bring about denial of access to victims. Indeed, Kosovo is the exception that proves the rule: In most contemporary conflicts there is no political will either to oppose a process that is underway or to relieve the suffering of victims. In certain cases, NGOs are the last ones to remain in the field, after the diplomats and United Nations personnel have been evacuated. It is in such situations that the witness of humanitarian workers becomes vital and a crucial change of direction to be negotiated for NGOs with regard to the role they can henceforth play in the field of international criminal justice.

Indeed, an additional though secondary judicial element may have changed the equation. The various elements must be put in their correct places: It is not the testimony of expatriates that will be useful in a criminal court but rather the testimony of victims as gathered by expatriates who are in no way in charge of the inquiry and are no substitutes for the courts' investigators. And, above all, humanitarian agencies take no position whatsoever on the personal responsibility of the alleged authors of the atrocities. When NGOs are themselves required to denounce situations of violations of the law in their areas of operation, they are going much further than they would have by merely collecting testimony for the ICC for the former Yugoslavia.

On the other hand, this method may have consequences for the perception of others of what is being done. Indeed, the present order may be affected if excessive media coverage tends to present humanitarian workers as modern day "white knights" and creates new confusion, since the association between NGOs and the defense of human rights would necessarily lie at the end of the road. Even if a measure of complementarity does indeed exist and needs to be further refined, it does not amount to a total identification of one with the other.

There has in fact been no fundamental change, since, in principle, humanitarian workers by their very presence are ultimately undesirable witnesses. This is so because witnessing is an inherent part of their mission. Everything will therefore hinge on how to adapt their discourse and translate it at the operational level, which at the moment often wavers between assistance and protection without genuinely wishing to closely scrutinize what the term *protection* actually covers.

Neutrality and Impartiality:
Relevant Criteria for Humanitarian Action?

How a relief organization is granted the status of "humanitarian" is defined in international humanitarian law.[3] An organization is humanitarian if it seeks, with complete impartiality, to relieve human suffering. The humanitarian protection provided to victims has first a quantifiable aspect: assistance to enable survival in a desperate situation, for example, temporary refuge for a refugee or access to food and to care for noncombatants during periods of conflict; it has second a legal aspect that derives from legal provisions that grant rights to specific groups: refugees, noncombatants, and so on.

Impartiality is the real Hippocratic oath of a humanitarian organization. This is an operational principle that seeks to match relief to need, in situations in which available resources are always limited. Impartiality finds expression in a rule of distribution that is proportional to needs and their urgency, established according to a standard analytical grid. Providing assistance to populations (and not to governments or heads of factions, of course) on both sides of a front line does not mean mathematical equality. The "beneficiaries" are identifiable from evaluations that are objective and not imposed by governments. Impartiality is therefore assured by the principle of nondiscrimination, and it is for states to guarantee these humanitarian principles, in other words, to guarantee the implementation of the Geneva Conventions. In practice, NGOs are subjected daily to pressures and other tensions that violate with complete impunity these principles and reduce even further the protection given to the victim populations.

The tools used for the analysis of needs are themselves objective, and an information grid for collecting testimony is not different from a food security questionnaire. Impartiality will consist in having conducted evaluations with the same analytic grid and the same methods on both sides (Serbs and Albanians, for example).

Neutrality is not prescribed by international humanitarian law but is set out instead in the charters of numerous humanitarian organizations. It characterizes organizations that claim neither political color nor religious membership. It also has an operational and security objective: In the Geneva Conventions, security must be provided for persons and property on humanitarian missions as well as for victims. Neutrality is also necessary for the International Committee of the Red Cross for its mediation activities.

This therefore is the definition of neutrality for a humanitarian organization. Indeed, since the vocation of NGOs is to bear witness, denouncing atrocities against protected groups amounts to the same thing as accusing the party that commits the atrocity. In Rwanda, Tutsis have been the victims of a genocide. In Kosovo, Albanians have been the victims of a policy of ethnic cleansing. In Burma, the Rohingyas are condemned to forced labor, prohibition from traveling, and various other forms of discrimination. We can therefore cite countless examples on which NGOs have widely reported. Neutrality pure and simple, which consists in remaining silent about a crime being committed, would amount to connivance with the oppressor, to being an accomplice to the injustice committed. Bearing witness is thus also a form of assistance to populations. Publicizing their fate can also be a means of relieving their suffering, by drawing attention to the violations of rights of which they are the victims. The debate over whether testimony is irreconcilable with access to victims is an old one, which sometimes poses intractable dilemmas within humanitarian organizations. Particularly so as this type of debate inevitably focuses on the security of humanitarian personnel on mission in the field and on the situation of the victim populations. Our presence in the field is thus in itself a form of protection, and yet, in the absence of any means of coercion inherent in the term *protect,* we must accept with all the required humility our status as "disposable" humanitarian workers. But this is not the only form of protection: Bearing witness in order to more effectively prevent crises, by resolutely refusing to let humanitarianism be used merely as dressing for gaping wounds and sometimes to complete the dirty work in situations of an unacceptable status quo, illustrates our vocation to never remain neutral in the face of violations, especially when these are massive violations of human rights.

Notes

Carole Dubrulle is head of the Human Rights Project of Action Against Hunger in France.

    1. A very similar case arose recently (6 July 2000) when the Belgian authorities issued a warrant against the foreign minister of the Democratic Republic of Congo, Abolulaye Yerodia, indicting him for crimes under international law. If the minister travels abroad, he could be arrested, and Belgium will request his extradition.

    2. Jacques Julliard, *Ce fascisme qui vient* (Paris: Seuil, 1994). Jacques Julliard is a member of the board of directors of Action Against Hunger in France.

    3. The argument in the section that follows is taken from Gaelle Fedida, "Emergency Humanitarian NGOs, New Subjects of International Law?" (doctor of law thesis, University of Paris X–Nanterre, 1998, under the supervision of Emmanuel Decaux). Fedida was formerly Action Against Hunger head of the mission in Pristina, Kosovo.

22

Combating Man-Made Famine: Legal Instruments

Marie-Josée Domestici-Met

As I have written earlier,[1] positive law does not at present guarantee any legally enforceable right to food; the primary legal instrument remains the objective obligation to act against hunger used as weapon. That instrument applies to everyone in positions of power—the power to make decisions, control information, or exert pressure in a given situation.

Efforts are now underway to perfect legal instruments. Strenuous efforts are being made to secure the recognition of a universal right to food, and a code of conduct is emerging. Furthermore, the instrument of positive law that we already have for situations in which hunger is used as a weapon seems to be gaining in legal importance.

Recognition of a Universal Right to Food

Studies on this subject are based on article 11 of the International Covenant on Economic, Social, and Cultural Rights, which proclaims "the right of everyone to an adequate standard of living for himself and his family, including adequate food, clothing and housing" and recognizes in paragraph 2 "the fundamental right of everyone to be free from hunger."

This article has become part of positive law, since the covenant has been ratified by a large number of states. It has more programmatic than operational significance, as indicated in the language of article 2: "Each State Party to the present Covenant undertakes to take steps ... to the maximum of its available resources, with a view to achieving progressively the full realization of the rights recognized in the present Covenant."

Even though we no longer believe that only states that have reached a certain level of development should be bound by these obligations and even though the obligation to act arises immediately, its tangible results cannot be felt until after a long period of work.[2] Article 11(2) cited above concludes, moreover, with reference to the adoption of "specific programs."

While the United Nations' bodies charged with promoting economic and social progress have made considerable efforts to refine the concept, the synergy being witnessed today transcends this framework and draws in civil society. This is, of course, a very encouraging sign, even if a number of legal problems still remain to be resolved.

Concerted Efforts to Develop a Code of Conduct

The World Food Conference convened in 1974 resulted in the adoption of a universal declaration on the eradication of all forms of malnutrition. Since then, numerous official documents have deplored the persistence of hunger and malnutrition and insisted on the need for "adequate food."[3]

But a difference in ideological approach has characterized this emerging synergy. One approach sought to make the right to adequate food an enforceable human right that, when not respected, gives rise to an obligation to compensate. In 1987, a Special Rapporteur of the Subcommission on Prevention of Discrimination and Protection of Minorities tried this new approach. The Committee on Economic, Social, and Cultural Rights was also created in 1987.

The other approach, which was officially adopted by the World Food Summit held in Rome in 1996, was geared to needs rather than rights. Its perspective was long term and its content more programmatic than decision driven: Its goal was to reduce by the year 2015 the number of malnourished people to 50 percent of what it had been in 1996. It is a specific, material objective, and any criticism for failing to achieve it would be unjustified. Nevertheless, the Plan of Action adopted at the Rome Summit on 17 November, with its Declaration on World Food Security, consists of seven commitments, some of which include a number of objectives. The one that most directly concerns our subject is Objective 7.4, which invites the High Commissioner for Human Rights, in collaboration with the specialized agencies, the United Nations programs, and various intergovernmental mechanisms, to better define the right to food set out in article 11 of the covenant.

Concurrently with the World Food Summit, a meeting of NGOs was held at which the most active representatives debated the fundamental question of a global approach, that is, need versus right.[4] As a result of these extremely productive discussions, groups of NGOs opted for a position based on the "human rights" approach.[5] The Food First Information and Action Network (FIAN) was the strongest advocate of this approach. In September 1997, together with the International Human Rights Organization for the Right to Feed Oneself, the World Alliance for Nutrition and Human Rights, and Il'Istituto Internazionale Jacques Maritain, FIAN established a Code of Conduct for the human right to adequate food.

The NGOs that had opted for this approach participated in the follow-up process organized by the High Commissioner for Human Rights. While this process was taking place, the Commission for Human Rights had also advanced the notion of the "right to food." At its fifty-third session, it adopted resolution 1997/8, which reaffirmed that hunger was a violation of human dignity, and pledged to work for a better definition of the right. The topic remained on its agenda. In 1998, the United Nations High Commissioner for Human Rights submitted a comprehensive report to the Commission for Human Rights, which highlighted the following points:

1. While clear rules have been established as regards the meaning of civil and political rights, the meaning of economic, social, and cultural rights remains vague (point 10);
2. A "human rights" approach should be adopted defining responsibilities and legal remedies—or rights of substitution—in case of violation (point 11);
3. However, switching from a "needs" approach to a "rights" approach cannot be done from one day to the next.

Many issues therefore remain to be resolved.

Remaining Problems

A quotation from the High Commissioner for Human Rights is indicative of the incomplete nature of the project: "The right of a person to adequate food is firmly established in international law, but its operational content and its methods of application are universally misunderstood."

The work that remains concerns mainly the definition of (1) a precise content, without which the "right to assistance" has no normative value, and (2) specific obligors charged with specific obligations, without which the "right" in question has no legal value.

The Problem of Content

The notion of a right to adequate food is beginning to emerge. But what does adequate food consist of? Is it sufficient food? Food that is free of harmful substances, that is culturally acceptable, that satisfies a person's nutritional and dietary needs? These formulations appear in the Code of Conduct of FIAN, which acknowledges that it offers only general principles and guidelines for the enforcement of this right.

The Problem of the Obligor

A general consensus seems to have emerged that each state will have obligations toward its own population; there is general reluctance to provide for any commitment toward the population of a third country. But what is the nature of these obligations?

The Problem of the Specific Obligations of Obligors

Obligations derived from the International Covenant on Economic, Social, and Cultural Rights are grouped in United Nations documents into four categories, which the FIAN Code of Conduct attempts to clarify:[6]

Obligation to respect.   This is the passive obligation to take no action that violates the right of citizens to food. Article 6 of the FIAN code lists various specific rights that must be respected: physical and economic access to food, ancestral rights to land, and the right of women to breast-feed their babies for at least six months. These are very specific obligations, which would make certain practices punishable if the code became positive law.

Obligation to protect.   This is an obligation of jurisdictional protection against any kind of violation (including violations committed by private persons) and specific provisions for protection against public disturbances (for example, looting, which violates the right to property).

Obligation to promote.   This obligation refers to the enactment of new internal legislative provisions and establishment of new institutions whose purpose is to facilitate access to food and to promote human rights from the perspective of the right to food.

Obligation to ensure enjoyment of the right. This obligation does not necessarily fall upon the moral person of the state, contrary to the belief popular in the 1970s. It is now acknowledged that the right to food is facilitated through the improvement of general conditions under which the right to food could be effectively enjoyed. This is what the report of the High Commissioner for Human Rights termed the "obligation of results," a formula that has been criticized by French jurists.[7]

In the FIAN Code of Conduct, however, it is no longer a question of the right to food in general but the fight against hunger's being used as a weapon, and here the formulation is less bold: Food "should not be used as an instrument of political and economic pressure" (article 5.5). But man-made, deliberate famine is an easily identifiable practice, and the guilty parties could be easily denounced. The answer then is not the Code of Conduct, which is not prescriptive enough. Other approaches must be used to combat this scourge.

A Growing Place in the Juridical Order for the Objective Obligation to Fight Against Man-Made Hunger

In *Geopolitics of Hunger, 1998–1999,* we discussed the legal foundations of this obligation on the part of states, notably by demonstrating how the peremptory norms that guarantee the right to life, physical integrity, and a minimum of dignity include, among their guarantee mechanisms, the mechanism of objective obligation. Whether or not this is explicitly stated—Article 1 of the Geneva Conventions[8]—the obligation to work for the protection of human rights is intrinsically linked to the question. We also cited some examples of actions that could fulfill the objective obligation, either through material assistance, multilateral or bilateral diplomacy, or media intervention.[9]

The Geopolitics of Hunger, 2000–2001 emphasizes two strategies that exemplify recent international efforts toward the realization of objective obligations. The first concerns a modality of action that evokes the objective obligation but not specifically the problem of hunger. The second is more closely related to the problem of hunger but in the very specific context of man-made hunger justified by law. In the first case, we cite the conflict in Kosovo; in the second, the economic sanctions imposed in the name of peacekeeping.

Objective Obligation and Force

Recent events lead us to question the possibility of enforcing—*manu militari*—an objective obligation. Whatever the debates over the operation of the Allied Forces in Kosovo and the methods employed—or more precisely, the nonobservance of the procedures of the United Nations, officially the only ones authorized for coercive action for the past fifty years—the operation creates a major precedent for continued humanitarian intervention in contemporary international society. This technique was widely used in the nineteenth century and the first half of the twentieth century. In the era of institutions into which international society entered following the United Nations Conference on International Organization in San Francisco in 1945, only a few sporadic episodes—Stanleyville-Paulis, Entebbe, and Kolwesi—could be cited in favor of such a technique. And many observers viewed these episodes merely as operations to extract the nationals of the power taking the action, although this view may be disputed.

Even if the precedent of Kosovo is far from enjoying a unanimous *opinio juris*, it at least revives the idea that absolute necessity may prevail over the observance of procedures.[10] And if the major powers and a part of public opinion are of the view that the prompt use of force was justified by the need to enforce respect for the rights of minorities, it would not seem out of place to advocate use of the same procedure to put an end to an ongoing situation of famine.

Objective Obligation and the
Legal Challenge to Economic Sanctions

The problem of man-made famine imposed in the name of "peacekeeping," that is, economic sanctions, is now of major concern. Although Article 41 of the United Nations Charter was included in the hope of maintaining peace at less human cost than by force of arms, we now know that its application over a long period leads to scarcity. An embargo, even in its "selective" form, seriously affects the health status of civilians. The case of Iraq is particularly illustrative, perhaps to be followed by that of Serbia.

Legal research addresses this problem with abundant caution, given that the cause of man-made hunger is not—exceptionally in this case—a violation of international law. Instead, it is a norm that supposedly maintains the higher values of international law.

Mention is made in particular of the colloquium organized in Geneva, from 23 to 25 June 1999, by the Institut Universitaire des Hautes Etudes Internationales. The colloquium subjected these sanctions to a four-point test of their legality, that is, through the prism of humanitarian law, human rights, the United Nations Charter itself, and the mandates that protect individual rights—whether under multilateral agreements or through unilateral decisions—that might be invoked to oppose the implementation of a Security Council decision. The exercise was dominated not only by the idea of a hierarchy of norms but also by the application of the specificity of "moral persons." In light of these findings, the specialized agencies of the United Nations would not have competence to agree to abide by decisions taken by the Security Council to impose sanctions. The objective obligation would dictate here a certain form of constructive disobedience.

Thus we now find coexisting around the legal problems associated with food, a certain militancy in favor of a universal right to food and a carefully constructed legal argument in favor of an objective obligation to act against man-made hunger. The first battle is already won: Hunger is no longer the "banal tragedy" denounced by Sylvie Brunel.[11]

Notes

Marie-Josée Domestici-Met is professor of international law at the Faculty of Law and Political Science of the University of Aix-Marseille III, director of the Diplome d'Etudes Superieures et Scientifiques (DESS) "International Humanitarian Aid Emergencies and Rehabilitation," and director of the diploma of international law (field studies).

1. Marie-Josée Domestici-Met, "Against the Use of Hunger as a Weapon—Legal Instruments," *Geopolitics of Hunger 1998–1999* (Paris: PUF, 1998), pp. 137–154.

2. The idea that human rights were a luxury that could be demanded only of the developed states is no longer defended officially, even among the least developed states. The Limburg principles adopted by a group of experts at Maastricht in 1986 interpret article 2 to mean that all states that are parties, whatever their level of economic development, have an obligation to ensure that every one enjoys the right to a minimum level of subsistence.

3. There have been specific declarations on the handicapped (1975), the prohibition of all forms of discrimination against women (1979), and the right to development. Also addressing this issue have been the final acts of the Conference of Vienna on Human Rights (1993), the Conference of

Copenhagen on Social Development and the Conference of Beijing on Women (1995), and finally the Convention on the Rights of the Child (1985) and the International Labor Organization (ILO) Convention No. 169 on the employment of indigenous peoples.

4. Nearly one thousand organizations from eighty countries participated in the meeting. Among the most active, mention should be made of the Jacques Maritain Institute, the South African Rights Commission, and the International Council of Jewish Women.

5. Food First Information and Action Network, the World Alliance for Nutrition and Human Rights, and the Global Forum on Sustainable Food and Nutrition Security were involved. These organizations sometimes assist the Committee on Economic, Social, and Cultural Rights and submit communications on violations of the "right to adequate food."

6. Cf. "Committee on Economic, Social and Cultural Rights," Information Bulletin No. 16, distributed during the United Nations World Public Information Campaign on Human Rights, p. 9.

7. The reference to the "obligation of results" is in Item 5 on the agenda of the commission on Human Rights, 15 January 1998 (Doc. E/CN.4/1998/21, p. 4, §15). The formula has been criticized even though this formulation also appears in the French version of documents of the same type (cf. "Committee on Economic, Social and Cultural Rights," Information Bulletin No. 16, distributed during the United Nations World Public Information Campaign on Human Rights, p. 9). It must be noted that this is not the obligation of result that is established in French law, that is to say, the obligation to obtain a certain result from a given activity in time and in space. Here, it is rather a "finality," as stated in the above-mentioned Information Bulletin No. 16, which draws a distinction between obligations "of conduct" (action or inaction) and obligations "of result" (finality). In the French law of obligations, the finality does not serve to categorize obligations, but rather causes them. Consequently, under this law, obligations of result would be classified under obligations of conduct and would form a particularly demanding category: obligations whose discharge must absolutely result in a specified outcome.

8. States have an obligation to respect and to ensure respect for humanitarian law in all circumstances.

9. Material assistance is that in the form of delivery of foodstuffs. Diplomacy can consist of submissions to the Security Council and submissions to the various oversight bodies: Commission on Human Rights; Committee on Economic, Social, and Cultural Rights; and (why not) the Committee Against Torture, since the infliction of a state of hunger may be considered to be ill treatment. Media intervention can take the form of public campaigns to denounce violations, which may have a powerful effect. Public opinion in Western states, alerted by the press, "decided" in the case of Biafra that, while a government may lawfully put down an attempt at secession, it cannot do so by using famine as a weapon. Under that pressure, the federal government of Nigeria lifted the embargo against deliveries of food.

10. In other words, it strengthens the belief that the precedent of Kosovo is indeed the application of international law, or—to use a formulation that is less typical in legal parlance—a sort of acquiescence to its lawfulness.

11. Brunel, Sylvie, *Une tragédie banalisée, La faim dans le monde* (Paris: Hachette Pluriel, 1991).

23

Why Embargoes?

Romain Coti and Anne-Laure Wipff

Embargoes are ineffective, supporting instead of weakening the very regimes they target.[1] But it is easy to see how embargoes allow the nations that impose them to maintain the illusion that they are taking action against criminal regimes.

Recognized as an international sanction by Article 41 of the United Nations Charter, the embargo is an old technique of reprisal that seems relatively simple to apply. The nation imposing the embargo prohibits imports into its territory from the country whose government it wishes to sanction and even prohibits exports from its own enterprises to the country in question. The flaw in the plan is evident in the very essence of an embargo: It has a political objective, namely, to influence a government or to instigate the fall of a regime, but uses economic constraints. This fundamental distinction between the end pursued and the means employed undermines the legitimacy of this instrument as an effective tool.

It should be noted that none of the United Nations Security Council embargoes—against Haiti, Iraq, Libya, and the former Yugoslavia—have achieved their goals. All of the regimes in those countries have remained in power and in some cases have even strengthened their grip on civil society. In seeking to understand the justification for and results of sanctions, we must first question the embargo's effectiveness as a tool for resolving conflicts and ask what real purpose it serves for those countries that choose to use it.

In order to clarify the issues in this debate, we will examine how the embargo has been used in real situations and demonstrate how this sanction, which is coming under increasing criticism, has been searching for new legitimacy in recent years.

Limited Effectiveness

The desired effect of an embargo is to force a government to change its policies under pressure from the population or to destabilize the regime in power. This ideal and democratic concept of how an embargo should function often turns out to be quite naive because the regimes chosen for destabilization are nearly always strong. Two conditions are necessary in order for the population to play its expected role: First, the regime has to be responsive to popular opinion and concerned about the fate of the population; second, citizens must have the ability to demonstrate their discontent. Furthermore, the economic environment determines the degree of effectiveness of sanctions as a function of three parameters: (1) the degree of dependence on the outside world, (2) the weight of the state—a state that is heavily involved in the country's economy would manage the scarcity of resources more successfully—and (3) the key resources under government control.

But even when all of these internal factors—these conditions and parameters—are present, there is no guarantee that an embargo would succeed; there are additional circumstances that nations imposing the embargo cannot ignore. During the first embargo against Iraq, Jordan did not agree to join the coalition, and its deliveries greatly diminished the effectiveness of the sanctions. It is clear that, in order for an embargo to be successful, a united political commitment is required.

Nor must we forget the economic impact of the embargo on the nations imposing it. In order to preserve the political coalition and discourage contraband activities, this economic impact should not be too severe. The high volume of illegal exports from the Dominican Republic to Haiti during the 1991–1994 embargo against Haiti is hardly surprising when one considers the degree to which these two economies are interdependent. Moreover, the embargo on Iraqi oil would have been impossible to enforce if world supplies had not been plentiful. In 1990, Saudi Arabia, under financial pressure from foreign debt, was producing oil at maximum capacity. Such an embargo would have been unimaginable in 1980. Favorable economic conditions are therefore a requirement if an embargo is to be strategically effective.

Ineffectiveness and Negative Effects

An embargo can have many unwanted side effects that cannot be easily dismissed as "collateral damage," since they fundamentally undermine the effectiveness of the sanctions.

The political pressure that results from the economic hardship in the target country depends on two factors that are difficult to control: public opinion and the duration of the embargo.

Hopes of a popular revolt are often thwarted by the turn of events. In a disrupted economy dominated by criminals and the black market, civil society is also destabilized. Under these conditions, the regime frequently regains some degree of legitimacy. As the only stable authority in an otherwise chaotic situation, the regime may pose as the protector of the national identity through effective propaganda that blames the embargo for all the evils suffered by the people and cultivates the psychosis of the nation as victim. Moreover, the link between the population's discontent and its influence on the government is more tenuous in countries in which the government pursues a political objective that is unrelated to the satisfaction of the broad interests of the public. In truth, an embargo against a democracy would surely be more effective than one against an authoritarian regime. But why should anyone need to decree an embargo against a democracy?

Embargoes, moreover, often cause human suffering on a disastrous scale, exacerbating the impoverishment of the most destitute. The case of Iraq is a good example of these tragic effects: a rising infant mortality rate, a prosperous black market, and official denunciations of the embargo as responsible for the country's problems.

An embargo must be long term in order to bring about any political change. This creates further problems in terms of the cohesiveness of the nations imposing the sanctions and gives the embargoed country the time to organize its defenses. South Africa, for example, which was under an arms embargo, developed its own arms industry. Moreover, by confiscating humanitarian aid, the regime is able not only to organize corruption and thereby to attract more support but also to regulate supplies to the population. Doing so allows it to favor its supporters and punish its opponents, who have difficulty in organizing themselves for resistance, since their chief concern is to secure the means for their daily subsistence (this is the case of the Kurds today).

Alarmist humanitarian assessments could also fuel propaganda and encourage feelings of guilt among the citizens of the sanctioning countries. The continuation of the embargo therefore becomes more difficult, since the countries imposing it are usually democracies that are accountable to their citizens for their actions.

Ironically, an embargo can completely reverse the situation. Although originally it may have sent a clear message, informing the nation under sanctions that the embargo would not be lifted until it changed its policy, the embargo can become a diplomatic bargaining chip in place of the change in policy that is expected. Its lifting may be the precondition for the resumption of negotiations. The Serbs, for example, demanded a halt to the North Atlantic Treaty Organization strikes in April 1999 as a condition for the resumption of dialogue.

Despite the many factors that can cause an embargo to fail, not all embargoes are complete failures. The embargoes against Rhodesia in 1965 and against South Africa may be considered to have been relatively successful. The first softened the white authorities, while the second was a symbol of the international community's support for the black liberation movement.

A Legitimacy Called into Question

In light of the scant political results of recent embargoes and their numerous damaging effects, we should ask why Western countries have not given up the practice. The question is particularly apt since an embargo is totally unsuited to cases of imminent danger, such as Iraq and Serbia, because it is effective only in the long term. Embargoes may also be used in support of military action, as in the case of the oil embargo against Serbia. But this measure can have only limited impact if Russia continues to supply Belgrade; only a blockade, which constitutes military action, would then make any sense. Moreover, an oil embargo would deprive Montenegro of its oil resources and further weaken its government, which is doing all it can to remain out of the conflict.

If the embargoes are not really used to force certain governments to change their policies, as we were initially led to believe, then what is the point of imposing them? It is because the embargo also functions as a symbolic condemnation, an international diplomatic message. This can be seen from the recent U.S. practice that, to say the least, has been ambiguous. The United States uses the embargo to demonstrate its power in the international arena. Its use also permits the United States to test the loyalty of its European allies, which have repeatedly violated agreements by selling wheat to the USSR or supplying arms to Bosnia. A certain antagonism led to an open crisis between the European Union and the United States when the latter enacted the Helms-Burton bill in 1996, providing for penalties for companies in any country that had business relations with Cuba. This extraterritoriality of sanctions, a blatant display of power, was not acceptable to Europeans. President Clinton was inclined to forgo the application of this law, but domestic political considerations forced him to take a stronger stance than he would have preferred.

Doubt about the effectiveness of the embargo arises largely because it is used for domestic political ends, including at times to gain an advantage at election time. It is a signal aimed at domestic public opinion. In the 1980s, the public in the United States was impressed by the administration's efforts to promote democracy—that is, the embargo against South Africa—and in the 1990s it felt protected by the vigorous attempt to combat terrorism—the embargo against Libya.

These domestic policy messages offer citizens the illusion of action and effectiveness. The embargo therefore poses a real ethical problem for democracies: Can domestic policy considerations justify using an often inefficient weapon, with damaging effects as serious as the political strengthening of the target regime and as painful as the suffering of the populations of the countries under embargo?

Seeking a Clear Conscience

In order to counter this criticism, democracies have tried in recent years to take into consideration the humanitarian problems that are a consequence of embargoes by introducing the notion of the "selective embargo." The principle is simple: The embargo prohibits trading in the goods necessary for the repressive apparatus of the embargoed state while allowing trade in the supplies that are absolutely essential for the population's survival (food, medicine, clothing) or humanitarian items (minimum energy supplies, hospital equipment, and vehicles such as ambulances). This new concept was tested during the embargo against Iraq in 1990.

The idea seems simple, but its application is more difficult. The sanctions committees created to review applications to export to countries under sanctions are overwhelmed with work. They also regularly face ethical dilemmas that are difficult to resolve. During a colloquium organized by Action Against Hunger on 15 October 1996, at the Sorbonne, Mario Bettati described the case involving a shipment of anesthetic products to Iraq for cesarean operations. Such an item should not, in principle, have posed the slightest problem, but the quantity was far greater than the country's needs and the active ingredient could also have been used for making chemical weapons.

However, sanctions committees have now gained more experience in their work, and they undeniably help to make embargoes more humane and tolerable. The real problem lies elsewhere. By diminishing the population's suffering, the embargo jeopardizes the attainment of its political objective. By keeping civilians alive, it does not push them to the limit, which might lead to a popular uprising. Even more serious, in granting the regime in the embargoed country a monopoly over the distribution of basic food items, the embargo gives the regime the most reliable means of gaining the support of certain groups and of repressing its opponents, who would spend their energies in trying to survive and therefore not have the time to organize themselves for effective political opposition. The political use of food supply is well documented: It has proven its fearful power in the Ukraine (1929–1933) and in North Korea today.

If therefore embargoes are only rarely effective, how can democracies justify their use? Other than the wish to show the population that something is being done—without taking too many risks—this sanction should perhaps be seen as one more step on the ladder of dissuasion. Democracies must demonstrate that they will not stay idle when faced with the provocations of certain regimes. Embargoes offer the least costly means of taking action.

Notes

Romain Coti and Anne-Laure Wipff are students at the Institut d'Etudes Politiques de Paris in the seminar "The Geopolitics of Hunger," organized by Sylvie Brunel.

1. This text is the result of research conducted by students at the Institut d'Etudes Politiques de Paris for the seminar "The Geopolitics of Hunger," organized by Sylvie Brunel.

24

The Birth of
Responsible Humanitarianism

Sylvie Brunel

Humanitarianism triumphed in the late 1980s. Growing international cooperation and the collapse of the Berlin Wall seemed to herald a glorious future for humankind, henceforth peaceful and interdependent and thus necessarily on the path of further progress.

Ten years later, disenchantment had set in: Humanitarianism would be exploited, used as a tool, and become more harmful than useful for some—generally speaking, those who also question even the notion of development.

The turning point between these two eras can be dated precisely: The U.S. intervention in Somalia, in December 1992, which ended a few months later in a rout, in violence and chaos—from which that country still has not emerged—seemed to sound the death knell for humanitarian hopes. No, the world is not benefiting from the peace dividend. No, intervention is not putting an end to the tragedies of certain peoples. The so-called global village, far from leveling differences, is in reality widening the gap that separates nonconsumers from consumers.

Today, to cultivate hopelessness, even hatred, for humanitarianism seems to have become fashionable among those who had been its advocates (see several publications written by Rony Brauman, former president of Medecins sans Frontières). The generation that gave birth to the notion of a borderless world, that was the most enthusiastic backer of humanitarianism, even when its methods and choices were still undefined and naive, now turns its back on it and criticizes it at precisely the moment when it is beginning to play an essential role in international relations. Indeed, just when it might be said that humanitarianism is entering into responsible adulthood.

Never, in fact, has humanitarian action had so many reasons to exist. Never has it had such an important role to play. This is a time when states are in crisis. French writer Jean-François Bayart points to the extent to which they are overpowered from above, by financial transnationals and multinationals; frontally assaulted by international financial institutions with their disastrous theories of structural adjustment; and attacked from within by the rise of regionalism, demands for recognition of distinctive identities, and criminalization of the economy. This is also a time when the United Nations is being increasingly rejected as incapable of even playing its role as the "interstitial power," to use the phrase coined by Ghassan Salame, when the real powers, the United States first, but also China, decide the contrary.

The question, then, is how to counterbalance the weight of global corporations, the drive for profit, and the decisions made for the short-term financial gain of a handful of international speculators. How do we counter the appetite of dictators for power, dictators who know that they face only democracies weakened by uncertainty and indecision?

Only citizens' movements, in both the North and South, can erect effective counterbalances because they are sufficiently informed and mobilized to strengthen the capacity of the political system to resist the power of the lobbies.

Some recent examples reveal the extent to which the power of nongovernmental organizations (NGOs) has grown. Take, for example, the failure of the Multilateral Agreement on Investment (MAI); the success, rewarded by a Nobel Peace Prize, of the campaign against antipersonnel landmines; the precautions taken by the European Parliament to guard against the introduction of genetically modified organisms into the European market; the indictment of Slobodan Milosevic by the International Criminal Tribunal for the former Yugoslavia on the basis, notably, of testimony gathered by NGOs from refugees from Kosovo (for more on this subject, see Chapter 21); and the cancellation of a significant portion of the debt of the poorest countries by the Group of 8 in Cologne in June 1999 after worldwide mobilization by NGOs.

The recognition of economic, social, or environmental rights or the adoption of ethical principles in international relations concerning child labor, for example, are thus also to be credited to the untiring efforts of citizen groups.

It is because the humanitarian movement has applied to itself the same moral rigor and firmness that it had used to denounce the ills of the world that it today finds itself in the hot seat. Nonprofit groups were the first to denounce the manipulation of which they were victims and the modest results that they achieved in more difficult situations. As a result, they have been vilified by those who were waiting for an opportunity to discredit them because the militant activism of nonprofit groups thwarted their desire for conquest or power. Even worse, they have been vilified by certain militants themselves, often the most idealistic or the most radical among them. These people, having expected too much from humanitarianism, could not stand to see their dreams disappointed and thus violently rejected what they had once revered.

Yet, it is precisely the movement's capacity for self-criticism and its desire for transparency that has pushed the humanitarian movement to publicly air the problems it has encountered in order to be better able to overcome them. NGOs have seen the need for increased efficiency and monitoring through a more professional approach to their activities and also the need for standards and codes to enable them to harmonize their methods and objectives. It is in this area that most of them are focused at this very moment, precisely to be able to avoid pitfalls in the future and to better target their interventions.

Why do we seem to be discovering today something that in reality has always existed? The notion of a world without borders appeared, in fact, at the same time as it began to be manipulated. In Biafra, in the early 1970s, General Odumegwu Ojukwu deliberately kept the Ibo people in a state of famine in order to rally public opinion to his independence cause. That was when Doctors Without Borders was born.

Today, how can we deliberately forgo helping a starving child when we possess the miraculous ability to prevent his certain death by intervening in time? How can we turn our backs on populations that are victims of deliberate oppression and unbearable suffering, which are in no way attributable to fate, on the pretext that we risk being manipulated?

It is for us, NGOs, to mount our best defenses so as not to fall into the sordid and cynical trap of those who cause starvation. That is precisely what we are now seeking to do, all of us together, which is why we are the object of such virulent criticism.

The only thing that is dead, now that humanitarianism has entered into a stage of responsible maturity, is the youthful illusions:

- That it was sufficient to disembark somewhere with the halo of the aid worker's goodwill in order to be welcomed as a benefactor of humanity and also to be useful.
- That citizens could by themselves make the world better, bypassing states and politicians, all "thoroughly rotten." On the contrary, it is through the strength of citizen commitment and the translation of that commitment into political action that the nongovernmental movement can achieve lasting reforms.
- That "Western civilization" had a model of universal progress to offer the rest of the world, transforming itself into an eager propagandist for techniques that it claimed would improve the quality of life sufficiently to spread development.

To be sure, the hope of transforming the world solely by the strength of its good will, by its generosity and its "kindness," died on the beaches of Mogadishu one day in December 1992. And so much the better: It is ultimately preferable for there to be a return to realism, when the only humanitarianism that can survive is the kind that fulfils its role from within the "global society," without allowing the notion of good and evil to be used as justification for ineffectiveness.

Notes

Sylvie Brunel is strategy adviser, Action Against Hunger.

PART THREE

FOOD POLICIES
TO ERADICATE HUNGER

Humanitarian assistance alone cannot pretend to save 800 million people worldwide from malnutrition. However, the role of such assistance also encompasses proposing analysis and solutions to allow for poverty eradication and advocating for efficient food policies. These things should be done not only for North-South cooperation, but also for countries affected by this silent hunger that primarily threatens the most vulnerable segments of the population.

In this regard, food aid, the apparently obvious remedy against hunger, is far from being the best solution enabling people to feed themselves.

25

Feeding Ten Billion People?

Sylvie Brunel

The six-billionth human being was born in June 1999, demographers say. They are most probably right: Since the beginning of the 1970s, their predictions have been surprisingly correct.

The demographic curve has followed the path predicted. We were three billion in the 1960s. At the time, the population increase seemed terrifying, since every year the world population increased by 2 percent, or fifty-eight million people—the current population of France. For nearly twenty years, the world has panicked in the face of what some have not hesitated to call "proliferation." Cassandras on all sides spoke with one voice to demand vigorous birth control measures, which, however, seemed futile in most countries. Kenya became a case in point. In 1967 it became the first country in Africa to adopt a genuine family planning policy, but ten years later, it still held the African record for fertility—an average of nearly eight children for every woman.

After having decided that a rapidly increasing population was an asset for their country, many governments, frightened by the endless race between rising birthrates and declining food production and investment in the health and education sectors for which they lacked the resources, decreed and sometimes enforced a pause. In the mid-1970s, India launched a vast program for limiting births with the implementation of draconian measures, such as the forced sterilization of women, and in 1979 China adopted the so-called one-child policy. But certain societies seemed resistant: Demographers described black Africa and the Near and Middle East as "irreducible."

A generation later, the diagnosis must be revised: The most pessimistic predictions have proven themselves to be wrong. We did not know it, but the 2 percent annual growth of the 1960s represented a peak: The present increase in world population is steadily declining year after year. The drop is noticeable: It was +1.5 percent in 1995, +1.4 percent in 1998. It is true that during this interval world population has doubled: from 3 billion to 6 billion, which explains why 1.4 percent still translates into an additional 87 million human beings each year, much more than in 1960. And the world has more young people than ever: more than a billion fifteen- to twenty-four-year-olds. What is referred to as demographic momentum, that is, the high birthrate associated with this large proportion of young women of reproductive age, therefore means that population growth will remain high, even if on average each of these women has no more than three children in the course of her life, or half the number her mother brought into the world.

Of the six billion human beings on the planet, nearly five billion live in the so-called developing countries. The latter account for 90 percent of the current population increase because women in these countries still bear on average 3.5 children (compared with 1.6 in the so-called developed countries). But considerable differences separate South America and Asia, on the one hand, and Africa, on the other. In the first two continents population growth has fallen to 2.6 children per woman (although if China is subtracted from Asia, this figure climbs to 3.5); in Africa, the fertility rate is still 5.3 children per woman. And that is an essential factor: If the peak of population growth is behind us in Latin America (where it was attained in 1965–1970) and in Asia (where it was attained in 1970–1975), it is also behind us in Africa as well: On that continent too, a significant drop is today being noted in the number of children per household, particularly in urban areas, where a third of Africans now live.

Projections of population growth have therefore been revised downward: Most demographers now agree that world population will climb to 8 billion people by 2025. After that, opinions differ, depending on whether one adopts a "low" (9 billion people by 2050) or intermediate hypothesis (10 billion people, also by 2050).

Nonetheless, experts all agree on one thing: World population will stabilize at around 10 or even 11 billion people by the year 2100, but not more. The current world population of 6 billion will therefore never double.

After that, the key question is whether the earth will be able to feed these 10 or even 11 billion human beings at the end of the twenty-first century. This question leads very naturally to questions about two essential factors:

- On the one hand, does the earth have the "technical" capacity to feed these 11 billion people? What is the potential for increasing the current agricultural production? In a word, can the world feed the world?
- On the other hand, will humanity have the desire, the political will, to feed its own, all of its own? Or will the world want to feed the world?

This second question is just as legitimate as the first. Is there not a risk that there will be increasing numbers of people who will not eat when hungry, because they will no longer have access to food that has become scarce and, thus, more contested?

This concern is not new: Crises of subsistence, which have resulted in deadly famines, have punctuated the history of humanity. In 1798, Malthus wrote in his "Essay on the Principle of Population" that all populations tend naturally toward a maximum, which is determined by the level at which it can subsist. According to him, the excess can be regulated only by the mortality rate. This idea that there must necessarily be "regulators" of population growth continues to be implicitly acknowledged. In the nineteenth century, confronted by recurrent famines in India, the colonial administration concluded that it was extremely difficult, even futile, to attempt to save an entire section of the population that was composed of the most wretched individuals or those whose status placed them at the very bottom of the social ladder: These "starving sections" were in any case condemned to disappear. They, however, represented 20 percent of the Indian population at the time, or one out of five. One cannot help but notice that that is precisely the proportion of malnourished people in today's Third World.

The question may well be asked of whether there are still "starving sections" today. These would be the poorest of the poor, social misfits, those marginalized in the wave of liberalism and globalization sweeping the five continents (and particularly black Africa), a kind of surplus population, an excess that some a little too readily resign themselves to letting die of hunger. Saving them, some might feel, would place too heavy a burden on ecosystems rendered increasingly fragile as a result of demographic pressure and on non-renewable resources that are increasingly in demand.

Each human being could easily eat his or her fill if the world food production were equally distributed (enough food is available today to provide 2,700 calories per person per day). Why then does the world seem so resigned to the fact that some 800 million people in the developing countries are malnourished? During its World Summit held in Rome in November 1996, the United Nations Food and Agriculture Organization proclaimed that its goal was to cut in half the number of malnourished people over the course of the next thirty years. While this goal is laudable and will require enormous efforts to increase agricultural production and ensure better distribution of food supplies, is it not at the same time an implicit admission that there will still be 400 million people—a massive "starving section"—for whom nothing material will be done?

Chapter 26 will therefore address two fundamental issues:

1. Production and distributive capacities in the context of globalization, with special emphasis on sub-Saharan Africa.
2. Food justice and its various components: how to guarantee the right of each human being to adequate and sufficient food, a right explicitly enshrined in the Universal Declaration of Human Rights, which was fifty years old in December 1998. Article 3 of the declaration stipulates clearly that "everyone has the right to life, liberty and security of person."

Notes

Sylvie Brunel is strategy adviser, Action Against Hunger.

26

Increasing Productive Capacity: A Global Imperative

Sylvie Brunel

Can the earth feed its inhabitants? Despite the most alarmist predictions—those of Lester Brown in his State of the World published each year by the World Watch Institute of Washington; those of Paul Ehrlich, author of *The Population Bomb;* or those of the Club of Rome—there is no doubt that world food production, if equally distributed among all the world's peoples, is enough to meet the needs of them all. It is true that the increase in world agricultural production has slowed in recent years, a situation that has led to an immediate flood of alarmist predictions. The world, however, is not heading toward famine. And this is for a number of reasons.

The Increase in World Agricultural Production Continues to Outpace Population Growth

Only persons who are ill informed or of bad faith can argue that the trend is toward a decline in food production. They may even succeed in proving that claim. It is enough for them to select as the base year one in which harvests were particularly good and a second year in which they declined steeply in order to show a "disturbing" trend. Hervé Kempf demonstrated, for example, how a comparison of 1984 and 1991 would show an increase in cereal production of only 0.7 percent per year, which would be "disturbing," since it is far below the 1.7% annual rate of population increase.[1] By selecting the preceding years, one can show, on the contrary, that world agriculture has never been more productive: A comparison between 1983 and 1990 shows an increase in cereal production of 2.7 percent per year. These two statistics are clearly equally deceptive, and Joseph Klatzmann, in a refreshing little book, repeatedly warned against the danger of blindly trusting statistical data taken out of context.[2]

If we examine world agricultural production over a long period, it becomes clear that the production curve exceeds the population growth curve. While world population did indeed double in one generation, grain production increased more than threefold, from 600 million to approximately 1,900 million tons per year. Each human being has available in theory 20 percent more food than in the early 1970s, or 2,700 calories per person per day, which is far more than a person's estimated need of between 2,000 and 2,200 calories, depending on the sources. However, half of the current grain production does not directly benefit people: Approximately 20 percent is used to feed cattle, 5 percent is kept for seeds, and the remaining 25 percent is quite simply lost as a result of poor storage or destruction by rodents, insects, and so on, especially in developing countries. It is therefore not the impossibility of increasing agricultural production that threatens mankind, but rather the way in which this increase is achieved and for the benefit of whom.

Indeed, it is in fact not in the countries of the so-called Third World but rather in the developed countries that agricultural production has slowed, in other words precisely where the problems of hunger have been overcome. (At least they have been overcome in quantitative terms; in qualitative terms, obesity, on the one hand, and malnutrition caused by the economic and social marginalization of certain categories of persons, on the other, have become real societal problems.) The developed countries have chosen to voluntarily limit their agricultural production in order to adapt it to the level of demand at which production would be profitable, in other words, to the consumer market. The fact that there are some 800 million people suffering from malnutrition in the world in no way changes this calculation, since those persons are too poor to buy food.

The reduction or slowdown in the rate of increase in world food production is thus attributable mainly to the developed countries, for reasons that have nothing to do with ecological limitations. Pierre Le Roy estimates at 20 million tons the reduction in supply that results from Europe's policy of limitation of production (land left fallow), an amount that represents twice the total of all food imports by sub-Saharan Africa.[3]

Food imports by the Third World are indeed increasing, rising from 20 million tons in 1960, or 2 percent of consumption, to 120 million tons in the mid 1990s, or 20 percent of consumption. Economic forecasts suggest that this dependency is likely to increase even further in the decades ahead and to rise to 160 million tons within two decades. The reasons for this growing dependence, which will create problems without precedent for the economies of poor countries that will face increasingly onerous food import bills, are both negative and positive.

The negative factor of continuing population growth and spreading urbanization in the countries of the South, where nearly half the population now lives in cities, explains why more and more people are consuming food that their farmers are incapable of providing. The positive factor of the increase in average living standards in the developing countries and the emergence of a middle class that consumes more meat and dairy products places increasing pressure on the demand for cereals, in particular secondary cereals for stock feed.

Two-Speed Agricultural Policies

Why cannot the Third World feed itself, even though self-sufficiency in food was the grand slogan of the 1970s and 1980s?

The "technical" impossibility of increasing agricultural production in the South is not the problem: The earth is far from reaching its maximum agricultural potential, and the Food and Agriculture Organization (FAO) has pointed out that the useful agricultural surface in developing countries (700 million hectares) could be doubled without encroaching on protected areas such as forests or areas in which people live. Latin America and Africa hold the greatest potential in this regard. In addition, the potential for increased production through more intensive farming methods remains considerable. Only 11 kilograms of fertilizer are used per hectare in Africa, compared with 66 kilograms in Latin America and 139 kilograms in Asia, and only 5 percent of land is irrigated in Africa (most of this in countries that are unable to take advantage of it, such as Sudan and Madagascar), compared to 37 percent in Asia and 14 percent in Latin America. This situation offers tremendous potential for growth.

But the political and economic choices made by the countries of the Third World have thus far been detrimental to agriculture, and in particular to small peasant farming. Investments in agriculture have been concentrated in regions in which purchasing power is greatest and are characterized by a concern to protect the income of farmers, which has been steadily declining. As a result, these investments are moving in the direction of a two-tiered world that is becoming increasingly unequal in terms of access to food.

On one hand, the developed countries enjoy rapid growth, and despite the fact that farmers represent on average no more than 3 percent of the active population, their food supply is abundant and diversified, prices are low, and import levels are low as a result of the massive support given to the agricultural sector (in the mid-1990s, Organization for Economic Cooperation and Development (OECD) countries each year spent more than two hundred billion dollars to support their agricultural sectors). In that part of the world, the concern is no longer the fear of shortage, but rather the quality of the food consumed. The agrofood industry, now powerful after being forced to steadily increase its output over the past decades in order to keep up with the steadily rising demand, is today facing another challenge, namely, shifting to production methods that focus less on quantity and more on the quality of the inputs used and on the quality of the final product. Producers are also concerned about the methods used to satisfy the demand of consumers, who now want food that is not only abundant but also varied and, above all, healthy. The successive scandals of mad-cow disease, salmonella poisoning in chickens, hormone-treated beef cattle; the rejection by consumer groups of genetically modified plants; animal feed that includes mud from cleaning stations; and the questions raised about the production of eggs by battery hens are indicative of a new era in which insistence on quality is now a greater challenge than the demand for quantity.

On the other side are the poor and vulnerable countries, where malnutrition is endemic and where a majority of the population still depends on agriculture. The food supply remains insufficient, however, because of the poor yields that result from the low level of technology used, the absence of incentives to produce because of economic policies that discourage agriculture, and unfavorable exchange rates that make the importation of agricultural imports expensive. It is therefore precisely in those countries that agricultural production needs to be increased. First, increased production would reduce the cost of food, particularly in the large urban centers, and thereby make it accessible to this large sector of the population that is too poor to eat properly. Second, increased production would reduce the food import bills of countries that are increasingly dependent on imports, mainly from the rich countries.

The Food Supply Is a
Regional, Not a Global Problem

At the global level, the food supply is increasing for reasons that are both positive and negative. On the positive side, the agricultural sector in Eastern Europe, which needed to be restructured following the collapse of the Iron Curtain, is now on the road to recovery. On the negative side, the economic difficulties of East Asia have led to a decline in food imports by that region.

At the regional level, the structural overproduction that the world has been experiencing for the past twenty years hardly prevents sub-Saharan Africa and South Asia from experiencing hunger. Of the approximately 800 million malnourished people in the world, more than 200 million live in Africa (nearly 40 percent of the population) and 530 million in South Asia (or one person out of five).

What is therefore responsible for this disastrous and paradoxical situation at a time when, in order to reduce the supply of food, rich countries are destroying mountains of surplus food each year and forcing their farmers to leave a portion of their land uncultivated, through subsidies for land that is left fallow?

One answer is wars and conflicts, particularly in Africa, that disrupt agricultural production. A second, even more important answer is mass poverty, which prevents an entire sector of the world's population (one out of every five inhabitants of the Third World) from obtaining adequate food. That sector is incapable of producing enough food to meet its needs and lacks the means to purchase it, even when the food is available and can be bought. Worldwide, some 1.5 billion people live below the poverty level. Mass poverty is all the more serious, as it is always combined with ignorance: It is always the poorest classes that commit the most harmful errors of nutrition, since they lack the advantage of basic education. The errors of nutrition committed by pregnant women and children, who make up the primary groups at risk of hunger, should be the focus of particular attention, since these errors have disastrous consequences for the future of the entire society.

According to the United Nations Children's Fund (UNICEF), half of the world's malnourished children live in Asia, which has 100 million of the 200 million total, including 70 million in India. That country alone has two and a half times more malnourished children than all of sub-Saharan Africa.

Writing about South Asia in Chapter 27, Gilbert Etienne remarked on the extent to which the problem of hunger remains unresolved because of mass poverty and the slowdown in investments in agriculture. This is despite the notable progress achieved on the Asian continent.

The case of Africa gives cause for even greater concern:

1. Unlike the situation in other continents, the rate of malnutrition is not declining. Quite the opposite, in fact, because chronic malnutrition still affects nearly 40 percent of the region's population.

2. The high proportion of young people in the population, a sign of a vigorous population still characterized by high birthrates, has led to a high proportion of unemployed in relation to the number of those who are in a position to contribute to production. The burden on the economies of African countries is therefore particularly heavy, especially since most of these countries suffer from an acute lack of financial resources.

3. The continent's dependency on food from foreign countries is due to the low productivity of its own agriculture and the growing number of Africans now living in urban areas (more than one in three compared with one in ten a generation ago). This dependency is effectively addressed neither by imports (9 to 10 million tons per year), because of the lack of adequate financial resources, nor by food aid (approximately 2 million tons), which has been falling drastically for some years now. Consequently, the food needs of Africans are not being satisfied, since the widespread poverty of a sector of the urban population does not permit that sector to obtain food at market prices. At the same time many rural dwellers are unable to provide for themselves during the period between harvests, on account of the low productivity levels and inadequate access to food.

4. A large number of people in Africa are affected by war or internal conflict. Even in countries in which the population could, in theory, be properly fed, there is an adverse impact on the food situation of the population because of the insecurity of the economic actors, the weakness of the State, and the destruction or confiscation of crops. In this regard, Africa is by far the continent most affected by conflicts, which also result in massive populations of refugees and displaced persons who depend on international aid for their survival.

5. Poverty and the pressure on land and resources of the high population growth rate are not matched by corresponding investments in agriculture that would bring about increases in yields. Africa is thus the continent in which the problems of deforestation, desertification, and soil erosion are most acute. It is also the continent in which access to drinking water and irrigation is still very limited.

The situation is not desperate, however: Despite the lack of investment in small peasant farming, agricultural production in Africa has risen by 2 percent per year since the early 1960s. Grain production has more than doubled, from 30 million to 66 million tons. This rate of increase is insufficient to meet the needs of a growing population (3 percent per year) because of the way in which it has been achieved (mainly by increasing the area of land under cultivation). Nevertheless it shows that more intensive farming methods are needed in Africa and that this approach has the potential to significantly increase agricultural output. When the FAO states that the "load capacity of the land" in many countries has now been exceeded, it is basing its conclusions on the use of traditional production methods, such as use of the hoe more often than not, lack of fertilizers, lack of irrigation, and use of a diverse range of traditional varieties of grain to compensate for climatic and pedological constraints, with but modest results. The average yield for Africa remains 1,000 kilograms per hectare of millet and corn, which shows how much room for improvement there would be if African governments were to decide to treat their farmers a little better and to invest in their agricultural potential.

What are some of the ways in which agricultural production can be increased? It is interesting to note that food problems do not occur in countries that are at peace, that enjoy democracy, and in which farmers operate under conditions of relative legal and administrative security, even when these countries are densely populated and located in unfavorable climatic zones. It is better to live in Burkina Faso than in the Democratic Republic of Congo, even though the Congo is infinitely better endowed than Burkina Faso in terms of rainfall and available land. Similarly, the "white revolution" in Mali is revitalizing those regions that produce rice, millet, and cotton and enriching their farmers, even as hunger still plagues Madagascar, the former breadbasket of southern Africa, which has been making error after economic error over the last quarter of a century.

In order to bring about peace and security in Africa, a resumption of cooperation is necessary. However, the level of official development assistance has never been lower. Will the renegotiation of the Lomé Convention relaunch the partnership between Europe and Africa for the concerted development of agriculture? Jean-Jacques Gabas drew attention in Chapter 33 to the obstacles that have been encountered in the search for food security since the signing of the first agreements in 1975.

Notes

Sylvie Brunel is strategy adviser, Action Against Hunger.
1. In *La Baleine qui cache la forêt* (Paris: La Découverte, 1994).
2. *Attention Statistiques!* (Paris: La Découverte, 1996). See also Joseph

Klatzmann, *Nourrir l'humanité, espoirs et inquiétudes* (Paris: Inra-Economica, 1991).

3. *Agriculture et alimentation mondiales: des raisons d'espérer?* (Paris: Crédit Mutuel, 1996).

27

Overcoming Rural Poverty: The Lessons of Asia

Gilbert Etienne

Over the past half century, Asia has redoubled its efforts to overcome poverty, particularly in rural areas, where malnutrition is one of the principal manifestations of poverty. This concern is all the more justified as the continent today, from Pakistan to the Far East, is still heavily rural. With the exception of Japan, South Korea, and the island of Taiwan, the proportion of urban dwellers is between 20 and 35 percent of the total population. Some 50 to 70 percent of active workers are engaged in agriculture, which accounts for 20 to 30 percent of gross domestic product (although in the late 1990s the proportion of active workers engaged in agriculture in China fell below 50 percent).

The fight against rural poverty and malnutrition should therefore be placed at the center of any development strategy. In this regard, Asia offers us a series of contrasting lessons, some positive and others negative, depending on the period.

The Golden Age of the Green Revolution

In most of Asia, reliance on traditional techniques had run its course by the 1960s. With few exceptions, hardly any undeveloped land still remained, and yields had already reached their limits. At the same time, the increase in the grain deficit and the massive famine in China (1959–1961) spurred governments to intensify their efforts by turning to new production techniques.

The Ford and Rockefeller Foundations, soon to be supported by the World Bank and the U.S. Agency for International Development

259

(USAID), provided valuable cooperation through high-level experts. The result was a period of research and dissemination of experiences within and outside the continent from 1965 to 1970 and, in China, from 1971 to 1972. (China recovered its seat in the United Nations on 25 October 1971 and resumed relations with the United States.)

The Green Revolution—consisting of irrigation, improved seeds, and partial mechanization—in Asia led to a decline in the importation of cereals and at times even to the cessation of imports and their replacement with exports. Visionary political leaders, agronomists, and rural dwellers identified the three points of the triangle that became the foundation of a coherent strategy. Irrigation, the cornerstone of the system, was strongly encouraged. The distribution of new varieties of seed, chemical fertilizers, and pesticides was accompanied by partial mechanization, such as motor-driven pumps, tractors, threshing machines, and so on.

In contrast to those areas that were characterized by unfavorable physical conditions and thus unsuitable for the Green Revolution (owing to lack of rainfall and/or irrigation), the vast alluvial plains from the Indus basin to the plains of northern China experienced a remarkable transformation during the 1965–1972 period. The marked increase in cereal production, especially that of wheat and rice, was accompanied by improvements in infrastructure, roads, electricity, commerce, and small industries. Other secondary activities, such as cattle farming, fruit and vegetable production, and fish farming also experienced significant growth from the 1980s onward. It was in fact a process of comprehensive rural development characterized by a twofold trend: growth and diversification of the rural agricultural and nonagricultural economy.

Large, small, and medium-sized landowners were all swept up by these currents, while large numbers of landless peasants saw their wages increase together with opportunities for employment both in and out of the agricultural sector. Studies conducted in countries including India, Java, and China (collectivist until 1980) pointed to a clear correlation between agriculture growth and poverty reduction.

As John Mellor, one of the most widely recognized U.S. experts on rural Asia, has noted, even accelerated growth in the secondary and tertiary sectors of urban areas has only a limited impact on the reduction of poverty at the national level. On the other hand, strong growth in the agricultural sector accompanied by improved living standards in villages has a greater multiplier effect both in the countryside and in cities, as a result of the expansion of rural markets for the products manufactured by city dwellers: cement, machines, semi-durable goods, and common consumer items. Growth and diversification of the rural economy lead to increased employment, often in the form of part-time jobs, while at the same time improving the lot of the poorest sectors. Mellor's observations are supported by other authors.[1]

Mistakes and Setbacks

The early results of the Green Revolution were obscured by the social-ist and populist currents, in some cases reinforced by Marxism-Leninism, which emerged in the late 1960s. The social impact of the Green Revolution was ignored or called into question. Sartaj Aziz, the Pakistani national who was at the time the deputy director of the Food and Agricultural Organization, went so far as to write: "In many countries, rapid growth has aggravated the problem of poverty."[2] The focus then shifted to ways of meeting "basic needs," attacking poverty directly through programs designed to benefit the most disadvan-taged sectors, with heavy doses of subsidies for food consumption, loans made from grants, measures solely for the benefit of the most disadvantaged social classes, and an increase in public works to create employment.

Opportunistic leaders, such as Indira Gandhi in India; experts from numerous international organizations, including the World Bank; and numerous nongovernmental organizations (NGOs), all to different degrees, took the same road.

The result was a decline in the level of technical and economic resources allocated to those activities that produce growth, namely, research and public investments in water supply systems and other rural infrastructural works. This trend was noticeable in several states as was the decline in the level of international cooperation.

This direct attack on poverty yielded mixed and even disappoint-ing results. While there were undoubtedly some success stories in a number of Asian countries, various official reports, including those from India, Bangladesh, and Pakistan, as well as private surveys revealed severe leakages in the system: misappropriation of funds, which ended up in the pockets of the rich instead of helping the poor; the bribing of officials in return for subsidized loans; substan-dard public works; and so on. Moreover, these programs had an impact on only a small proportion of the poor and, when successful, at a high cost in terms of program support, which precluded their replication on a large scale.

The leftist excesses were compounded or replaced in the 1980s by rightist excesses. Economic liberalization, privatization, and globalization were all promoted to varying degrees throughout the continent. These new approaches, while generally positive, suffered from a serious weakness. They tended to neglect agriculture while contributing to the reduction in public investments, as if the private sector could meet all of society's needs.

In the area of North-South cooperation, the share in official development assistance has been declining since 1980. The emphasis placed on agriculture by cooperation agencies, which was so noticeable in the early days of the Green Revolution, began to decline. "In U.S. aid programs, the number of agricultural experts declined by 80 percent in recent decades. The attitude of European donors underwent a similar change," according to John Mellor.[3] In debates on the Third World held in research institutes in Asia and in Western countries, the emphasis placed on agriculture declined significantly.

The subsidies allocated to production deserve special mention. There is no doubt that the start of the Green Revolution was facilitated by such subsidies. But, far from declining subsequently, the overall share of subsidies tended to increase, despite their elimination or reduction in some cases (including in Pakistan and Bangladesh for fertilizers and pesticides). In most countries, fees charged for water for irrigation purposes and the cost of electricity remained at absurdly low levels, which were often insufficient to pay for minimal maintenance of canals and electricity supply systems. Sales of subsidized grain by the state proved burdensome and failed in their stated aim of benefiting only the poor. Subsidies for inputs for agriculture benefited the less poor and the rich, as in the case of electricity for irrigation pumps and fertilizers. However, for reasons of narrow political interest, governments were slow to cut back these subsidies.

In some cases, the opposite was true. During the legislative elections held in 1997 in the Indian state of Punjab, the largest food producer in the country with the highest per capita income, the party that emerged victorious carried out its promise to provide free electricity to peasants. A similar trend can be seen in Maharashtra in the period preceding the next elections there.

These subsidies are partially responsible for the declining share of productive investments. In India, such investments represent 15 percent of gross domestic product. In India also, the share of public funds allocated to productive activities fell from 60 percent of all resources channeled into the rural economy in 1981 to 38 percent in 1994, while antipoverty programs and subsidies increased.

Mention should also be made of certain shortcomings that are only too rarely identified, except in the local press: fraud and the adulteration of seeds, fertilizers, and pesticides. Examples of this abound: in Anhui (China), 2,600 hectares yielded no harvest in 1998 as a result of the poor quality of the seeds planted.

As I pointed out in *The Geopolitics of Hunger, 1998–1999,* the lack of public investments contributes to the failure to develop better varieties of food crops, cotton, and oil-producing plants, trends that were confirmed in 1998 and early 1999, with some variations, depending on weather conditions and natural disasters. In Thailand, the poor state of the water supply system became evident in 1999 when rainfall was insufficient. Vietnam and Indonesia did not enjoy favorable weather in 1998, but Indonesia's harvests were better in 1999, thanks to more favorable weather conditions. China and Bangladesh suffered from exceptionally severe floods in 1998. In Pakistan, cotton, a major crop, suffered from excessive rainfall in 1998; the rain, however, was helpful to the rice crops. In 1999, wheat harvests were good in India, but rather poor in Pakistan and reduced in China as a result of the drought experienced by that country. The conclusion that may be drawn here is that improved water supply systems would help to limit the damage caused by the vagaries of the weather.

As of early 1999, no major change was foreseen in the export and import patterns of grain. A return to greater awareness of the importance of agriculture, which was noted in 1998, is now taking root in China, India, and Southeast Asia. China is trying to learn the lessons from the disasters of 1998 by improving its dikes, which had long been poorly maintained. Many other measures are needed, however, to expand the area under irrigation and to promote research and dissemination activities. The Indian budget for the year April 1999–March 2000 increased the share of public funds allocated to agriculture. Whether the objectives would be met was questionable, since the government is too weak to reduce subsidies. China and Vietnam are still suffering from the aftershocks of the East Asia crisis and will have difficulty in mobilizing the necessary funds. While operating in a different context, it is difficult to see Indonesia and Pakistan relaunching vigorous agricultural programs, since their financial situation is extremely precarious.

A widespread problem in Latin America, Africa, and Asia is the loss incurred during the transport and especially during storage of fruits, vegetables, and cereals. In the prestigious Indian Punjab, it was discovered that stocks of paddy with a value of at least $800 million were rotting either in poorly maintained silos or under roadside tarpaulins. Some of the grain had been harvested in 1992 and the rest in subsequent years. At the national level, nearly one-third of the stocks will not be fit for consumption. In China, losses are no less heavy at nearly 45 million tons, according to the *China Daily* of 26 June 1997.

Even though data for other countries are unavailable, the problem is no less common. Local efforts with outside support would help to reduce this tremendous waste.

Those Excluded from the Green Revolution

In the initial stages, governments were correct to focus their efforts on the regions that were most suitable for the Green Revolution, since this was the only way to increase national production of grain within the shortest possible time. This policy, however, favored zones that were already relatively advanced, to the detriment of the populations located in the less geographically advantageous areas. Now, several years later, it is possible to partially correct this approach, thanks to the progress made in the irrigated plains. But, let us not deceive ourselves: There will never be a Green Revolution in the high Afghan plateaus, in numerous districts of peninsular India, in the plateaus of northeast Thailand, in northwest China, or in many other regions where water is unavailable.

Two approaches may be used. The first is recourse to various techniques of dry farming and watershed development to reduce runoff from occasional rainfall, combat erosion, and, where possible, enrich the soil. The fruit of these measures, which are relatively costly and complex, are in no way comparable to those of the Green Revolution. They are not negligible, however, especially since these methods permit broad areas to be cultivated with a wide variety of crops or to be put to other agricultural uses, including the planting of sorghum, millet, and fruit trees or use as pasture land.

The work being done in this field should be pursued more vigorously. The Indian budget for 1999–2000 provides for one hundred districts to be covered over the next three years. The same concerns are present in China and Vietnam. Will the efforts being made be adequate to the needs that exist?

The second approach to improving the living standards of those who cannot benefit from the Green Revolution is through emigration: from the village to the city, from the village to foreign countries (as in the case of the heavy emigration from Pakistan to the Middle East), and from poor districts to districts that often need additional labor for large agricultural works. The social cost to the families concerned (one or two members abroad who remit their savings to the village) may be heavy, especially in the case of unstable migrations. But such solutions—which of course do not exclude all possible local development programs—are all the more inevitable as population pressure increases. In Europe, for example, migration from the Alpine valleys has played an important role in eliminating poverty, even though the rate of population growth in Europe has been lower than in Asia.

Positive Trends

Along with these phenomena that act as constraints to agriculture, there are other, more favorable trends that are common throughout Asia. Cereals and sometimes other main crops lose ground and are replaced by secondary agricultural activities: cattle raising, fruits, vegetables, fish farming, or even flower cultivation. These activities are much more lucrative than the cultivation of rice or wheat. Profits can be substantial even on a properly prepared plot a quarter of a hectare in area. Many jobs are created in and out of agriculture: The landless untouchable in India, for example, each day transports on his bicycle 50 liters of milk to the milk collection center. All of these products are a response to the increase in demand in both town and country. Some of the production is exported, which brings additional benefits to the economy. These activities all have a further advantage: They are not dependent on the state. Examples are a landowner who installs a drip system of irrigation on less than a hectare for his mango and orange trees or a peasant who raises chickens or, in East Asia, pigs. In these conditions, the need to be self-sufficient in grain becomes less urgent. First, it is more profitable to export more valuable products even if it then becomes necessary to import cereals. Also, and this trend is already very pronounced in China, the development of cattle farming makes it necessary to import stock feed that may not be available locally, based on the model observed in developed countries.

Account must be taken of the many small innovations about whose origins little is known. In 1992, we were struck in the Punjab region of Pakistan by the appearance of a large number of carts that had wheels equipped with rubber tires and that were pulled by smartly trotting donkeys. Despite the difference in the load carried, this means of transport was faster and less expensive than ox-drawn carts. Eight years later and 500 kilometers from Pakistan, in Uttar Pradesh, the same type of carts are being noted. In 1998, during another visit to Bangladesh, I came upon peasants who had abandoned the system of threshing paddy by beating the stalks of grain on a stone—a method that caused huge losses—in favor of a rustic pedal-driven machine. Several years previously, these same peasants had had the idea of diverting some water from their hand pumps, the source of their drinking water, to their plot of vegetables, a process that enabled them to multiply the number of crops harvested during the year.

However encouraging these trends may be, they are not enough to offset the difficulties faced in order to grow the principal crops in places where, despite the complaints of vested interests on the political right, the state still plays a major role. Even the most creative peasants cannot restore the canals that irrigate millions of hectares, repair roads that are poorly maintained, or improve electrical grids that are in pitiful condition. Nor can private initiative alone suffice to carry out the multiple tasks that need to be done in the area of agronomical research or extension services. There is an urgent need, for example, to improve the dosages in the components of chemical fertilizers and to conduct soil analyses, tasks that are now largely neglected.

What Conclusions Are to Be Drawn?

The shortcomings highlighted above have been known to the experts for the last two or three decades to no avail, and corrective measures have been slow in coming. The return of famines appears very unlikely (except in special situations such as in North Korea), given the progress achieved and the reserves of grain that have been accumulated. Diversification of the agricultural sector does not necessarily exclude the importation of cereals, but brings it within certain limits. Recent projections indicate that in India, if the decline in productivity is not reversed fairly soon, demand for grain may outstrip production by 24 million tons by the year 2020. If, on the contrary, agricultural policy is strengthened, India will have some 16 million tons of grain, rice, and wheat each year for net exports,[4] even as it imports stock feed for cattle and poultry. The situation in several other countries should not be very different.

More proactive agricultural policies and international cooperation that places greater emphasis on growth will have a more beneficial impact on the poor and undernourished than direct but less focused action against poverty.

Notes

Gilbert Etienne is honorary professor at the Institute of Advanced International Studies and the Institute of Development Studies in Geneva.

1. Cf. John Mellor, *Agriculture on the Road to Industrialization* (Baltimore, MD: The Johns Hopkins University Press, 1995); M. Ravallion and G. Datt, "How Important to India's Poor Is the Sectoral Composition of Economic Growth?" *World Bank Economic Review* 10, no. 1; G. Etienne, with C. Aubert and J. L. Maurer, *Feeding Asia in the Next Century* (New Delhi: Macmillan, 1998).

2. S. Aziz, *Learning from China* (London, 1976), p. xvi. This work gives a very biased account of Maoist China.

3. In his chapter in C. Auroi and J. L. Maurer (supervisor), *Tradition and Modernization of Rural Economies in Asia, Africa and Latin America* (Paris: Presses Universitaires de France, 1998).

4. R. E. Evenson, C. E. Pray, and M. W. Rosegrant, *Agricultural Research and Productivity Growth in India*, IFPRI Research Report 109 (Washington D.C.: IFPRI, 1999).

28

The Role of
Nutrition in Public Health

Claudine Prudhon

Nutrition plays an important role in our daily lives, a fact that we sometimes overlook because it seems so obvious to us. The food that we eat is necessary for life, and we also derive satisfaction from sharing a pleasant meal. Because for most of us eating every day is not a major problem, we too often tend to forget that a balanced diet is indispensable for life.

The key role of adequate nutrition is, however, becoming increasingly clear, not only in situations of food shortages but also in industrialized countries in the relationship between adequate nutrition and illnesses such as cancer and cardiovascular pathologies. It is now recognized that the individual's nutritional status is at the heart of the general well-being of populations.

Questioning the Common Wisdom

A Starving Individual Can Eat Anything

There is a common tendency to believe that individuals who are hungry can eat anything, provided they fill their stomachs. This is completely false.

Feeding unsuitable food to an individual who is suffering from malnutrition endangers that person's life. This was widely observed among deportees leaving concentration camps after World War II and more recently among malnourished populations of children and adults in Africa. Because a severely malnourished individual suffers from severe disruptions to his metabolism, feeding must be resumed using a careful balance of nutrients.[1] Malnutrition is a disease, just like a throat infection or a cold, and must be treated as such. The medicine in this case will be a suitable nutritional product, which works in the same way as an antibiotic.

The same is true for populations that are not malnourished. People cannot survive an unbalanced diet without causing harm to themselves. They will quickly suffer from numerous deficiencies that will have major repercussions on their health.

In Cases of Food Shortages, Only a Section of the Population Is Affected

Contrary to what is sometimes believed, in cases of severe food shortages, it is the entire population that is affected to different degrees and not only that part of the population that is shown to us most often by the media: the malnourished population.

The impact of food scarcity on the nutritional status of a population can take different forms that are more or less visible: loss of weight, appearance of edemas, stunted growth in children, and vitamin and mineral deficiencies that may range from marginal to epidemics of severe deficiencies. These different types of malnutrition will sooner or later all have repercussions on the health of the individual.

The results of anthropometric nutritional surveys carried out among children under the age of five clearly show that in the event of deterioration of the children's nutritional status, the entire population is affected. Preliminary studies tend to show the same phenomenon among the adult population. For example, in Chad, significant weight loss has been noted in children and their mothers during the "hungry season," the period preceding the harvest, during which stocks from the previous harvest are exhausted. However, only a part of this population is considered to be malnourished, measured by thresholds that are more or less arbitrarily defined.

Whatever the type of alteration of nutritional status that is observed in cases of food shortages, it will have a significant impact on the health of the individual.

People Do Not Die of Hunger

The link between nutritional status and mortality is often underestimated, since the cause of death will be imputed to a medical pathology rather than to the nutritional status of the individual. An individual's nutritional state, however, underlies his well-being; an individual who is nutritionally healthy will have a reduced risk of being affected by a disease and if affected runs less risk of having serious consequences.

The link between the percentage of individuals affected by malnutrition and the mortality rate in refugee camps is illustrated by the fact that the rate of malnutrition is followed by a corresponding increase in the rate of mortality.

The relationship between malnutrition and mortality exists not only among individuals who are identified as malnourished, but is present as soon as the nutritional status of an individual deteriorates even slightly. Whenever an individual exhibits a nutritional state that is even marginally below the normal range, that individual's risk of dying increases.

This is true not only in cases of food shortages. It has been demonstrated in France that the risk of dying among hospital patients increases significantly if these patients suffer from disruptions of their nutritional status.

Toward an Optimal Response to Food Needs

In situations of food scarcity, the provision of adequate food to prevent any deterioration of the population's nutritional status and to feed the malnourished population will therefore be crucial in terms of public health, in order to limit the number of deaths.

The provision of adequate food to an entire population is not easy to achieve, given the numerous constraints, and a special effort must be made in this area.

Food Needs

The needs of a population stricken by disaster are the same as those of any other population, or even greater if we are to address the underlying deficiencies and increased exposure to diseases.

Various references in terms of food needs have been established, including the European, French, and World Health Organization references, and the objective should be to meet these needs.[2] Although the nutritional requirements of a population have long been known, food aid does not always take these needs into account. The emergence of ration standards shows, however, that it is gradually being recognized that a refugee has the same needs as any other individual. Over the years, the minimum energy intake recommended by United

Nations agencies has increased.[3] Vitamin and mineral needs are increasingly being taken into account in establishing standards for rations.

Inadequacy of Response

Deficiencies in rations are often seen in the field: Follow-up checks among families after rations have been distributed have shown that the theoretical amount of the ration to be distributed is often not achieved. Over the last ten years, numerous epidemics of vitamin deficiencies have been noted among refugee populations, because food aid did not provide an adequate intake, and these populations had no other means of obtaining the missing elements.[4]

The food ration distributed in African countries consists mainly of cereals, legumes, and oil. Apart from the fact that this ration is monotonous, its analysis has shown that it is less balanced than pet food.[5] Since 1992, vitamins and minerals have been increasingly taken into account in determining what is a balanced ration. Meeting these requirements, however, remains difficult.

Strategies to Be Implemented in Order to Improve the Response

A ration must be balanced in proteins, carbohydrates, lipids, vitamins, and minerals. A balance in the first three nutrients is relatively easy to achieve with staple foods. On the other hand, an adequate intake of vitamins and minerals is more difficult, since some of these elements are present mainly in fresh produce and animal products that are often difficult, if not impossible, to distribute for reasons of conservation and cost. These same concerns affect populations living in precarious conditions in France that, because they consume low-cost products, are exposed to nutritional deficiencies.

Different approaches may be used to optimize food rations. Based on the products that are available in the market, foods can be classified according to the nutrients that they contain and their cost. This makes it possible to prepare optimal rations at lower cost, an approach first attempted by a group of researchers in France for populations living in precarious conditions.[6] This approach nevertheless has its limits, since, as mentioned above, certain nutrients are obtained only from fresh produce or animal products, which are not easy to distribute in the field.

Another approach consists in designing products containing vitamin and mineral supplements specifically for emergency food aid.

This approach has the disadvantage of being removed from normal food habits and does not address the need for diversification of the rations. It does make it possible, however, to obtain an adequate ration more easily and reduce the logistical problems of conservation and distribution.

The fortification of food products with vitamins and minerals is increasingly being discussed by nutritionists. Significant progress has been made in the treatment of severe malnutrition. The Scientific Committee of Action Against Hunger, which is composed of renowned researchers, has actively participated in the development of specific products supplemented with vitamins and minerals for the treatment of severe malnutrition. These products were perfected in 1994 and are now widely used by other humanitarian agencies and recommended by the World Health Organization.[7] It has been observed that the use of these products has led to improvements in the weight gain of severely malnourished children at a quite negligible additional cost: twelve percent of the total cost of the food.

The success of this strategy is due to a set of factors: (1) the pooling of the skills of scientists, humanitarian workers, and nutritionists, which has been instrumental in the development of an effective product, and (2) awareness-promotion and lobbying campaigns targeted to the international community and to donors in order to ensure that the value of the product is recognized and that the funds necessary to purchase it are made available.

The fortification with vitamins and minerals of rations consisting of cereals, legumes, and oil, which are intended for distribution to the general population, is more difficult to achieve. The quantities of food to be distributed are considerable, and enrichment should not present a risk of overdosing.

Various vectors of fortification have been considered, such as the enrichment of cereals and condiments and the distribution of enriched flour. Thus far, none of the strategies that have been tried has proven to be truly effective.

Much more remains to be done among humanitarian agencies, scientists, food technologists, and donors to ensure that the skills of some serve the needs of others and that the necessary funds are made available.

Last, one of the major constraints we have observed is the constraint of cost, particularly for the countries of the South. The food rations distributed to refugee and displaced populations in the countries of Eastern Europe are much more diversified, include processed products, and cost five times more than the rations distributed in African countries. It is therefore easier to obtain balanced rations.

The nutritional needs of all populations are similar, however, and the question of why such great differences exist must therefore be posed.

Adequate food must be seen as an essential factor for public health, and the basis of the physical integrity of the individual. Strategies aimed at providing populations with satisfying food must be developed both by technical measures to define appropriate strategies and by making the necessary resources available. We must also be careful to ensure that food aid has the same quality for all and that the same strategies are used for the countries of the South as for the countries of the North.

Notes

Claudine Prudhon was the head of the Nutrition Department of Action Against Hunger–France until June 2000.

1. M.H.N. Golden and A. Briend, "Treatment of Malnutrition in Refugee Camps," *Lancet* 342 (1993).

2. Reports of the Scientific Committee for Food, Brussels: Commission Nutrient and *Energy Intakes for the European Community* (of the European Community, 1993). H. Dupin, J. Abraham, and I. Giachetti, *Apports nutritionnels conseillés pour la population française* (Paris: Centre National de la Recherche Scientifique—Centre National D'Etudes et de Recommandations sur la Nutrition et L'Alimentation, 1992). *Nutritional Requirements in Emergencies* (Geneva: World Health Organization, 1997).

3. *World Food Program/UN High Commission for Refugees Guidelines for Estimating Food and Nutritional Needs in Emergencies* (Rome: World Food Program/United Nations High Commission for Refugees, 1997).

4. M. J. Tool, "Micronutrient Deficiencies in Refugees," *Lancet* 339 (1992).

5. C.J.K. Henry, "Comparison of Nutrient Composition of Refugee Rations and Pet Foods," *Lancet* 340 (1992).

6. N. Darmon and A. Briend, "Les aliments de bons rapports qualité (nutritionnelle)/prix," *Alimentation et précarité*, no. 5 (1999).

7. *Management of Severe Malnutrition: A Manual for Physicians and Health Workers* (Geneva: World Health Organization, 1999).

29

Is Food Aid to Russia Necessary?

Alain Giroux

Should Russia be given food aid? A review of the country's agrofood situation provides a clear response to this question: Aid first and foremost enables donor countries to resolve their problems of overproduction and does not provide Russia with the support it needs to restructure its agricultural sector.

This question can be approached from different perspectives: that of the United States and the European Union, which are the principal aid donors; that of the Moscow authorities; that of the Russian entities responsible for distributing the aid; that of Russian agricultural producers; and that of Russian political parties and pressure groups.

The responses of the different parties may all be quite different, since their interests do not always coincide. In order to evaluate the need for food aid to Russia, it is necessary to compare and contrast the positions and arguments of the many actors involved and also to ascertain the political motives behind the good intentions.

Why Food Aid?

The difficulties faced by the agricultural sector in Russia can be traced back not to 1991, the year of the disintegration of the USSR, but to the Soviet era. The fact that 80 percent of agricultural enterprises were in deficit in 1999, as the authorities have acknowledged, can be explained by the inertia of producers, which was the legacy of a long period during which direct state subsidies systematically averted the bankruptcy of the *kolkhoz* and *sovkhoz*. The consequences have been numerous: little or no interest on the part of peasants in the final results of their work, high production cost, poor quality of products, and absence of flexibility in production policies. Under market conditions, other problems have been added: the disparity in prices between agricultural products and the price of inputs, with the latter being higher; lack of competitiveness of national products; inability to react rapidly to changes in market conditions; and the technological backwardness of most enterprises.

For many years, after each bad crop, many Western observers have predicted severe food shortages and even famine at the onset of winter, without those somber predictions ever having come to pass. The situation in 1998, however, was very different, when drought severely affected crops. The 47.8-million-ton grain harvest was the worst since the 1950s and was more than 40 million tons less than the 1997 harvest. At the end of 1998, the Russian government projected shortfalls in grain production in approximately forty of the eighty-nine legal entities of the Russian Federation (republics, territories, regions) and a shortage of seeds for the 1999 planting season. Certain producer regions witnessed a return to the old reflex toward autarky, with governments prohibiting the shipment of grains outside of their territories. In addition, the serious financial crisis faced by Russia in mid-August 1998 led, from September onward, to a drastic drop in imports of food products on which Russia is very dependent. Thus, because of the steady decline in the size of livestock, the share of imports of meat and milk products rose to 43 percent (nearly 90 percent for Moscow and St. Petersburg).

These factors, combined with the suspension of international funding, led officials to fear that they would no longer be able to meet the food needs of the population, especially in the regions on the northern periphery and in eastern Siberia, which are poor in agricultural products and depend on cumbersome and expensive logistical networks. Russia therefore made a request for food and humanitarian aid to which the United States and the European Union responded in late 1998, with Canada and Japan also providing bilateral assistance. The Red Cross, for its part, made plans for an emergency program worth seventeen million dollars for the remote northeastern region of the country.

The agreement on food aid that was concluded in November 1998, and finalized in December with the United States, provided for the delivery of 1.7 million tons of wheat, 500,000 tons of corn, 300,000 tons of soya for animal feed and 200,000 tons for human consumption, 100,000 tons of rice, 120,000 tons of beef, 50,000 tons of pork, 30,000 tons of powdered milk, and 100,000 tons of miscellaneous products. In addition, it provided for a line of credit in the amount of $600 million for the purchase of U.S. food products, reimbursable over twenty years at the very favorable rate of 2 percent per year. For its part, the European Union proposed in 1998 to supply Russia with one million tons of wheat, 500,000 tons of rye, 100,000 tons of pork, 150,000 tons of beef, and 50,000 tons of powdered milk and an equal amount of rice, worth in total approximately $480 million. The final agreement was also signed in December.

The volumes and financing for these two programs far exceeded the food aid granted to Moscow in 1992–1993. The memory of the massive scale of the misappropriation of that aid and the questions surrounding the real needs of Russia gave rise to extensive negotiations that were carried on for nearly two months before agreement was finally reached. The Americans and Europeans demanded solid guarantees on the conditions for the distribution and sale of the products. The European Commission requested a monthly status report and monitoring of the operations by an independent authority. In the event of fraud, shipments would be suspended. The Russian government pledged to send the aid received to the regions in difficulty (North, Siberia, Far East) and to exclude Moscow and Saint Petersburg from receiving any of the aid from Europe. Sale of the foodstuffs at Russian market prices was to be done through state-controlled agencies, and the money obtained (approximately $680 million) was to be allocated to social welfare funds, with priority being given to the payment of arrears of pension, which amounted to twenty-three billion roubles, or nearly $1 billion. Some of the aid was to be allocated to hospitals, orphanages, and prisons.

Before any analysis of the wisdom of this aid to Russia and the problems that it creates in the country, it must be stated that the United States and European Union are the principal beneficiaries of the operation. In the 1980s Russia purchased millions of tons of grain. Since 1990–1991, however, it has been importing only very small quantities, thereby causing serious problems for Western farmers, who were faced with a situation of overproduction and consequent drop in prices. Behind this humanitarian gesture to a country in great difficulty, Americans and Europeans found a good opportunity both to get rid of unwanted surpluses and to reconquer, through the return of their products, a Russian market from which they had practically disappeared following the Russian economic collapse.[1] It may also be correctly assumed that the European Union and Washington in particular put pressure on Moscow to accept this aid in exchange for using their influence over international agencies such as the International Monetary Fund to disburse loans to a cash-strapped Russia.

While aid to Russia may be considered necessary by Western governments, its provision creates certain problems and has given rise to fierce debates within Russia, which have been picked up by the media.

Under the terms of the November 1998 agreement, food aid should have begun to arrive in Russia by the start of 1999, but that date was pushed back to the end of the first quarter. The reasons for this delay were many. First of all, it was only in February that Moscow presented the United States with a plan for the distribution of the U.S. aid to the Russian regions; the U.S. secretary of agriculture termed the plan incomplete and decided to suspend the shipment of pork and beef pending the submission of a more detailed plan.

For its part, the European Commission temporarily suspended its aid to Russia on 10 February to protest against administrative bottlenecks. In fact, the commercial operators chosen by Moscow to market the products made what were considered to be unacceptable demands in the areas of health standards and quality controls. They demanded, for example, that the quality of the products should be the same as that of products delivered in normal commercial exchanges and argued that, according to their standards, meat that had been stored for more than eighteen months in freezers was unfit for human consumption. Russian veterinarians responsible for health controls charged exorbitant fees that were tantamount to racketeering.

The fear of diversion of the shipment of food still exists in 2000. The Americans believed that the aid could serve the electoral interests of the governors of Russian regions. With an eye to the legislative elections of December 1999, some of them would receive more aid than had been planned because of their political strength.

In addition to the problem of the monitoring of distribution, Western operators feared the reexport of food products. Indeed, since the domestic prices of the products are lower than world prices, the temptation is great for the entities receiving aid to sell it abroad, and we have recently witnessed the resale of oil proteins, flour, and grains. The West therefore imposed on Russia, which accepted it, the suspension of its exports of grain and beef for a period of at least six months.

Questioning Aid in Russia

Since the end of 1998, the Russian media have given extensive coverage to the debates on Western food aid that have gripped the country's agricultural and political sectors and that have focused mainly on the issue of the wisdom of food aid in the form of grains. Each party knows full well that, as far as beef is concerned, it would take several years for Russia to rebuild its livestock sector, despite the increases in 1998 in the production of beef, pork, and chicken.

The main question concerns the real amount of grain stocks. Russian officials make the most contradictory statements on this subject. In January 1999, the Russian minister of agriculture and food, Victor Semienov, stated that the country had a grain deficit and that he was placing great hopes on Western aid. Only a month before the deputy prime minister responsible for food-related issues, Gennady Kulik, had declared that food reserves were sufficient for 1999 and that Russia was in no danger of shortages. This declaration, which was no doubt made for political purposes, was clearly intended to reassure a public opinion that was concerned following the very poor harvest and the trauma of the financial crisis.

The answer must be sought in the notoriously vague Russian statistics. Analysts who are critical of aid argued that Russia had reserves from its abundant harvest of 1997 estimated at 20–25 million tons. When added to the harvest of 1998, which was not as good, this would have enabled the country to cover its needs up until the next harvest. But other experts challenged these figures. For them, it was impossible to locate these "phantom reserves," since the silos were empty. If, as was likely, stocks did exist on farms, they would have been stored under conditions making them unfit for consumption. Data from early 1999, published after two months of polemics and silence on the part of officials, supported the arguments of the second group. For example, as of 1 April 1999, according to the Russian Statistical Committee, the grain company reserves stood at 16.8 million tons, or 51.4 percent less than they had been on the same date in the previous year. Imports would bridge the gap up until the next harvest. The Russian Grain Producers Union, for its part, projected for 1999 a deficit of 7 million tons and estimated that in order to meet its consumption and storage needs, Russia would have to harvest 90 million tons of grain, much more than the 68 million tons projected by the minister of agriculture.

As a whole, Russian political parties are critical of food aid. The leftist opposition—communists, agrarian party—regularly condemned earlier reformist governments, which they accused of systematic misappropriations. But the opposition has also consistently sought to exaggerate the bleakness of the agricultural situation in order to show the disaster to which the policies of the reformists have led. Their great fear is that the aid would take away the opportunity being offered to the Russian agrofood sector to benefit from the crisis and from the drop in imports in order to regain from national production the share of the market that it had abandoned to foreign exporters. For their part, the reformists insist that rumors of food shortages tend to be exaggerated and that the supply difficulties should be considered rather as problems comparable to the lack of liquidity among much of the population, which sometimes does not receive salaries for months at a time, or the difficulty of shipping products into certain regions, such as the great North. Nonetheless, they all share the same opinion, namely that the West, through its aid, is pursuing a twofold objective: to reduce its own stocks and to maintain a presence on the Russian food market.

This picture of the dissatisfied would not be complete without mention of the Western exporters and Russian importers who fear a restriction and disruption of markets because of the impact of this massive aid. Nor should we ignore Russian farmers, who are already experiencing considerable difficulty in selling their produce.

Other Forms of Aid?

From the perspective of the donors, the response to the question asked earlier on in this article is most certainly yes, Russia must be given food aid. The donors' position is based on a calculated humanitarianism. But, in absolute terms, one may say that food aid on these terms is not necessary. There are emergency situations that require the shipment of food products to populations in difficulty that are carefully targeted (evaluated by the Red Cross at some 1.7 million people) and the donation of grains to reconstitute stocks that are clearly inadequate. But quite apart from these emergencies, genuine aid to Russia would consist of using the funds disbursed to purchase Russian products from Russian agricultural enterprises and then redistribute them to the population groups affected by the shortages. This approach has been used by Canada with more limited resources (U.S.$1.6 million) given to the Red Cross to purchase food stuffs locally and distribute them using its own networks. It is an approach, however, that has drawn criticism from the United States and the European Union. The real question to be asked is: Are Westerners prepared to help Russia by participating in the rehabilitation of its agrofood sector so that it becomes more productive and capable of meeting the country's needs? The response would no doubt be a "no."

Notes

Alain Giroux is analyst at the Center for Studies and Documentation on the former USSR, China, and Eastern Europe in Paris.

    1. Jean-André Glavany, the French minister of agriculture, expressed satisfaction at this aid, which he saw as holding out hope for a solution to the pork crisis in France, while the president of the Union of Pork Producers of France referred in December 1998 to the need for a "humanitarian offloading" on Russia.

30

Food Aid to Russia: Welcome or Unwelcome?

Jonathan Littell

Aid?

In late October 1998, two months after the spectacular financial crash of 17 August, Michel Camdessus, director of the International Monetary Fund (IMF), asked the European Union to send food aid to Russia "so that hunger will not arrive in that country with winter, so that serious social unrest will not break out."[1] The Russian press immediately reacted rather badly: "Food is a good thing, but Russian authorities expected to get some money."[2] The initiative, however, had come from the Russian authorities: On 9 October, at the Moscow summit, Yevgeny Primakov, just recently appointed prime minister, had indeed asked Jacques Santer, president of the European Commission, for food aid. The question was raised again during the European Union–Russia summit in Vienna in late October, and negotiations started, not only with the European Union but with the United States as well. The negotiations were conducted by Gennady Kulik, vice-prime minister in charge of agriculture.

They evolved very quickly: By 6 November, the U.S. Department of Agriculture (USDA) was announcing that an agreement had been concluded. This agreement, which would hardly be modified from then on, had three parts:

1. Some 1.5 million tons was to be sold under a $600 million "soft loan" at 2 percent interest for twenty years. This allotment provided for the purchase by Russia of 0.5 million tons of maize,

0.5 million tons of soy beans, 120,000 tons of meat and powdered milk, and 200,000 tons of cereals.

2. In addition, 1.5 million tons of wheat were to be given to
Russia. From this amount, 1.1 million tons were to be sold in
Russia based on a monetization process in which profits were
to be transferred to the Pension Fund of Russia, which was in
severe deficit. The remaining 400,000 tons were to be distributed free of charge among various social institutions, such as
orphanages, hospitals, and old people's homes.

3. One hundred thousand tons of various food products were to
be distributed to needy beneficiaries by international humanitarian organizations.[3]

The total value of the program was close to $1 billion.

The U.S. agreement allowed the negotiations with the European
Union, fruitless up to that point, to be concluded. On 12 November,
the European Commission announced in turn an agreement bearing
on 1.85 million tons of products, valued at 500 million euros, which
would be given to Russia to be sold and monetized using a procedure
similar to that used for the U.S. 1.1 million tons. Again the profits
would be transferred to the Pension Fund and other social programs.[4]

All three parties to these agreements described them as a crucial
aid for Russia and needy Russians. However, from the very beginning
these two programs came under severe criticism, particularly from
the press, both international and Russian.

Food Aid: A Long History

International food aid has a long and ill-fated history in Russia. In
1921 and 1922, while a terrible famine devastated the Ukraine and
European Russia, the United States established the American Relief
Administration (ARA) and launched a vast relief operation that was
finally able to save some eight million of the thirteen million people
affected by the famine. A *Moscow Times* editorial written on the eve of
the 6 November 1998 agreement described the precedent in a positive
manner: "The ARA demanded and got complete control of the
process. ... This food aid program was a triumph."[5] Without diminishing the results achieved in 1921, one should look at the details. The
same article admitted that "the Soviet Union was quietly exporting
grain even as its own citizens starved."[6] But more particularly, as is
skillfully demonstrated by J. C. Rufin, the ARA was above all for Lenin

and the Bolsheviks the occasion for a gigantic political man,
the first historical manipulation of humanitarian aid:

> For the first time aid becomes the subject of large-scale po
> blackmail. ... The Russians ... lay down draconian conditions for the
> entry of aid: official recognition of Soviet Russia and exclusive con-
> trol over the aid which they will distribute. ... The donors, caught,
> realize that they cannot do anything for the Russian people without
> recognizing the legitimacy of those imposing their will upon them.

To conclude: "Whether or not misappropriation occurred is not the
point. The profit Lenin derived from this affair was essentially political."[7]

The terrible famine of 1932–1933, which the historian Robert
Conquest called the "terror-famine,"[8] was concealed from foreigners.
No aid was requested; on the contrary, Stalin, as far as possible, aggravated the famine in order to shatter the resistance of the Ukrainian
peasantry. In the 1960s, the USSR, confronted with the obvious failure of its collectivization policy in terms of effectiveness and productivity, was finally forced to resort to imports, to the delight of U.S.
grain producers. At the end of the 1970s U.S. agriculture was boom-
ing but had become very dependent on these exports. Jimmy Carter's
decision in early 1980 to cut them, in protest of the Soviet invasion of
Afghanistan on 27 December 1979, led to serious protest. Ronald
Reagan was able to play on this point during his election campaign a
few months later; the hostility of such a powerful lobby contributed to
Carter's defeat. Once in office, Reagan, despite his loud diatribes
about the Evil Empire, rapidly resumed exports.

In 1991 the USSR collapsed. Overnight the situation changed,
and the United States, once a major rival, became the main ally and
supporter of the fifteen new countries formed out of the USSR. The
chaos of the first stage of transition was accompanied by a sharp
explosion of criminality and inflation and by a slump in the living
standard of Russians. In 1992, panic set in: There was a great deal of
serious talk about famine the following winter. The United States and
the European Union offered food aid; the results were a disaster. To
quote again from the *Moscow Times* editorial of 5 November 1998,
"This time ... the Russia being helped was not in any real danger of
famine; the subsidized exports smothered Russian domestic producers; and the aid was ripped off on a massive scale." Innumerable
reports cropped up of bags still stamped "USA" or "European Union"
being sold in local markets; a part of the aid was even allegedly found
in Ireland, where it was being resold more cheaply than European
products. The negative impression left by this operation considerably

cooled down the donors. In the following years, operations of this kind were no longer carried out, except for small local ones. Thus, at the beginning of 1996, the Humanitarian Office of the European Commission (ECHO), accepted an Action Against Hunger proposal to distribute one thousand tons of food to victims of the war in Chechnya. But even such a small operation suffered from perverse distortions: Although food products for distribution could be purchased locally at advantageous prices, ECHO insisted that they should be bought in Europe. Doing so almost doubled the cost and inevitably entailed considerable delays for what should have been an emergency operation.

Thus, there were few reasons to be surprised at the scale of the negative reactions to the operation announced in November 1998. But the details of the operation and the criticism expressed—at least in the press—were extremely vague and caused numerous misunderstandings.

Is Aid Necessary?

Despite numerous available documents, it is very difficult to judge objectively whether the cries of alarm heard from the autumn of 1998 onward were well founded. As with every sector of the Russian economy, there are seemingly no reliable statistics in the field of agriculture. There are several reasons for this. One is the huge confusion and lack of communication among the various services responsible (the Ministry of Agriculture, the State Statistical Committee [Goskomstat], the regions). Another is the fact that a considerable portion of production is concealed by producers in order to avoid taxation and by regional governments in order to resell it outside of legal channels—either out of simple corruption or to increase the region's budget while bypassing Moscow. No expert is able to assess the proportion of this "gray agriculture," which may account for up to 20 percent of total production. Of course, the so-called private production, that is, the production from garden plots (thanks to which the majority of Russians survive), is not completely taken into account either, though estimates in this field could be a little more reliable. According to Goskomstat, the proportion of private plots in Russia's agriculture in 1995 accounted for 43 percent compared with 55 percent for former *sovkhoz* and *kolkhoz* (the remaining 2 percent being the rare private farms established under the 1990 law). For months, experts and ministries argued about the numbers, and these arguments were further complicated by the political biases of the supporters and opponents of food aid.

The question of how 147 million Russians would feed themselves during the winter was asked rhetorically by *Le Monde* in late October 1998 in an article that quoted numerous contradictory statements. One was by Primakov, who announced on 6 October that "there are at least enough potatoes and vegetables this winter."[9] On 20 October, the Goskomstat declared that total agricultural production had fallen by 9 percent compared with the previous year. As for cereals, by that date Russia had allegedly harvested only 50 percent of the 1997 production.[10] The chorus built: "These are the worst yields since 1953."[11] This statement quickly snowballed. The Emergency Appeal of the International Federation of the Red Cross (IFRC), on behalf of the Far North Territories, particularly impressed the international press.

However, as we have pointed out, journalists were generally skeptical. The article in *Le Monde* quoted "a Western expert" who spoke about "a large-scale disinformation campaign designed to influence world prices."[12] Russian newspapers were usually even more critical.

As for the Russian government, its official declarations were extremely contradictory. Victor Semionov, minister of agriculture (Kulik's subordinate in the Russian hierarchy), announced on 29 October that in the coming winter Russia would not suffer from food shortages.[13] Kulik, on 12 November, wrote to the European commissioner for foreign affairs, Hans Van Den Broek: "The objective analysis of the situation reveals that there will be real food shortages this winter in Russia."[14] Semionov at first persisted: "Many Russians grow most of their own food," he claimed. "They [will] not go hungry in the winter."[15] "Our problem," he announced in another interview, quite pertinently, "is not so much to fill shops but rather to make products accessible to consumers whose means have been reduced by the financial crisis" (we shall return to this point later on).[16] At last, on 24 November, he announced frankly: "There is no danger of famine this winter, contrary to statements playing into the hands of food importers and their lobbyists."[17] However, at the same time, his own ministry was pointing out that "Russia needs approximately seven million tons of cereals."[18]

In fact, as soon as the foreign aid was agreed to, Kulik himself quickly backed off from his alarming statements of October, afraid, perhaps, of provoking panic: "Russia possesses sufficient food reserves to last through 1999. … There won't be any food shortage, to say nothing of famine," he declared on 26 December to a major weekly linked to the Communists.[19] Yuri Maslyukov, one of Primakov's first deputy prime ministers and also a Communist, added that "due to the rapid efforts of the Cabinet and contrary to initial apprehensions, there is no and will not be any famine in Russia."[20]

It is difficult to objectively claim, as some people have done, that the Communists cried for help to receive aid. However, as late as April, *Izvestia* was headlining: "Why Kulik frightened the country with [talk about] famine."[21] While it is certainly true that Kulik and Semionov generally represented conflicting interests—Kulik being closely connected with the importers' and intermediaries' lobby, while Semionov, a pragmatic former businessman, supported the farming lobby—their shifting positions on the issue of "famine" and aid were often contradictory and have evolved over time.[22]

In the end, what about this so-called famine? First, it should be noted that all the threatening statements dealt with winter. However, most experts recognize that the most difficult period in case of food shortages, for people living mainly on their own produce (as is often the case in Russia), is not in fact winter but the "food gap" that occurs when all stocks are exhausted and runs until the following harvest.

In European Russia this period begins approximately in April-May and is curbed only during summer, when vegetables come onto the market in July.[23] A prison director whom Action Against Hunger staff met in the Republic of Tyva (southern Siberia) explained that during winter he managed to meet the targets, but that this became difficult from April until July. By that time his food stocks, which were supplied mainly by prison farms, were down to nothing.[24]

By the spring of 1999, the aid had only just begun to arrive and one was forced to admit, to quote Maslyukov, that there had not been and would not be any famine. But could one still speak of shortages? Even here, it is difficult to support one or the other point of view. The USDA claimed in May: "If you count our aid and the European aid, current food stocks in Russia are at zero; without the aid there would have been a deficit."[25] A World Bank expert, however, believed there were no exact figures: "No one can say whether there is a deficit or not. Taking into account the purchasing capacity of the population, I personally think there is no deficit: consumption is very low—nutritionally inadequate—but in any case lower than supply." According to this same expert, the economists of the Ministry of Agriculture seemed to reason in terms of "profiteers" who allegedly withhold stocks in order to drive prices up. The aid, according to this logic of the planned economy, counteracts such attempts and keeps prices down.[26]

Furthermore, Russia in 1998 exported nearly as much produce as it was due to receive in foreign aid. Official exports ran to more than

1.5 million tons, but there were also a considerable amount of illegal, "black market" exports. Stavropol and Krasnodar producers, in particular, were said to have sold hundreds of thousands of tons through Azerbaijan to Iran and Iraq.[27] The explanation is simple: World prices for wheat in late 1998 were approximately $100-110 per ton, while Russian prices were only $30-35. Export profits in hard currency from Russian wheat sold abroad were enormous. Despite the demands by the United States and the European Union that Russian exports cease as a precondition for aid, it is still difficult to speak of a real deficit, at least in overall terms. As for regional deficits, as the *Moscow Times* observed, "If the U.S. Government is so worried about hunger in Russia's regions, why doesn't it give Russia loans to buy Russian wheat—at a third of the price? That would let Russia feed three times as many people. It would also let Russia build up its domestic agriculture sector." But, the editorial concluded, "the last thing Kansas farmers want is for the U.S. Government to help their competitors."[28]

In fact, two elements should be identified, which has rarely been done during these debates. One is the "macro" situation of a country's agriculture, which is mainly an economic question in which reductions of stocks lead not to a humanitarian problem but to price fluctuations, which are always affected by a number of other factors (demand, exports, domestic distribution networks, speculation, and so on). The other is the problem of food security in Russia, which certainly affects a considerable part of the population but which is primarily the problem of the accessibility of food, that is, of people's ability to buy food, at whatever price. We shall return to this point later.

Is Aid Harmful?

Beyond the question of needs, critics of food aid place particular emphasis on the harmful effects of the operation on Russian farmers. The general situation of the agriculture and food industry in Russia could indeed be described as catastrophic. Prior to the crisis of 17 August 1998, Russia imported large amounts of food products.[29] Overnight, with the collapse of the rouble, these products, which had dominated the market and very often had been cheaper than their Russian equivalents, disappeared from the shelves. In the chaos of the ensuing months, numerous analysts considered that the crisis had given an unexpected impetus to the Russian agriculture and food industry: Foreign competitors had been eliminated, and rouble prices remained relatively stable. Suddenly the Russians could hope to increase sales and thus, thanks to an inflow of capital, modernize and develop their equipment and future productive capacity.

The case of chicken is typical: Before the crisis, according to the USDA, Russia imported more than one million tons of chicken from the United States. The demand was very strong, as chicken is a good source of protein and the price was much lower than that of beef. But local supply could not meet this demand, mainly owing to a dearth of investment to increase production and to the lack of grain and fodder.[30] An article in *Libération* described the experience of the Zarechnaya factory, a large chicken factory in Penza, 800 kilometers from Moscow:

> Founded in 1986, it became one of the ten best [factories] in its sector in the USSR. ... At its height, it produced 6 million chickens a year. But at the beginning of 1992, the Government ... began its "shock therapy." Subsidies were abruptly cut. ... Without the State purchases, the factory no longer had a market. Shortages of eggs, fodder and grain for the chickens began.

By 1992, local chicken cost twenty roubles per kilo compared with five roubles for chicken from the United States.

> From 1995 on, the factory no longer paid its taxes or its social security payments. Wages were paid erratically, whenever a customer paid in cash. ... The last chickens were slaughtered on April 1, 1998. The workers were placed on "forced holiday" [and] pilfered everything that could still be useful.[31]

This is just the kind of business that will most profit from the financial crisis:

> American chicken disappears. The factory, meanwhile, is making good deals: It buys eggs on credit, at pre-devaluation prices, and sells its chickens at post-devaluation prices. By the end of September the staff receives its first wages ... and the factory is producing 50 tons of chicken; by December, seven times more. "The meat is sold the day it leaves the factory," the deputy director says happily: "We are still working at only 35 percent to 40 percent of capacity. And we cannot meet the demand." ... However, due to the lack of cash flow, the factory cannot invest in order to achieve "European quality." Its enormous debts—for gas, electricity, etc.—have been "rescheduled," i.e. frozen. ... Zarechnaya could double its production within a year. But with the threat of a return of foreign imports, its future remains uncertain."[32]

Chicken producers were not the only ones who feared aid. In May, Mr. Zhukov, director of the Russian Association of Grain

Producers, published an open letter to the minister of agriculture on the front page of a major Russian agricultural journal: "We cannot even sell our own seeds which are cheaper and of better quality. We don't need foreign seeds."[33] Leonid Kholod, former deputy minister of agriculture, thought the same: "Just when Russian farmers have a chance to take advantage of market trends and get off the ground, [the Government] goes and whacks them."[34] Andrei Sizov, an expert working for the Russian agricultural consultancy SovEcon, claimed: "From the point of view of traders, it deprives them of a market. These volumes, 500,000 tons of corn and 250,000 tons of soya beans, are enormous. They're twice Russia's annual imports. ... Traders also stand to suffer if Russia introduces measures to limit exports, as donors have insisted they do."[35] It should also be mentioned that the German government expressed similar reservations during the negotiations on European aid.

Supporters of the food aid, of course, rejected these arguments. As Asif Chaudhry explained, the USDA "selected only those products for which there are deficits; these products will be supplied to specific regions where they are not available. They will therefore not compete with Russian products anywhere." With regard to chicken, he pointed out that the United States was planning to provide Russia, as part of the aid program, with only fifty thousand tons, an insignificant amount compared to previous exports.[36] The agricultural attaché of the European Union in Moscow, Tom Wiley, explained that

> it is the Russian Government that has asked us for aid for winter because there were deficits. Taking into account the duration of the production cycle, in any case, Russian producers could not reduce these deficits till the beginning of the next season. Of course, if the aid lasted for several years, it would reduce incentive to produce; but we hope that by next season Russian farmers will already have produced more.[37]

Neither Kulik nor Semionov made, as far as we know, any public statements on this subject, though rumors in Moscow pointed to serious internal disagreements.

Whom Does Aid Profit?

This massive aid operation produced far more questions than answers. The opponents of the aid had just as few hard facts as its supporters. There were few truly convincing or even completely convinced answers to the critics' questions of whether this aid was really necessary or whether it would be harmful to Russian producers. There were assertions, but no proof. No one carried out any food security surveys or "vulnerability analysis mapping" that could concretely assess the food needs of the population. In fact, it seems clear that, given that the Russian government had asked for the aid and that for mainly political and economic reasons the request was granted, no one was interested in a genuine debate about these issues. Thus one should perhaps ask the following questions: Why was the aid requested? And why was it granted?

On the donors' side, things are clear. The U.S. secretary of agriculture, Dan Glickman, stated quite frankly: "This understanding is good news for the Russian people who might otherwise face the possibility of food shortages this winter and it is good news for America's farmers and ranchers, who are facing economic hardship related to abundant supplies and low prices."[38] The Europeans were more discreet in public, though the stakes were the same. The European aid, as an article in the *Guardian Weekly* pointed out, came out of

> surplus stocks that the EU buys from its farmers under the common agricultural policy (CAP) to keep prices high. [These products] are then stockpiled at considerable cost to taxpayers. The grain mountain is currently around 17 million tons—about 10% of the EU's annual production—and Europe was delighted at the prospect of Russia taking 1.5 million tons off its hands. Russia was also to take a third of the current stocks of 480.000 tons of beef, and most of the milk powder stocks too. [Furthermore] pork prices have collapsed to the point where farmers are selling the meat for less than the cost of raising a pig. So the European Commission thought it would be a good wheeze to buy pork on the market, thus raising the price, and send it off to Russia."[39]

And, in fact, the aid agreement was negotiated by the Commercial Service of the External Relations Department of the Commission, and the money to finance it came from the European Fund for the Orientation and Guarantee of Agriculture (EFOGA), the bureau within the Direction Générale VI of the European Commission (DG-6) that functions as the executive arm of the CAP.

The fact that these considerations were predominant does not mean that they were the only ones. "This aid," explained Gilbert Dubois, deputy head of the European Commission delegation in Russia, "is an important gesture to Russia from the political standpoint. It is a concrete expression of our aid. Our partner asked us for help and we gave it. This was reinforced by the situation in Yugoslavia: The Russian Government was afraid we would cut the aid, but we did not. On the contrary, it enabled us to send a clear message that even if there are local difficulties, we will not abandon Russia."[40] In any event, as the *Guardian Weekly* observed, "there was precious little else that Europe or the international community could do to assist Moscow. Because of the Russian default on its loans last August, the International Monetary Fund has decreed that there will be no Western loans or credits until the debt situation and the fate of Russian economic reforms have been settled."[41] It is no accident that one of the first Western voices to call for aid was that of the IMF.

On the Russian side, the stakes, on the contrary, were more obscure. To listen to the Russian press, the entire question simply came down to one of these affairs Russia has accustomed us to: Kulik would have launched and pushed this program simply to help some of his influential friends get richer. This is where the intermediaries come in: agents appointed by the Russian government to carry out the customs clearance, storage, and distribution of the aid. The background and method of selection of these agents are, to say the least, troubling. They were named in both the U.S. and European agreements: Roskhlebprodukt for wheat and rye, Raznoimport for rice, and Rosmyasomoltorg and Prodintorg for meat and powdered milk (the latter two, incidentally, have the same address and are considered by some observers to be one firm).

How were these firms selected? Curiously, Leonid Cheshinsky, the director of Roskhlebprodukt, was a member of the Russian delegation to the first aid negotiations, in October 1998. Immediately after the preliminary agreement with the United States, Kulik announced that Roskhlebprodukt and three other firms had been selected by the government to serve as intermediaries—a very lucrative function, as they were to receive a 3 percent commission on the amount of goods entrusted to them, amounting to roughly thirty million dollars in kind. Criticism was immediate. "Neither Prodintorg nor Myasomoltorg," according to Leonid Kholod, "are market leaders in the wholesale food trade." As for Roskhlebprodukt, its bad reputation preceded it: It had already "overseen the distribution of Western humanitarian aid in the early 1990s, when millions of dollars' worth of aid ended up in the pockets of private companies linked to corrupt officials."[42]

At first, Kulik stated that no open tender would be held: "A tender has to be announced one month in advance. The process itself will take one more month, and then we will have another two months of blah-blah." But according to a 1996 presidential decree, this type of federal contract must be put up for tender. Kulik answered that "a law could be passed to authorize the new scheme."[43] After strong pressure from the Ministry of Agriculture, and probably from the

Americans and the Europeans, a "closed" tender was issued, the terms and procedures of which were not disclosed: The same companies were selected.[44]

The accusations against Roskhlebprodukt, in particular, started piling up in the press. Grigory Yavlinsky, leader of the political party Yabloko, publicly accused Gennady Kulik of corruption. The tender also seemed to have been irregular. According to *Izvestia*, "only organizations that have no debts to the State are allowed to take part in such a tender. ... [However, Roskhlebprodukt] still owes 1.3 billion roubles to the budget."[45] The same article quoted a *Newsweek* article that, in discussing the diversions and other manipulations that overshadowed the 1992–1993 aid program, specifically fingered Roskhlebprodukt and opposed its participation in the current operation. For part of the Russian press, there could be no doubt: Kulik cried famine and requested the aid simply in order to hand it over to his friend Cheshinsky and to draw an enormous profit from it—at least one hundred million dollars, without even stealing any of it, but simply by playing on price differentials in the regions.[46]

Russian journalists were not the only ones who worried about the fate of the aid. Four days after signing the European agreement, Jacques Santer, president of the European Commission, confessed on Luxemburg television:

> But I tell you now, as I told the European Council, I cannot guarantee that the food will end up in the right hands. We don't have the staff to do it. With the mess that currently reigns in Russia, I'm sure that the EU Court of Auditors will come back in three or four years, when it makes its report on this, and conclude, "There were irregularities. Santer let it happen again." ... But how do we control that? We cannot guarantee ... that the money won't end up in the hands of the Russian mafia, or the beef we send them won't be exported back to us. How on earth can we control that from Brussels?[47]

The obsession with diversion, however, seems to us (as J. C. Rufin noted in his discussion of the ARA; see Note 7) a false problem. It mattered little, in fact, that Roskhlebprodukt might sell the food a bit more expensively than the prices fixed in the agreements and pocket the profits, as long as the sums agreed upon in fact reached the Pension Fund. It mattered little whether Cheshinsky or even Kulik was corrupt or not, as long as the aid achieved its goals. We shall see further on if this is the case.

The paranoia of the Russian media is quite understandable, given the current climate in the country. However, it seems difficult to believe that corruption was the primary motive behind the request for aid—a request that, let us not forget, initially came from Primakov, who has never been accused of corruption by anyone, even if the negotiations were then conducted and concluded by Kulik. The West, in spite of—or perhaps because of—all the blunders made in Russia, is not naive. Yes, the cries about famine were grossly exaggerated, but the issue of agricultural deficits was real, as was the issue of the aid's effect on local production. If the aid were truly harmful, the West might well think that the Russians would not have asked for it. It was for them, after all, to determine their needs.

It is probably easier to understand Kulik's motives if one understands his logic. "Kulik is not a man of the market," a World Bank expert explained, "he is a man who still thinks in terms of a planned economy. And according to this logic, 'the more you have, the better.' This foreign food aid policy was simply not thought through. Kulik has very little knowledge in this field and he was very ill-advised."[48] Thus, the problem of the producers was not seen as a problem of the market, but simply as a problem of lack of the resources that the state should provide. For Kulik, as for his Communist allies, such an operation could only be profitable. From a personal standpoint, it enabled Kulik to personally plan and allocate massive amounts of food. It boosted his image and consequently his authority and power. All of Russia's governors, in order to receive a part of the aid, would have to go through him. From a political standpoint, this operation could be presented to the electorate as a great success of the Communists. Numerous sources confirmed that during the negotiations, Kulik's first priority was the Pension Fund, meaning the monetization of the aid in order to feed the special account opened for this purpose.[49] Pensioners, of course, are the main source of Communist support. The "humanitarian" aspect of the aid could also be used by the Communists, who could portray the distribution as a result of their efforts (although this seems to have been a lesser priority for Kulik than the Pension Fund).

Large Numbers of Vulnerable People

As we suggested earlier, over and above all these debates, the needs remain. And needs there are. Food insecurity is considerable and widespread throughout Russian society. It is not, of course, a matter of famine, like that of 1921–1922 and 1932–1933. It is rather a question of chronic undernutrition, of deficiencies in micronutrients, and so on. Such problems nationwide can have a serious impact: severe problems of growth and development for children; increased vulnerability of adults to opportunistic infections, especially tuberculosis, which has reached epidemic proportions in Russia; increased mortality rate for elderly people, clearly seen in the abrupt drop in average life expectancy.

Who indeed are the main victims of these problems? First, the elderly, who are strongly dependent on their pensions. The purchasing power of those pensions has collapsed (the average monthly pension of about 300 roubles in August 1999 was worth less than fifteen dollars); furthermore, the pensions are rarely paid on time. The next group of victims is people living in institutions: prisoners (more than one million in Russia), orphans or abandoned children, insane patients, and others. In hospitals, patients have to provide not only their medicine, but also their own food. And even when the food available in such institutions gives enough or nearly enough calories, it lacks variety: no meat, no fresh vegetables, no dairy products, only cabbage, potatoes, and *kasha* (groats of various grain). The prisons and children's institutions somehow survive, coping in different ways: bakeries to produce goods to sell and to produce their own food, potato farming, small businesses running at 10 percent capacity. Worse still is the situation of vulnerable persons living among the general population: millions of sick or isolated elderly people without a garden plot, without a family, without friends. This is to say nothing of people without documents and of homeless people, whose situation is catastrophic: Last winter more than 116 of them died of cold in the streets of Moscow, by far the most affected city in the country.

The food aid program, according to Asif Chaudhry, had two objectives: to help reduce deficits in the regions and to build up the Pension Fund through monetization.[50] We have seen that while the first purpose remained ambiguous, the second one was less so. The main criticism in this area concerned the Russian government's ability to collect the money and the donors' ability to monitor and guarantee the operation. The most pessimistic, such as *Izvestia,* went so far as to suggest that most of the money would be stolen or siphoned off by the regions. But the system set up by the donors to guarantee the transfer of the money to the two special accounts opened by the Ministry of Finance (from which it would be transferred to the Pension Fund) seemed—as far as is possible in a country such as Russia—well thought out and transparent.

Let us consider the U.S. arrangement (the European one does not differ much). First, a set price would be fixed for each allotment: That is, for a given region and a given amount of food products, a joint U.S.-Russian commission would fix the "value at the port of entry," the sum to be transferred to the special account. Storage and transportation costs would subsequently be bedded. The final price would be the one paid by the "first purchaser" in each region, usually a state company, sometimes a wholesaler or a private food processing factory. Each receiving region would sign a guarantee with the Ministry of Agriculture, certifying that the money would be paid back to the special account. In addition, given the nonpayment problems that plague Russia, the Ministry of Finance agreed to set a "hook" on this money: For any region that did not pay by a set deadline, the sum of the debt would be deducted from the money that the Federal government owed to that region for its budget payments and would be transferred directly into the special account. The American Embassy was to check all bank transactions, and at some point an independent firm would carry out an external audit.

According to Asif Chaudhry, the first payments were paid into the special account by May 1999.[51] And the Russian government seemed so sure of the income to be obtained under this system that in May it borrowed a large sum from Sberbank to pay pensions, an amount that would be reimbursed from the revenues obtained from the food aid. It seemed that the government's anxiety over the Pension Fund was real and that the system adopted certainly did not rely on the good will of the regions to collect the money.

But even the timely payment of pensions lagged far behind the needs. We have already mentioned the issue of food accessibility: Even with 300 roubles, how can one hope to survive if a loaf of bread costs 5 roubles and a subway ticket is 3 roubles? The fact that statistically speaking there might be enough sugar or powdered milk in a given region did not mean that people could buy such products: A third of the population was thought to lack the necessary purchasing power. Only direct and free aid held out any hope for helping these people. And as far as we are concerned, this remains the only criterion by which one can judge the aid operations.

The United States, as we have seen, planned from the very start to distribute a considerable quantity of free food: five hundred thousand tons in total, twice as much as the aid distributed by the World Food Program in North Korea, where a genuine famine raged. Considering the bad experiences of previous aid operations, one could fear the worst for the 400,000-ton allotment to be distributed directly by the government. "When [the products] get to the regions," said Arkady Zloshevsky, the director general of OGO, a major firm on the Russian seed market, "there will be governors who will provide [Western] officials with the documentation about the aid distribution. But they will only give them access to select information. No Western observer will ever really be able to ascertain how the aid was actually distributed."[52] We have also seen Jacques Santer's opinion on this point. Finally, as Roman Serbyn, a historian at Quebec University, pointed out: "To reach the needy population, control must be exercised by the donating agency and not be left to the [local] authorities."[53] Yet U.S. officials offered assurance that strict control mechanisms would be put into place, with complete lists of beneficiary institutions and U.S. monitors who would carry out spot checks in almost every region concerned. The remaining 100,000 tons were to be distributed directly by reliable international organizations such as the IFRC.

The European Union had not planned any direct aid within the framework of this operation. Of all the issues raised, this one seems to us to be the most open to criticism. Why is it that the EU is not planning direct aid? In fact, the European aid agreements at least considered the possibility of direct aid;[54] and some European officials, in particular those within the European delegation in Moscow, would like to have seen a humanitarian component in their operation. At the beginning of March 1999, the deputy head of delegation went so far as to propose quantities of food to a number of humanitarian organizations, such as the IFRC and Action Against Hunger. This offer was rejected, however, because the European Union was unable to pay the high costs of transport, distribution, and monitoring involved in such a program. The problem was mainly of a bureaucratic nature: The food aid was managed by the DG-6, or more precisely by the EFOGA, which (unlike the USDA, which is structured differently) has no budget for humanitarian aid. ECHO, for its part, explained to the humanitarian organizations that, since DG-6 had given Russia so much food, ECHO could not do anything extra.

Financing a program to distribute food under DG-6 control was also impossible. The question was raised in mid-March by IFRC and Action Against Hunger at a meeting with a European parliamentary delegation in charge of relations with Russia: Constance Krehl, a member of the European Parliament and head of the delegation, promised to try to find a way out of the impasse in consultation with Emma Bonino, the then–European commissioner for humanitarian aid. Unfortunately, the very next day the latter had to resign along with the entire commission. This final attempt therefore remained fruitless.

The European Union did not even try to push the Russians to distribute part of the aid themselves, as the Americans had done. Neither the high-ranking European officials from the Commercial Service of the External Relations, who negotiated the agreements, nor the DG-6, which was concerned only with getting rid of CAP stocks as cheaply as possible and agreed to pay transport only up to the Russian border, paid any attention to the question. The Russian side also showed limited interest. That is regrettable.

A balanced assessment of this massive and costly operation has yet to be carried out and will undoubtedly take some time. It is still too early to follow in the footsteps of numerous critics and to assert that the economic interests of the donors were incompatible with genuine and effective aid. At this point we simply deplore the fact that the European Union, a victim of its own bureaucratic restrictions, was unable to take into account not only its own interests and those of Yevgeny Primakov's government, but also those of the most vulnerable and disadvantaged populations of Russia.

Notes

Jonathan Littell is head of mission, Action Against Hunger–Russia.

1. Kirill Koriukin, "IMF Calls for Food, Cabinet for Cash," *Moscow Times*, 21 October 1998.

2. Quoted in ibid.

3. All U.S. agreements are available on the USDA Web site: http://www.usda.gov.

4. The two core documents are the Memorandum of Understanding on Implementation of Free Delivery of Food Products, dated 20 January 1999 and the Operational Memorandum of Understanding Concerning the Implementation of Free Delivery of Food Products, dated 19 February 1999, which complements and clarifies the first one. The 19 February agreement listed the food products to be given: wheat, 1 million tons; rye, 0.5 million tons; white rice, 50,000 tons; beef, 150,000 tons; pork, 100,000 tons; and dry milk, 50,000 tons.

5. "US Aid Saves Face, Not Russia," *Moscow Times*, 5 November 1998.

6. Ibid.

7. Jean-Claude Rufin, *Le Piège humanitaire* (Paris: J. C. Lattes, 1986), pp. 39–40.

8. Robert Conquest, *The Harvest of Sorrows* (Oxford: N.p., 1985). This is a key book on the history of collectivization and the manipulation of famine in the USSR.

9. François Bonnet, "Moscow Wants to Negotiate Massive Food Imports at Very Low Prices," *Le Monde*, 29 October 1998.

10. Associated Press dispatch quoted in the *Moscow Times*, 21 October 1998.

11. Bonnet, "Moscow Wants to Negotiate Massive Food Imports at Very Low Prices."

12. Ibid.

13. Kirill Koriukin, "Minister: Food Will Last Winter," *Moscow Times*, 30 October 1998.

14. Igor Korolkov, "Zachem Kulik pugal stranu golodom," *Izvestia*, 12 April 1999.

15. Koriukin, "Minister: Food Will Last Winter."

16. "Russia Rejects the Dumping of Foreign Food Aid," *Agence France Presse,* 29 October 1998.

17. "No Danger of Famine This Winter, According to Minister of Agriculture," *Agence France Presse,* 24 November 1998.

18. "Russia Lacks 7 Million Tons of Cereals," *Agence France Presse,* 30 November 1998.

19. Declaration in *Komsomolskaia Pravda,* reprinted in "Russia Claims It Has Sufficient Food Reserves for 1999," *Agence France Presse,* 26 December 1998.

20. "No Hunger in Russia," *Interfax,* 2 February 1999.

21. Korolgov, "Zachem Kulik pugal stranu golodom."

22. Personal discussion with a European Union expert. Moscow, n.d.

23. During the great famine of 1932–1933, for example, peasants only really began to die on a mass scale from March 1933 onward. Cf. Conquest, *The Harvest of Sorrows.*

24. Discussion with Ruslan Musaiev, director of the pretrial detention center of Kyzyl, Mowcow, n.d.

25. Discussion with Asif Chaudhry, minister-counselor for agriculture of the United States Embassy in Moscow, Moscow, n.d.

26. Private discussion with a food security expert of the World Bank, Moscow, n.d. In the end, the Russian authorities simply fixed the prices of basic food items in most regions, driving a number of businesses, including bakeries, close to bankruptcy.

27. Ibid.

28. "Poor Hungry Russia Sells Food to the West," *Moscow Times,* 14 November 1998.

29. In 1997, Russia imported thirteen billion dollars worth of food, that is, a third of the total consumption of the country. See "Does Russia Need Food Aid? Even Donors Ask," *Reuters,* 26 November 1998.

30. Discussion with Asif Chaudhry, USDA.

31. Veronique Soule, "La 'cuisse de Bush' donne la chair de poule," *Libération,* 28 December 1998.

32. Ibid.

33. Quoted in *Selskaia Jizn,* 5 May 1999.

34. Kirill Koriukin, "Russia Takes Up EU Offer of Aid," *Moscow Times,* 13 November 1999.

35. "Does Russia Need Food Aid? Even Donors Ask."

36. Discussion with Asif Chaudhry, USDA.

37. Discussion with Tom Wiley, agricultural attaché, delegation of the European Commission in Russia, Moscow, n.d.

38. "Statement by Agricultural Secretary Dan Glickman on Food Aid for Russia," Release no. 0459.98, 6 November 1998 (press release available on the USDA Web site: http://www.usda.gov).

39. Martin Walker, "EU Aid to Russia Gives Food for Nought," *Guardian Weekly,* 28 February 1999.

40. Discussion with Gilbert Dubois, deputy head of delegation, European Commission Delegation in Russia, Moscow, n.d.

41. Walker, "EU Aid to Russia Gives Food for Nought."

42. Kirill Koriukin, "US Trusts Russia's Aid Distribution," *Moscow Times,* 10 November 1998.

43. Koriukin, "Russia Takes Up EU Offer of Aid."

44. Kirill Koriukin, "Tender for Food Aid Picks Insider Trio," *Moscow Times*, 11 December 1998.

45. Korolkov, "Zachem Kulik pugal stranu golodom."

46. Ibid. The arguments about price differentials are rather complicated and cannot be summed up here. However, considering the system that had been set up for fixing prices ahead of time, such discrepancies should not occur, though a certain profit could still remain theoretically possible.

47. Walker, "EU Aid to Russia Gives Food for Nought."

48. Private discussion with a food security expert of the World Bank.

49. Discussion with Gilbert Dubois, European Commission Delegation in Russia.

50. Discussion with Asif Chaudhry, USDA.

51. Ibid.

52. Quoted in Yevgenia Borisova, "Devil Is in Details for European Food Aid," *Moscow Times*, 12 February 1999.

53. Quoted in Leonid Bershidsky, "Russia Agonizes over Accepting Aid," *Moscow Times*, 22 October 1998.

54. The Operational Memorandum of Understanding Concerning the Implementation of Free Delivery of Food Products actually notes in article 3.7 that "in exceptional cases, a portion of the products may be distributed free of charge to the most vulnerable part of the population in these regions." But no serious measures have been taken to carry out this provision, either on the Russian or the European side.

31

Hunger in the United States

Trudy Lieberman

Randall Mueck's job at San Francisco's meal clearinghouse is to decide who will get food and who will wait. Hundreds of the city's homebound elderly are on Mueck's waiting list, and the number grows each month. All qualify for a hot, home-delivered meal under the federal Older Americans Act, but there isn't enough money to feed everyone.

Seniors who move up the fastest are those in the custody of adult protective services, the dying, and the very old. Twenty-five percent of the people asking for food are over ninety. "I try to think of all 411 [on the waiting list] and fit someone in accordingly," Mueck explains. "Age is going to bump somebody way up."

Audrey Baker, age seventy-nine, waited more than four months for food. When she first asked for help, Mueck assigned her 750 points out of the 900 or so she needed to qualify for a meal. By the time she reached 877, she was almost at the head of the queue. (Each day on the list adds a point.) Baker, a thin woman, is blind, falls a lot, and broke her back. She also has hypertension and diabetes. "I've outlived everybody else in my family," Baker says. "I don't have any friends." Her only help is an aide who comes for two hours on Friday. Like many seniors, Baker is vague about what she eats. "It's whatever I can afford," she says. One night it was only an apple

This chapter is an adaptation by the author of "Hunger in America" from *The Nation* (30 March 1998) and "Hunger Watch: America's Elders Are Waiting for Food" from *Aging Today* (January/February 1999) by Trudy Lieberman.

and some nuts. She had a chicken in the freezer, but no strength to cook it.

Food isn't far from her mind, though. On the table beside the armchair in her tiny living room is a copy of the food magazine *Cooking Light*, in braille. "She's clearly struggling," says Frank Mitchell, a social worker with San Francisco's Meals on Wheels program. "How do you say, 'I know you're hungry. We'll serve you in three months?'"

But that's the reality all across the country. Thousands of elderly men and women too infirm to cook or even see the flames of the stove are put on ration lists for food in the most bountiful country in the world. A 1993 study by the Urban Institute found that some five million elderly have no food in the house, or worry about getting enough to eat. They experience what the social service business calls "food insecurity." In Miami alone, two thousand people are waiting. Says John Stokesberry, executive director of Miami's Alliance for Aging, "By the time we clean up the waiting list, some will be dead." Another study, done for the federal Administration on Aging, looked at food programs during the 1993–1995 period and found that 41 percent of the country's four thousand providers of home-delivered meals to the elderly had waiting lists. Malnutrition among the elderly is commonplace; researchers at Florida International University estimate that 63 percent of all older people are at moderate or high nutritional risk. Some 88 percent of those receiving home-delivered meals are at similar risk, according to a study by Mathematica Policy Research.

In the face of shifting demographics, the picture is not likely to improve. The number of people 60 and older has increased from 31 million in 1973 to 44 million today. And the number of the oldest of the old, those over 85, for whom assistance with meals is crucial, is growing even faster: Nearly 1.5 million people were over 85 in 1970; in 2000, their number will exceed 4 million.

The homebound elderly are largely invisible. They are not glamorous, and giving them food is not at the cutting edge of philanthropy. They are the antithesis of the "greedy geezer" who has come to represent all of the elderly in the public mind. They have no lobbyists—the interests of senior organizations lie elsewhere. Politicians neglect them: They do not vote or make campaign contributions. Often their children have moved far from home, leaving them without caregivers, a dilemma more keenly felt by women, who usually live longer than men. In 1970, 56 percent of the elderly over age seventy-five lived alone; by 1995, 76 percent were living by themselves.

For many, there are no meal lists to get on. In Big Springs, a speck on the Nebraska prairie, 134 of the town's 495 residents are eligible for a meal. But there is no money to start a program. Vic Walker, director of the Aging Office of Western Nebraska, does not even have enough money to feed those outside the city limits of Scottsbluff, the largest town in the area. One man living on a ranch three miles over the line "needed a meal so desperately," recalls Irma Walter, Walker's case manager. "He was so debilitated, but there was no access to food."

The Federal Commitment

Thirty-five years ago, in 1965, Congress recognized the lengthening life span and the infirmities that come with old age and enacted the Older Americans Act to help seniors live out their last days at home with essential support: transportation, household help, and personal care. The act is not a welfare program; anyone over age sixty is eligible for services if there is room.

In his 1972 budget message, President Nixon noted that a "new commitment to the aging is long overdue," and two nutrition programs were added that year: (1) centralized, or congregate, meal sites—now numbering about sixteen thousand—where seniors could eat a hot lunch and socialize and (2) a delivery service to serve a hot meal to the homebound elderly. Meals prepared by a cadre of local churches, social service agencies, and nonprofit organizations, many with similar names, were meant to reach mobile seniors and the homebound in every nook and cranny of the United States.

The food programs were supposed to promote "better health" among the older population "through improved nutrition" and offer "older Americans an opportunity to live their remaining years in dignity." Nixon pledged that the federal commitment would "help make the last days of our older Americans their best days."

At the beginning, Nixon tried to make good on that promise. When the Office of Management and Budget thought the initial funding should be $40 million, and Nixon's adviser on aging, Dr. Arthur Flemming, suggested $60 million, Nixon upped the amount to $100 million. Throughout the 1970s, funding kept pace with need. After that, however, it did not. Adjusting for inflation, per capita appropriations for all Older Americans Act programs in 1995 should have been $39. Actual per capita funding was only $19. Although total annual spending for services has gone from $200 million in 1973 to almost $900 million today, that money not only has not kept up with inflation but has not kept pace with the number of people who need help. The 1995 appropriations were down by about 50 percent relative to what the government spent in 1973. Money spent on the two food programs shrank by a similar amount.

Though payment is not mandatory, three-quarters of the elderly who get a home-delivered meal and almost everyone who eats at the congregate sites contributes, sometimes as little as fifty cents, toward the roughly $5.30 it costs to provide a meal. Half of those receiving home-delivered meals and about one-third of participants eating at congregate meal sites have annual incomes of less than $7,900. "Those least able to pay won't eat unless they put something in," says Larry Ross, the chief fiscal officer for San Francisco's Commission on the Aging.

The Vanishing Commitment

By today's standards, Nixon's game of one-upmanship seems so out of place it could have happened in another dimension. If anything, the federal commitment to the elderly has diminished, partly because the antigovernment ideology that has so permeated the public psyche has taken its toll on such basic programs as providing food for old people and partly because no congressional hero has emerged to champion the needs of the elderly. Indeed it is now fashionable to heap scorn on organizations like the American Association of Retired Persons (AARP) and to address all of the elderly as rich geezers who take money from the public table.

So it was hardly surprising that when the deals were cut on the omnibus appropriations bill that went through Congress in the fall of 1998, programs for the elderly came up short. The amount allocated to congregate meals remained at $374 million; the sum for home-delivered meals was $112 million—the same funding levels as the year before. To make matters worse, $390 million was cut from the Social Services Block Grant, on which many local food programs rely in order to feed the homebound elderly.

It was a long shot that more money would be coming. The Clinton administration budget did not call for an increase. When the proposed budget for that year was announced, Secretary of Health and Human Services Donna Shalala was asked by a reporter why no increase had been requested for programs aimed at older people, given the growing number of people who need help. Shalala replied: "Obviously we had to make some choices. What we recommend is sufficient for next year."

In the meantime, waiting lists have grown longer in some parts of the country even though there has been a federal budget surplus of more than seventy million dollars.

The budget gave bipartisan rewards to current and former members of Congress. Mitch McConnell, Patrick Leahy, Claiborne Pell, Paul Simon, and Robert Dole received a total of $21 million from taxpayers to preserve their legacies at various libraries and institutes—a sum that would have bought more than four million meals. There was also plenty of money for the military—for instance, the fifty million dollars for parts for a helicopter that the Navy did not request.

Programs in Health and Human Services that compete for funding with the food programs got gigantic increases. The National Institute of Health got a $2 billion raise, the Head Start budget rose by $300 million, and the Centers for Disease Control received a $200 million increase.

Why does research on mundane subjects like grasshoppers rate higher than hunger when it comes to congressional largesse? Probably because if the government pays the research and development costs of finding a new treatment for some disease, or if it helps farmers grow better lettuce, private business can benefit from the technology and make money. Nobody profits from feeding the elderly.

In the 1999 budget, the Clinton administration asked for a modest $35 million increase in the budget for home-delivered meals. By fall 1999, the Senate had approved the increase, boosting the total allocated to home-delivered meals to $147 million. However, a House appropriations committee recommended no increase, leaving the funding at the same level as the year before. It is not clear whether more money will be going into home-delivered meals in the final budget bill that passes Congress. Competition for funds in the Labor, Education, and Health and Human Services appropriations bill (where funding for the food programs resides) is tough. Food programs do not have forceful lobbyists or congressional champions; biotechnology firms do.

Furthermore, the Older Americans Act itself is in trouble. For the last several years, Congress has refused to reauthorize the act, which provides the only federal framework for services to the elderly. Without the act in place, various programs could be parceled out to the states in the form of block grants, and the states could decide whether or not to fund them. Services, however scarce today, could become even scarcer.

The dispute over reauthorization involves money that goes to organizations such as AARP, Green Thumb, and the National Council of Senior Citizens, which accept federal money to administer job-training programs for the elderly. Conservative members of Congress and right-wing organizations want to end federal grants and send the programs to the states. For some of the groups that receive funds, federal money is a matter of survival.

One Meal a Day

It is not that the elderly who are currently receiving meals are living high on the hog. In fact, they get only 260 meals a year, or one meal a day five days a week (most Americans eat three meals a day—1,095 a year). Usually no food is delivered on weekends or holidays unless a program has raised outside funds to provide it. Only 4 percent of food providers routinely offer more than one meal a day, five days a week, and few offer weekend meals. In San Francisco, some eight hundred people lucky enough to receive their food from Meals on Wheels, one of the city's nine providers, get two meals seven days a week. The rest of the city's sixteen hundred food recipients get only one. If the city's Commission on the Aging paid for two meals per person, as many as four hundred people now served would not get any food. The trade-off is constant and stark: Do more people get fewer meals, or do fewer people get more meals?

The Salvation Army, which serves the meals in San Francisco's Tenderloin district, resolves the question in favor of the former, but there is pain whichever way it is answered. Richard Bertolovzi lives in a single-room-occupancy (S.R.O.) hotel. He is a skinny, bearded man with greasy hair, missing front teeth, and one red eye that looks infected. "You don't deliver tomorrow, do you?" "Bert" asks the young woman delivering his noon meal of fish, coleslaw, fruit cocktail, corn bread, and milk. A curtain of disappointment falls over his face, and he looks away in disgust. "I'm hungry," he says. "I can eat anything. I have a loaf of bread, that's all. That's all I got. And I got some instant coffee." The Salvation Army is able to offer him only a can of Ensure, a nutritional drink, to get through the weekend.

The Limits of Philanthropy

The conventional wisdom these days is that philanthropy should do more and government as little as possible, or, as Heritage Foundation senior fellow Dan Mitchell puts it, "If it's worth doing, the private sector can do it."

When it comes to feeding the elderly, private-sector funding works a little bit in a few places, not at all in most others. In San Francisco, Meals on Wheels can raise thousands of dollars each year, thanks in part to fancy dinners cooked by the city's top chefs. Its New York counterpart can raise eight or nine million dollars through direct mail campaigns, social events, grants, and corporate contributions to provide some weekend meals and to whittle down the city's waiting list. Celebrities like Lena Horne and Diane Sawyer think nothing of plunking down two or three hundred dollars to attend a Meals on Wheels event.

But towns like Ramona, California, population thirty thousand, high in the hills northeast of San Diego, have no such benefactors. Chuck Hunt, board president of the town's senior center, tells how he placed ads in the *Ramona Sentinel* and *North County Times* asking one thousand people to pledge $100 or two thousand people to give $50. He collected exactly $1,600—twelve people gave $100 and got on the center's "honor roll"; eight donated $50 for a place on the "silver honor roll." Hunt also wrote to Allied Signal Aerospace, where he had worked for twenty-six years, asking for $25,000 to pay down overdue food bills and take care of repairs on the vans that deliver meals. He says he felt "let down" when his old employer said no.

Raising private money in places like Ramona or Big Springs or even San Diego is not easy. There are few large corporations and foundations to tap, and if there are any, they have little interest in feeding the elderly. "If you flat-out ask people for food for seniors, you don't get much of a response," said Daniel Laver, who headed the Area Agency on Aging in San Diego. "Private foundations are looking at cutting-edge programs—new and innovative. Basic human needs programs are not as sexy."

State and Local Aid

States must contribute at least 15 percent of the total cost of the two federal meal programs. Some states go beyond that. Pennsylvania, for instance, contributes its lottery proceeds to services for the elderly. Local governments sometimes kick in money, and where they do, those funds help keep the food programs afloat. County funds, including a dedicated portion of San Francisco's parking tax, make up about 38 percent of the California budget for home-delivered meals. The city of New York contributes 55 percent of the food program budget. Voters in Cincinnati have twice approved a property tax levy to support a variety of services for the elderly, most recently in the fall of 1998 by a margin of 65 to 35 percent. Eighty-three percent of Cincinnati's Council on Aging's $4.1 million budget for home-delivered meals is funded by the tax levy. "It's a myth that people don't want to help their elderly," says Bob Logan, director of the council, the agency serving the Cincinnati area. He says the levy "was overwhelmingly supported by the young, the old, Republicans, Democrats, minorities and nonminorities." But even a generous stream of local money cannot stop waiting lists from mounting: In Cincinnati, local money just means those on the lists do not have to wait as long.

Penny-Wise and Pound-Foolish

The United States has no national policy on aging. Instead, an unwritten policy directs resources to the most expensive care in the last places the elderly reside—nursing homes and hospitals. When malnourished seniors go to the hospital, they may end up staying longer and costing more money. The Massachusetts Dietetic Association estimates that for every dollar spent on nutrition programs, $3.25 is saved in hospital costs. A study in Little Rock, Arkansas, compared two groups of hospitalized seniors who were the same age and had the same diagnosis. One group had received home-delivered meals; the other group had not. Patients who got food stayed in the hospital half as long as those who did not. Ronni Chernoff, associate director of geriatric research at the Veterans Administration hospital in Little Rock, who supervised the research, figured that the cost of eight extra days in the hospital—some $4,800 at Little Rock rates—was the equivalent of providing someone with a meal a day for two and a half years.

An acute episode, such as breaking a bone, healing a surgical incision, or the flu, makes demands that a poorly nourished body cannot accommodate. "The people I'm not serving but know in my heart of hearts I should are those just coming out of the hospital," says Gail Robillard, a nutritionist with the Jefferson Council on Aging in Metairie, Louisiana. Without such assistance, they often go back to the hospital, a vicious cycle that Robillard believes can be prevented with good nutrition. Medicare's home health care benefit covers the services of nurses, aides, and a variety of therapies, but not food.

Without food, the elderly also go to nursing homes prematurely, adding to what is already a huge national expense. The United States spends about $80 billion a year on nursing home care, nearly half paid by taxpayers through Medicaid. A year in a nursing home averages around $40,000; a year's worth of meals, $1,325. Lack of a coherent national policy on aging stems partly from a deep collective denial that our population is aging and will need services. We may all need home-delivered meals someday, but it's best not to think about that now. Part of the public's apathy results from a basic lack of sales appeal, important in a country that responds more easily to sound bites than to alleviating human suffering. Sickness caused by hunger does not have the same cachet as sickness caused by disease. That's why research at the National Institute of Health is seen as more glamorous and more worthy than everyday assistance provided by area agencies on aging.

It is indeed ironic that the United States is willing to spend billions on treatments to prolong life but gives short shrift to basic human needs such as food and transportation that make that longer life worth living. In 1963, President Kennedy, quoting the historian Arnold Toynbee, noted in a special message to Congress that "a society's quality and durability can be measured by the 'respect and care given its elderly citizens.'" So far, we are not measuring up.

Notes

Trudy Lieberman is director of the Consumers Union's Center for Consumer Health Choices.

32

Food Aid and Grain

José Bidegain and Astrid Filliol

> *We cannot say we did not know.*
> *We cannot say there was nothing we could do.*
> —Action Against Hunger Campaign, 1998–1999

Recent events have demonstrated as never before the extent to which food aid remains an essential form of assistance, even in Europe. It is useful to recall this as we note the steady decline in recent years in global food aid (from 17.3 million tons in 1993 to 8 million tons in 1998, with grain accounting for 90 percent of the total) both for economic reasons and as a result of the doubts that have been expressed in some quarters concerning the effectiveness of this instrument.

This situation, however, contradicts the results of a survey that ranks hunger in the world as one of the main subjects of concern to French public opinion at the century's end.[1] This ranking is justified, as surveys conducted by the Food and Agriculture Organization clearly show: More than 830 million people in the world suffer from chronic malnutrition; 30 to 60 million, victims of disasters, suffer from severe hunger.

The projected increase in world food needs does not hold out hope for any visible improvement in the situation. Moreover, this malnutrition is not a result of insufficient production, since the food that is available is quite enough, and the planet is perfectly capable of producing more food. Many countries that request aid are also exporters of food products (for instance, Sudan and Burma).

We at Action Against Hunger have been taking effective action in the field for some twenty years now to combat the problem of food shortages in forty countries spread across four continents. We are aware of the causes of hunger that are first and foremost man-made:

war, crises that are predominantly economic, absence of reserves to be used when conditions are temporarily unfavorable, embargoes, and so on. Indeed, food has become the weapon of choice in modern conflict.

In situations of crisis, which require solutions of a political, economic, or social nature, it must be noted that food aid, unfortunately, still remains today the response that is best suited, at least in the short term, if the aim is to limit the consequences of man-made disasters.

It remains clear, however, that this instrument can in no way replace what must be the principal objective of governments and of the international community: rebuilding the capacity of the populations to feed themselves. In this area, Action Against Hunger, unlike other international organizations specializing in the field of food aid, such as the World Food Program, offers more than a humanitarian logistics network.

Indeed, our activities are based on two highly complementary pillars: translating into action the fundamental ethical principles enshrined in our charter and using the technical and professional expertise of our technical departments at headquarters and of our teams in the field. Independence, neutrality, and nondiscrimination are the core principles of our demand for free and direct access to victims. The distribution of food products is carried out directly by our teams, which comprise residents of the receiving country under the supervision of expatriate professionals. We are able to monitor the effectiveness of our work, since we maintain an active presence among the vulnerable populations as we implement our programs.

It should be pointed out that this task is carried out with complete transparency, and we are accountable to our donors and partners.

Before any intervention, we of course undertake a review of the socioeconomic situation of the country so that our activities would respect the balance that exists; we learn the food and family habits of the populations concerned as well as their coping mechanisms with the aim of supporting them. This preliminary study enables us to undertake a sound evaluation of needs and to focus accurately on vulnerable populations.

The programs are based on a comprehensive and well-tested methodology that comprises various methods of food distribution, re-nutrition protocols for at-risk groups, and the use of foods that are specially suited to children and adults most severely affected by malnutrition. Notable among these foods is the therapeutic milk F100, developed in collaboration with the laboratory Nutriset, by the

Nutrition Department of Action Against Hunger and now used by all organizations throughout the world.

There are two types of programs: emergency programs that provide care for crisis victims (residents, displaced persons, refugees) and long-term programs, particularly in the field of agricultural rehabilitation. The latter seek to enable populations living in precarious conditions to reestablish their means of production and regain self-sufficiency (distribution of seeds, irrigation, and agricultural improvements).

While the long-term objectives remain essentially the same, the methods employed can and should be adapted to the particular characteristics and to the nature of the emergency. On the one hand, food aid through local purchases offers the advantage of being totally integrated into the structure of the local market and thus has a spin-off multiplier effect on the economic mechanisms. On the other hand, the use of food aid in the form of physical stock is indispensable when local purchases of food are likely to cause undesirable increases in price, especially in times of severe shortages. This mode of intervention also facilitates the monitoring of rations and permits greater flexibility.

Since the embargo imposed by the United Nations on Sierra Leone in 1997, which has prevented the shipment of essential food aid, we have sought to obtain the capacity to conduct this type of food aid operation by ourselves and in complete independence. We would do so in the form of physical stocks of food for situations in which the World Food Program is subject to very severe political pressures.

Given the important role of cereals in food aid, Action Against Hunger needed to sensitize grain producers to the food emergency. Cereals, supplemented by rations of oil and proteins, are in effect the key foods that should be provided in emergency situations because of their extraordinary nutritional qualities. Ultimately, it will also be useful to develop technologies for the enrichment of the grains themselves. The conditions under which grains are transported and stored also determine the effectiveness of distribution arrangements.

The know-how is already available in France, a major grain producer, which sees itself as having the "vocation to feed the world" through its substantial exports. It was therefore logical that Action Against Hunger should turn toward grain producers to obtain the indispensable support of their undeniable professional and organizational skills. Our partnership has demonstrated its effectiveness in two quite different types of emergency situations:

- temporary or situation-based emergencies, for which it is essential to intervene within a few days, as was the case in Kosovo.
- chronic and therefore more predictable emergencies, for which a longer-term response is required, as was the case in Sierra Leone.

Some 740 tons of wheat flour were thus used to supply bread to 50,000 refugees in the camps in Macedonia for one month before the "official" aid arrived; in Sierra Leone, 990 tons of dry rations were supplied to approximately 3,700 families over a three-month period to enable these families to bridge the gap until the next harvest. The director-general of the Grain Producers Association of France, Georges-Pierre Malpel, traveled to Kosovo and Macedonia with Action Against Hunger in July 1999. After the twenty-five truckloads of flour supplied on an emergency basis to the affected populations, Kosovo's needs for seeds for the next crop were estimated at some 6,000 tons. The French seed production sector was thus requested to provide, in partnership with Action Against Hunger, rustic varieties, capable of thriving with few inputs and fertilizers.

Therein lies the value of the concept of partnership that brings together complementary skills. In this case the partners were an NGO specializing in food distribution that is already on the ground, namely, Action Against Hunger, and a professional group from the French agricultural sector, the Grain Producers Association of France, pledging to commit itself on an ongoing basis to emergency and long-term humanitarian activities.

This approach is innovative in France. For the first time, emergency food aid operations and agricultural rehabilitation programs are conceived and organized by an integral chain of solidarity, from the donation to the distribution phase after shipment.

What is more, the arrangement has proven itself to be particularly effective because of the coordination that takes place before the crisis erupts. Our two organizations have beforehand coordinated their know-how and their different areas of competence—nutrition, food security, food collection, packaging, stocking, quality control, transportation, logistics, distribution—and put in place procedures for accelerated action that have greatly reduced the time taken to deliver emergency aid.

This integration of food aid, from the producer to the beneficiary, enables us to significantly reduce the risks of loss or inappropriate distribution. It strengthens our capacity to provide appropriate balanced rations on a timely basis in forms that are suited to the target populations and that respect local production structures. Such a coordination of efforts is vital to the success of food aid operations, as the experience of humanitarian crises in the past decade has shown.

In this spirit, the circle of collaboration that we have established with grain producers will continue to grow and attract other partners, such as local collectivities, transporters, financial institutions, and consultants, so that its beneficial impact would multiply not only beyond our frontiers, but also in France, where donors are happy to have the certainty that their gift has yielded the maximum benefit.

Notes

José Bidegain was the chairman of Action Against Hunger–France from 1990 until his tragic death in the fall of 1999. Astrid Filliol is director of the Partnerships Department of Action Against Hunger.

1. Cf. *Baromètre SOFRES* (Paris: SOFRES [a French statistical institute], May 1999).

33

The Lomé Conventions
and Food Security

Jean-Jacques Gabas

In 1981, the European Community proposed a Plan of Action to Combat Hunger in the World. In 1984, Edgard Pisani, the European commissioner for development, wrote the following: "The struggle against hunger is the struggle for a new international economic order and the struggle for food aid." [1] Sixteen years later, it is time to assess the developments that have taken place in the area of food security, from its conceptualization to its implementation, both through national policies and through the approaches advocated by donors, chief among which is the European Commission. It was only in 1996 that the European Commission finally elaborated its "community program for food security and food aid."

Indeed the problem of hunger is still unresolved: Even though the summary indicators of the Food and Agriculture Organization of the United Nations (FAO) or of the United Nations Development Program (UNDP) show some very slight improvement over a long period, these results must be looked at much more closely than the averages indicate. Situations of famine still exist and cover very different realities. Those related to conflicts (civil wars) are increasing in number, while the means of preventing them remain quite ineffective. Those related to a succession of poor agricultural harvests compounded by the exhaustion of the coping strategies of households are better known, and a review of the indicators, which go beyond agricultural and weather-related conditions, sheds greater light on the serious risk of food shortages. Natural disasters (flood, hurricanes, El Niño), for their part, result in chance famines whose scope is very often a result of poor coordination between the many external actors and national authorities. It should be noted, finally, that local situations of malnutrition are seen in countries that have grain surpluses and that zones of acute food insecurity, in both urban and rural areas, are found in many countries with fragile ecosystems, such as in the Sahel region.[2]

There is no longer talk of a new international economic order, as economic globalization takes hold, and food aid is no longer the only response to crises. The very nature and characteristics of aid itself have changed profoundly, and in many situations a variety of tools is available to better predict the occurrence of food crises.

What are the political responses of Europe to the African, Caribbean, and Pacific (ACP) states on the question of food security? What major constraints are likely to emerge, and how can the Commission respond to these constraints?

The Lomé Agreements: Notable Changes Since 1975

It is important to recall first of all the spirit of the Lomé Conventions, since the goal of cooperation that inspired them does not ignore the question of food security. Moreover, there is not a single Lomé Convention but several. Even though they share a common purpose, each of them has had a different focus that gives it a certain specificity.

The element that is common to the Lomé Conventions is the dialogue between the European Union and the ACP states as blocs and not as individual countries. It is the regional approach that has been adopted by the conventions. This first characteristic is important, since the interregional economic relations that are established will have at least two consequences:

- the contribution by the European Union to the establishment of regional economic subgroupings within the ACP;
- the effects of European agricultural policies on the development process in the ACP States.

The second element is the mechanism for financial cooperation, namely, the programming of assistance in phases, which gives a certain predictability to resource flows and reduces the volatility of official development assistance flows that are provided in the form of grants only (which distinguishes the Commission from other donors).

The third element is trade and the establishment of a system of nonreciprocal trade preferences between the European Union and the ACP that discriminates against non-ACP states, thereby opening up the European market to ACP products and protecting ACP countries from the potential competition of European Union exports to the ACP. This trading arrangement is based on protocols of agreement on products such as bananas, rum, beef, and sugar. For the ACP countries, which are highly dependent on their export income, any losses due to the instability of world prices are tempered by the triggering of price compensation systems: STABEX for agricultural products and SYSMIN for mineral products.

A final major element has been the creation of a complex and original institutional system. The Council of Ministers has the power to amend or to supplement various provisions of the convention, but it is the Joint Assembly (articles 29 and 32 of the Lomé IV Convention), composed of an equal number of members of the European Parliament and of parliamentarians designated by the ACP countries, that sets the Lomé system apart. The very existence of this forum for dialogue and discussion of ideas between ACP countries and the European Union is unique.

The contractual obligations and the political dialogue to which those obligations give rise are in fact the defining characteristics of all the conventions, together with the search for coherence and coordination between policies (trade and cooperation in particular), even if the latter aspect has been given greater emphasis since the signing of the Maastricht Treaty.

From these core elements, the conventions themselves have evolved in terms of their objectives, the volume of financial resources, and the number of ACP partners (initially forty-six, the total is now seventy-one countries). Their objectives have evolved just as the conventions' priorities have changed together with the actors with which the cooperation policy is being pursued. This evolution in the dialogue is interesting insofar as it is closely related to the changing view of what constitutes a "developing economy."

This may be seen from the Memorandum on the Community Development Policy published in 1982, which states the following:

> In its development activities, the Community will seek channels of political dialogue that go beyond mere negotiations on projects to be funded. While respecting the sovereignty of the beneficiary countries over the use of the resources provided to them by the Community, the latter considers that it has the right and the obligation to engage with the Governments of these countries in a dialogue on the effectiveness of the policies that they pursue. Such a dialogue was initially conducted on the specific subject of food

strategies. In order to support the adoption of coherent food strategies, the community will use means, including food aid, which, except in cases of emergency, should be integrated into its development activity instead of being an end in itself.

Economic growth will be achieved through the development of one sector: agriculture. Political dialogue will be tested on the experiences of "food strategies" (to be discussed below) that would later be applied to the strategies of industrialization and energy. This shows the key role played by the agricultural sector in the process of development: a source of wealth through the achievement of gains in productivity, but also the occasion for a new form of political dialogue. An analysis of the relationships of cooperation leads to conclusions that are still valid today: Between the strict conditionalities of funding agencies and the irresponsible absence of conditions, we must absolutely find channels of a political dialogue between those who provide external resources and local decisionmakers, and this political dialogue should go beyond mere haggling over terms or mere technical debates on projects to be financed. This focusing of funding resources on the objective of food security, the fundamental role of political dialogue, and better integration of food aid into other rural development programs were combined with the necessary strengthening of coordination between donors and of harmonization of the different policies of the European Commission. The first conventions contained very few references to regional integration; the most recent, on the contrary, insist on the regionalization of economies as a condition for their development.

If we analyze the objectives of the Lomé IV bis Convention (an extension of the Lomé IV Convention), we see that the convention puts absolutely no priority on any particular sector, and certainly not on the agricultural sector. There is movement toward other priorities that could be described as horizontal, which concern more the modalities of aid than priority activities in any given sector. The modalities, moreover, are very clearly set out.

Strengthening of democratic conditionalities, respect for human rights, the notion of good governance, and strengthening of the rule of law all become essential criteria for selection. The suspension of cooperation may even take place in the event of serious violation of these principles.[3] Niger after the coup d'état of 27 January 1996 was the first case in which aid from the European Union was suspended. This mid-term revision of the convention introduced programming by phases, which marked a partial departure from the system of automatic allocation of aid in which any aid promised to every ACP state, after the convention was signed, was payable. The "novelty" in the system of Lomé IV bis is thus based on an assistance that is not only founded on needs but also on "merit," since the selectivity of aid is much more delicate to implement than in previous conventions. Because of this additional criterion,[4] the policy dialog between the Direction Generale VIII of the European Commission (DG VIII) and each ACP state is strengthened. Special emphasis is placed on the partnership and on ownership.

From Food Strategy to Food Security: Changing Concepts, Unchanged Practices

The European Commission's approach to food strategies outlined in the 1982 memorandum was innovative in at least two areas: It placed development projects in a coherent sectoral policy, and it sought to better integrate food aid into a long-term development policy. The third Lomé Convention, signed in 1984, had as a key element this approach to food strategies. Four ACP countries—Rwanda, Zambia, Kenya, and Mali—by way of experimenting, developed food strategies with the support of the European Community. In Mali, a commission for the development of a food strategy was set up to prepare a study of the following aspects: ecological zoning, agricultural statistics, research and development, processing of materials, logistics, marketing, consumption, health, and nutrition. This strategy covered all the parameters using a systemwide and comprehensive approach. The project approach, whose limitations were already generally known, was abandoned.

But, from the outset, the food strategy was confused with the technical awareness of the problem and never conceived as the translation of political will. The results of these attempts to implement "food strategies" were modest, for a number of reasons, as Serge Coelo points out in the case of Mali.

> The changes and reforms which the strategy requires are politically dangerous for the government in place. In these circumstances, temptation is great to relegate it to a technical level and a sectoral framework that renders it meaningless. In addition, a number of donors continued to prefer funding for highly capital intensive initiatives and projects; this meant that the sectors where the strategy was applied did not always coincide with the areas commonly preferred by development practitioners.

The entrenched practices of cooperation agencies were marked not only by the absence of any real dialogue on agricultural and food policies between governments and donors as a group, but also by the very conception of the food strategy that was still aimed at achieving food self-sufficiency (defined as the capacity of a country to provide all of its population with adequate food and a good nutritional level through national production alone). In a number of countries, this definition of food self-sufficiency was most frequently understood as self-sufficiency in grain production, a concept that was even more restrictive.

This concept that was so narrow in its interpretation, that was perceived with many reservations by governments, and that disrupted the practices of cooperation agencies gave way in 1985 to the concept of food security. Three components describe the food security approach (see *Geopolitics of Hunger, 1998–1999*):

- The availability of food (production, commercial imports and food aid, stocks);
- The stability of these supplies in time and space;
- The access to food for all (demand that can be met).

This concept of food security, defined in terms of the production of food but especially in terms of access by the population to food, will be compressed or even severely watered down by the structural adjustment programs. These programs will result in weaker domestic demand by placing emphasis on the economic and financial balances of the state (balancing of the table of financial operations) and by liberalization of the economy that changes the respective roles of the state and market in the elaboration and implementation of agricultural policy. The market plays a central role in the food supply policy. However, development policies aiming at economic adjustments have had negative effects in a number of countries on the food security of their populations. More specifically, grain departments have seen their role diminished in the marketing of grains, since they no longer contribute to the regulation of the grain market even though they continue to manage the national reserves of grain. On the other hand, they are responsible for the management of information on food security (early warning systems, agricultural surveys, monitoring of market prices of grain and cattle): During the 1980s, the Commission funded continuing diagnostic projects in the agricultural sector in the Sahel by providing support for agricultural surveys, information systems on grain markets, or early warning systems, among others.

In March 1994, the European Community began a comprehensive review of the policy of food aid management as an instrument of food security. A modest balance sheet of the European Union's food aid programs was prepared in 1997: limited success of counterpart funds, modest impact on the nutritional status of vulnerable groups, doubtful cost-effectiveness ratio, and so on.[5]

In 1996, the European Commission established a Food Security and Food Aid Program for the seventy-one ACP countries. Of these, nineteen were considered high priority and constituted group I: the least developed countries, which are heavily dependent on food aid and which have a high index of food insecurity.[6] The ten countries in group II are countries in crisis or postcrisis situations.[7] The Commission uses specially tailored instruments in dealing with these groups. For group I, support is provided for sectoral reforms, security stocks, and reserves and for the production, processing, and marketing of grains. Food aid in kind is limited and is used only if the needs are clearly identified. Programs are designed for three years rather than on an annual basis. The countries undertake to elaborate a coherent and long-term food security policy. For the countries in crisis in group II, the approach used is to provide food aid in kind, rehabilitation programs, funding for information systems and food or cash for work operations. The Commission therefore makes available to states aid instruments that are different depending on the situations: financial or technical assistance for the reform of sectoral policies on production, processing, marketing, or storage; aid for the importation of basic food products through foreign exchange facilities; support for the constitution of security stocks and seed policies.

These measures are accompanied by efforts to ensure better coordination with other donors and a concentration of food aid for the so-called vulnerable groups. Moreover, the Commission's policy is to give preference to local purchases or triangular operations, and the new regulations reforming the PAA (Regulation 1292/96) encourage the private sector by allocating foreign currencies for food imports, still within the framework of national food security strategies.

This recent approach has the advantage of existing, of having been formalized, and of being coherent. The Commission therefore has a food security policy, which was not the case a few years ago or which had been implemented in the 1980s very timidly in a few countries, with a food aid policy based on transfers in kind.

It would be premature to make any judgments as to the effectiveness of the implementation of this policy that has been adopted. It is apparent, however, that one should not underestimate the major constraints, or even contradictions, that the Commission must face in order for the policy to be effective in achieving the established objectives. At least seven obstacles may be identified on which the Commission has a relatively wide margin of maneuver:[8]

1. Reduction in commitments to provide aid to the agricultural sector;
2. Coordination with other aid donors;
3. Compatibility with the rules of the World Trade Organization (WTO);
4. The instability of the commodities markets;
5. Consistency with other policies;
6. The implementation of the political dialogue;
7. The question of a reduction in the level of solvent demand.

Declining aid for the agricultural sector.   The trend in aid commitments is toward a reduction in official development assistance for agriculture. This reduction is accompanied by a redirection of aid to other sectors that are outside the scope of projects (structural adjustment, program assistance) and a drop in food aid programs generating counterpart funds (since these are unmanageable in practice). The shifts are generally in favor of emergency and project assistance but include a new strategy of food security in several African countries.[9] The evaluation of the PAA confirms that donors will have to reduce their commitments to the International Convention on Food Aid in order to focus on more efficient forms of aid.

In statistical terms, one notes a marked tendency toward lower levels of aid for integrated rural development projects since the mid-1980s: sixteen percent on average during the period 1986–1990 compared with less than 2 percent for the period 1991–1995.[10] The same is true of projects in the agricultural sector: a little over 9 percent in the period 1986–1990 compared with 4 percent from 1991 to 1995. However, a statistical bias may appear, since the definition of agricultural aid is changing from year to year in the same way as the development priorities identified by the European Commission; activities that may indirectly assist rural development fall under programs such as "infrastructural development." This neglect of the agricultural sector is part of the general trend characterized by the relative increase of aid for structural adjustment, of humanitarian aid, and of emergency food aid, while overall official development assistance resources (from all sources) are declining. This reduction of aid for agriculture raises questions about elements that might help to improve its effectiveness.[11] At the same time, the Commission has identified priority countries, whether or not these are in crisis, on which aid programs will be concentrated. How will this global allocation be carried out?

Coordination in terms of wishes rather than reality: What leadership? The question of coordination among donors has various dimensions. First of all, in the field, all donors do not follow the same policy. It should be noted that the Commission is not the leader in the area of food security even though the resources it makes available to its priority countries are considerable. For example, in a number of Sahelian countries, evaluations of the implementation of the food aid charter show that several donors, such as Japan or certain members of the Organization of Petroleum Exporting Countries, have their own food aid policy, which is often in contradiction to that of the Commission. The same is true of the U.S. policy for Ethiopia. These different policies are decided upon and implemented without being part of a more global plan or dynamic. It is well known that these divergences in policies and practices are elements of which beneficiary governments take advantage. Any policy that is not coordinated with other donors leads to distortions that in fact reduce the effectiveness of the measures.

In the area of coordination that harmonizes food security programs, the Commission plays a role that is still not clearly defined. It follows programs of liberalization and accepts the structural reforms proposed by the Bretton Woods institutions (do we not risk seeing measures that contradict each other?). More important, what is the philosophy of the Commission regarding the redefinition of the respective roles of the state and market and the division between public and private? Why, despite the substantial resources allocated by the Commission, does it not play this leadership role?

Another aspect of noncoordination, and not the least, is that of the priorities of cooperation policies. Each donor should announce on a fairly regular basis new priorities of its cooperation policy.[12] Food security today competes with the struggle against poverty. How do we position these two priorities? Is the struggle against poverty a subtheme of food security or the reverse? Is a comprehensive framework for the struggle against poverty necessary, as the World Bank argues? This debate on priorities is not sterile, since it determines the nature of the resources today mobilized in countries by aid agencies. On the very concept of food security, the divergences are quite profound between donors both bilateral and multilateral, as well as on the notion of vulnerable population, target population, at-risk population, and so on. These semantic differences reflect fundamental differences that have not been sufficiently expressed. It is a characteristic of aid in general to use concepts that are considered to be perfectly transparent and applicable to all situations, but that never-theless conceal very different understandings and interpretations, both between donors and with ACP states or representatives of civil society (nongovernmental organizations [NGOs], village associations, and so on).

Nor is coordination with NGOs a prospect that is any more imme-diate. Many of them see a reduction of their activity in this diversifica-tion of the instruments of European aid and therefore argue in favor of food aid in kind, even though the agricultural situation and nutri-tional status do not justify it.[13]

Compatibility with the rules of the WTO. One of the innovative features of the Lomé system is the existence of nonreciprocal trade preferences in favor of the ACP countries. The trade performance of these states have on the whole been unspectacular. During the period from 1988 to 1997, the increase in the volume of exports from ACP countries to the European Community was less than 4 percent, at a time when other developing countries enjoyed increases in the order of 75 per-cent. Five countries recorded growth in their export levels that was higher than that achieved by other developing countries on account of the margin of preference: Mauritius, Jamaica, and, to a lesser extent, Madagascar in the textile sector; Kenya and Zimbabwe in cut flowers, vegetables, and fruits.

In the sector of agricultural products, the margin of preference is significant. Half of all exports no longer benefit from preferences as of the year 2000 (mainly coffee and cocoa); the other half now bene-fit from preferences in the order of 10 percent. Exports of agricultur-al products (not including products covered by the protocols) have increased by 60 percent in those sectors in which the margin of pref-erence is higher than 3 percent. The sectors that have enjoyed a sig-nificant margin of preference and that have posted the highest growth are flowers (+230 percent), vegetables (+132 percent), fish processing (+110 percent), tobacco (+83 percent), and vegetable and fruit processing (+70 percent).

Less than 50 percent of the amounts allocated under the beef protocol was exported in 1997, compared with nearly 80 percent in 1995. In 1996, European prices were 50 percent higher than world prices, thereby generating additional income for ACP countries of 30 million ecus. As part of its Agenda 2000, the Commission proposed a reduction in the price of beef of approximately 30 percent. This would result in a commensurate reduction in export earnings.

The question has arisen of compatibility with the rules of the WTO. There is a direct relationship with food security in each of the states. The Commission is proposing to enter into regional economic partnership agreements (APER). Is not this free trade arrangement between the European Union and the regions inconsistent with a policy to stimulate national food production? Is there not a contradiction in wishing to enter into free trade agreements with Europe, given the risks of reduced competitiveness for several of the region's products (which is likely to be the case within the Southern African Development Community)?[14]

The problem of the instability of commodity markets remains unaddressed and unresolved. The STABEX mechanisms for the stabilization of earnings from agricultural exports have been the object of much criticism. Even though optimal use has not been made of these mechanisms to promote economic diversification, certain experiences have been favorable.[15] Moreover, elimination of the system will leave unresolved the problem of market instability and, in particular, how to deal with the uncertainty over the level of income to be derived from agricultural exports. There is no opposition between food crops and cash crops. Decisions about which crops to plant are very complex, and farmers do not choose between these two types of crops. In many regions of West Africa, in particular, cotton cultivation, for example, has a favorable effect on crops of millet or sorghum (use of fertilizers), guarantees the income of farmers, and thus contributes to their food security.

The question of coherence with other policies. During the 1990s, the incoherence between the promotion of cattle farming in the Sahel region and the massive shipments of frozen beef from Europe to ports on the West African coast was widely criticized.[16] Imported meat was sold on the market in Abijan at prices much lower than those at which locally produced meat (poultry) or beef from the Sahel region was sold. Some progress has been made in harmonizing the aid and trade policies of the European Union, but the situation still gives cause for concern, since it is linked to the orientation of the Common Agricultural Policy. Little account is taken of the impact of the latter policy on other countries, notably countries of the South.

The question also arises with respect to coherence between instruments of aid for food security and the process of macroeconomic reform. Contradictions may arise between the orientations of an agricultural policy that seeks to intensify agriculture and the macroeconomic targets that are part of the agricultural structural adjustment program, since it is precisely the subsidies for fertilizers or improved varieties of seeds that can promote this intensification.

A third level of coherence relates to national and regional development priorities. While the objective of the regionalization of economies has been established in the Commission's development program and has also been identified as a priority by states, particularly those in Africa, contradictions may nevertheless appear, and these must be resolved. For example, the objective of developing regional cattle trade between the Sahel region and the countries on the coast of West Africa may lead to inflationist pressures in the exporting countries because of the reduced supply that also reduces access by the most disadvantaged populations and thus the satisfaction of their nutritional needs. The same is true for cereals such as millet and maize.

Initiation of a political dialogue and of a dialogue on policies. Even though the European Commission has developed a mechanism for action in countries in crisis, the question about conflict prevention remains unanswered. How can the conflicts that cause famine be prevented? What stand should Europe take in these conflicts? The political dialogue remains delicate, since the happy balance between interference and nonintervention is not easy to achieve.

While dialogue on policies, especially agricultural policy, exists at the level of public statements, implementation of these policies is not without difficulties. How do governments participate in this exercise for the development of a food security policy? Is it really the expression of a political will or a means of responding to the Commission's demand that countries should elaborate a food security policy as a condition for obtaining financial resources? How, moreover, are the "actors of civil society" (NGOs, village associations, communes) involved in the elaboration and formulation of policies?

The question of the reduction in solvent demand. Many countries among the nineteen high-priority states that are eligible are experiencing not problems of the supply of food products but severe problems of accessibility. In the context of the shrinking purchasing power of populations in both cities and rural areas, coping strategies are developed that include traditional solidarity networks, diversification of activities, a change in patterns of consumption, and so on.[17] How can external aid influence a complex set of social relations while at the same time strengthening demand? How can account be taken of household coping strategies? How does one deal with the problem of poverty?

Notes

Jean-Jacques Gabas is professor at the University of Paris XI.
   1. Edgard Pisani, *La Main et l'outil* (Paris: R. Laffont, 1984).

2. Johnny Egy (under the supervision of Jean-Jacques Gabas), *La Prevention des crises alimentaires au Sahel* (Paris: Organisation pour la Cooperation et le Developpement Economiques (OCDE)/Sahel Club, 1997).

3. Article 366 bis of the Lomé IV bis Convention, in conjunction with the revision of article 5, identifies the three fundamental elements: democracy, human rights, and rule of law. If one party considers that another has failed to live up to its obligation concerning one of these elements, the first one should begin, except in the case of emergencies, consultations to address the problem. If the consultations fail to remedy the situation, the convention may be suspended.

4. From what moment does a country no longer respect the processes of democratization and human rights? The assassination of the president of Niger, General Ibrahim Baré Mainassara, did not lead to a suspension of aid from the European Union. The holding of elections of doubtful honesty in Togo resulted in no condemnation or even an expression of reservations on the part of the parliamentarians from the ACP countries in the joint EU-ACP Assembly. This shows that the implementation of measures based on merit, while a priori attractive, is rife with serious ambiguities or even impossibilities.

5. *Joint Evaluation of the Food Aid Program of the European Union* (Brussels: European Commission, 1997).

6. The countries in group I are Armenia, Azerbaijan, Bangladesh, Bolivia, Burkina, Cape Verde, Ethiopia, Faso, Georgia, Haiti, Honduras, Kyrgyzstan, Madagascar, Malawi, Mauritania, Mozambique, Nicaragua, Niger, and Yemen.

7. The countries of group II are Afghanistan, Angola, Liberia, North Korea, Palestine, Rwanda, Sierra Leone, Somalia, Sudan, and Tajikistan.

8. We will not address the question of drugs in West Africa, but production of illegal drugs has a considerable negative effect on the implementation and impact of agricultural policies and on the food security of populations. Despite the lack of specific data showing the scope of the problem, according to the NGO Geopolitical Unit for the Monitoring of Drugs (Observatoire Géopolitique des Drogues; OGD) it appears that in several regions of West Africa in particular (Côte d'Ivoire, Gambia, and Casamance) the production of cannabis is increasing very rapidly. The advantage for the producers is the very high prices it commands; although the consequences have not often been measured, they are not negligible.

9. Deliveries of food aid in the world increased from 14.8 million tons in 1988 to 16.8 million tons in 1993. Since then, deliveries have declined steadily to less than 8 million tons. These deliveries have thus been below the annual target of 10 million tons established in 1974 by the World Food Conference. The global distribution has changed markedly. There is a very clear drop in program aid (10 million tons in 1993 compared with approximately 3 million tons in 1996), but relative stagnation in project aid and emergency assistance.

10. Aidan Cox and Antonique Koning, *Inventaire de l'aide fournie par la communauté européenne* (London: Overseas Development Institute, 1996).

11. A study conducted at the request of the European Commission on Rural Development Policies in ACP countries is being carried out by the ADE/ODI offices. See the Web site http:\\www.rurpol.org.

12. J. J. Gabas and A. Sinidzingre, *Aid in the Context of Globalization: The Lomé Convention in Question* (Paris: Khartala, 1998).

13. See annual evaluations of the implementation of the Charter of Food Aid to the Sahel conducted by COBEA for the Sahel/OECD Club between 1993 and 1999.

14. On regional competitiveness in southern Africa, see Jean Coussy, *Quel espace de coopération entre l'Europe et les Etats ACP?* (Paris: University of Paris XI, 1999).

15. The experiences of "citizen regulations" of international trade in the name of fair trading are much too marginal to be an alternative to the operation of international markets and the introduction of other rules.

16. See the work of the French NGO Solagral at www.SOLAGRAL.org.

17. Ancey Véronique, *La consommation alimentaire à Ouagadougou* (Paris: Sahel/OECD Club, 1998) and *La consommation alimentaire à Niamey* (Paris: Sahel/OECD Club, 1999).

34

Twenty Years of Struggle Against Hunger: From Voluntarism to the Reality Principle

Sylvie Brunel

Action Against Hunger was born twenty-one years ago out of a growing awareness of the scandal of hunger. A handful of intellectuals refused to accept that scandal and sought to mobilize the maximum number of people in France around the need to combat it.

1979—"We Shall Conquer Hunger"

1979 was the year of the birth of International Action Against Hunger (Action Internationale Contre la Faim; AICF), the original name of Action Against Hunger. That was a black year for what we now refer to as "humanitarian tragedies." The entry of Vietnamese troops into Cambodia, which had been closed to the outside world for four years, revealed to the world the results of the Khmer Rouge's murderous utopia. Dreaming of a new society, they had starved, butchered, and deported thousands of people, killing more than a million. Humanitarians mobilized on the country's border in a great "march for the survival of Cambodia."

At the time, no one was afraid of verbal excess. Marco Panella, one of the organization's founders (together with Jacques Attali, Françoise Giroud, Marek Halter, Bernard-Henri Lévy, Guy Sorman, and Marc Ullman, among others), denounced the "fifty million deaths from hunger each year," despite the efforts of demographers to show that the annual number of deaths in the world—from all causes—was below that figure.

Be that as it may, one billion people, or one out of every three people in the Third World, still suffered from hunger at that time. The great famine in Biafra from 1967 to 1970 and the famine in the countries of the Sahel in 1973–1974 were still on people's minds, particularly since another severe drought was looming in Africa. For the French public, hunger has always been the greatest tragedy of our contemporary world.

Bernard-Henri Lévy drew up a charter that made Action Against Hunger a genuine federation of local committees, charged with mobilizing people and creating public awareness of hunger in the world. The first field programs were born. At the time, the organization acted on a modest scale in partnership with local organizations, through development programs in medical care, water, and agronomy as well as income-generating activities. The premise was that populations weakened by hunger could only regain their autonomy if they were able to earn their living and not depend on aid.

The organization began with one full-time staff member and a part-time secretary in a borrowed room on the rue de Rivoli. As the years passed, it grew slowly. The savoir faire of its founders enabled the organization to enjoy a reputation that was disproportionate to its real activity. In 1984 the slogan 500 million nonconsumers, accompanied by a giant open hand and a wide-open mouth, appeared on the walls of Paris accompanied by the logo of the organization. Famine had again struck the Sahel, and AICF issued an appeal for aid. Two years later, the faces of Michel Drucker, a French television sports commentator, and Isabelle Adjani, a French movie star, were plastered everywhere in the subways after they had agreed to support AICF as goodwill ambassadors. "We shall conquer hunger," AICF defiantly proclaimed, with the word *shall* written in red above a crossed-out *can*.

1989—The Dashed Hopes of Intervention

Let us pause along the way, in 1989. By then, AICF had relocated and now occupied an entire floor at 34, avenue Reille, in the 14th arrondissement of Paris. It now had a budget of $7 million and had 85,000 donors, 20 full-time staff members, and no fewer than 50 volunteers in the field for some thirty programs, which were still geared to the long-term goal of development.

It was a time of optimism. The slogan "We shall conquer hunger" seemed more topical than ever. Thanks to voluntary action by the major international development organizations on behalf of the poor and the agricultural sector, the number of malnourished people in the Third World had declined significantly to "no more than" 800 million, or one person in five, rather than one in three. And yet, population growth was at its peak: Each year, the earth's population increased by 100 million.

For the organization, the disappearance of hunger from the West and the fact that all famines were henceforth considered "political," which meant that they could easily be overcome, since neither overpopulation nor nature was involved, raised high expectations. In 1991 AICF published its first study of the subject.[1]

The United Nations had for the first time unanimously adopted a resolution on "humanitarian assistance to victims of natural disasters and similar emergency situations." A new era seemed to be dawning, that of the "duty to intervene" to assist victims.

What the heads of AICF could not have guessed was the extent to which the collapse of the Iron Curtain would change the existing order. Just when the world believed it would collect the "peace dividend," the opposite happened. Deprived of outside support, many regimes collapsed, thereby setting the scene for murderous civil wars. Nationalisms that had long been suppressed were exacerbated and led to fratricidal conflicts among peoples who until then had been constrained to live together peacefully. Official development assistance, which lost its geopolitical usefulness with the end of the Cold War, began to decline, forcing warlords to seek new means of subsistence: trafficking of all kinds, including the most dangerous such as drugs; pillaging of civilian populations; securing international aid by orchestrating what were beginning to be called "humanitarian tragedies."

The Gulf War in 1990 and the great exodus of the Kurdish people driven into the mountains on the border with Turkey ushered in a new season of hunger. Famines received attention depending on the coverage they received in the media, whose selective mobilization channeled Western compassion and overshadowed other more silent tragedies. High points—Kurdistan in 1991; Bosnia and Somalia in 1992–1993; Rwanda in 1994 and again in 1996, when the refugee camps were emptied by force; and Kosovo in 1999—occurred against the backdrop of long-term crises: civil war in Sudan and Angola, conflagrations in the Great Lakes region, and the slow strangulation of Afghanistan after the Taliban gained power. "Intervention" became a tool manipulated by the great powers based on their internal and external economic and political interests. The greatest tragedies unfolded with live coverage and with humanitarians unable to do much to alter the course of history. The United Nations, after having given the impression at one point that it was a superpower committed to the maintenance or even the restoration of peace everywhere, has had to face up to the fact that it is powerless to stop the tragedies.

Hunger has now returned to center stage more violently than ever. Famines multiply because hunger, an instrument of control over the population, has also become a weapon of war to enrich oneself, to obtain international recognition, and to benefit from the new manna of conflict—media visibility and its corollary, the outpouring of international compassion.

As a consequence of the phenomenon of exclusion, rising unemployment, and a new kind of poverty, hunger has reappeared in the developed countries of Europe and the United States and above all in an economically collapsing Russia.

Agronomic research into ways of increasing agricultural production for the benefit of the poor is slowing for lack of funds. The world is now divided between "consumers," who capture all the attention and all the privileges, and "the surplus population," which is ignored by the trade networks and which has been the hardest hit by the decline in cooperation activities and official development assistance.

The size of the malnourished population is increasing, rising from 800 million to 830 million according to the United Nations Food and Agriculture Organization (FAO). At the World Food Summit held in Rome in 1996, the FAO recognized that it would be difficult for that number to fall below 400 million, even with the willing commitment of all states.

1999—"We Cannot Say We Did Not Know"

For specialized humanitarian organizations such as Action Against Hunger (the word *International* was dropped along the way to illustrate the haunting presence of hunger everywhere, even in those countries that had believed they had banished it forever), the challenges to be overcome have multiplied.

Emergency interventions have become both more frequent and more difficult to carry out because access to victims is controlled by criminal regimes that use humanitarian aid as an instrument of manipulation.

Hunger is everywhere, but the resources of charitable organizations are necessarily limited. Thus, since 1989, Action Against Hunger has focused its attention on issues that are directly linked to the treatment of hunger and emergency situations (nutrition, water supply, and food aid). Such a focus has been to the detriment of development programs, which are more difficult to implement and whose results are less obvious because they are indirect.

Private donors in Europe, who are themselves subject to numerous solicitations and affected by unemployment and economic difficulties, have become less receptive at the same time that the "market for generosity" has become more and more competitive. For their part, states, following the example of the European Community, are seeking greater visibility in order to play a more important role in these "live" humanitarian activities. Substantial budgets are therefore placed at the disposal of nongovernmental organizations that, by accepting them, run the risk of becoming "service providers" for states or aid agencies pursuing geopolitical objectives, among which the fate of the starving is not a priority.

Humanitarian organizations artificially swollen by the massive amounts of public funds made available to them become enormous machines, difficult to manage and slower to react than in the past. Even if their technical level and logistical capacity are infinitely higher than before, they come up against political constraints that hinder access to the victims.

Hunger can therefore exist in a world of abundance, and humanitarian organizations become more effective in their operations without benefiting the hungry as much as they would wish.

In 2000, Action Against Hunger has become a respectable institution: Its budget has increased tenfold in ten years, as has the number of its volunteers present in the field, augmented by national teams totaling more than four thousand people. Action Against Hunger has certainly lost the federative character that distinguished it at the start, but it has exchanged that for a professionalism of action that sets it apart from the confusing proliferation of local microprograms. Moreover, the nucleus in Paris has expanded, and sister organizations have been established in London, Madrid, and New York.

Still, the organization can no longer continue the triumphant talk of its early days. Its latest campaign is drawing to a close in a subdued tone that perfectly illustrates its dilemma: "We cannot say we did not know; we cannot say there was nothing we could do." Never has information been so readily available. Never have the means of ending hunger been so numerous and so varied. But while, in principle, we can do something, it is also necessary to have a consensus on the absolute need to aid the starving, because the first among human rights is the right not to die of hunger. Now that is precisely our weakness. We may have the means to conquer hunger, but will we succeed?

Notes

Sylvie Brunel is strategy adviser, Action Against Hunger.

    1. *Action Internationale Contre la Faim (AICE), Une tragédie banalisée, la faim dans le monde* (Paris: Hachette, coll. Pluriel, 1991).

Index

About the Book

Widespread hunger continues to exist at the turn of the century, despite the efforts of scores of international relief organizations. Why? The authors of *The Geopolitics of Hunger, 2000–2001* draw on both research and their firsthand field experience to explore the use of hunger as a weapon in food crises around the world. They also discuss strategies to counter inequitable food distribution in complex, manipulative situations and review food policies to combat hunger and attain food justice.

Founded in 1979 to fight against hunger and advocate for the legal right to food, **Action Against Hunger** is one of the leading international organizations working to assist victims of man-made famines.

To Learn More About
Action Against Hunger

Visit our Web site: http://www.aah-usa.org

You can contact us:

In the USA: Action Against Hunger   phone: (212) 967-7800
875 Avenue of the Americas e-mail: aah@aah-usa.org
New York, NY 10001

In the UK: Action Against Hunger   phone: 0171 831 58 58
1 Catton Street   e-mail: aahuk@gn.apc.org
London WC1R 4AB

In France: Action Contre la Faim   phone: 01 43 35 88 88
4, Rue Niepce   e-mail: acf@acf.imaginet.fr
75014 Paris

In Spain: Accion Contra el Hambre   phone: 91 391 53 00
C/Caracas 6-1°   e-mail: ach@achesp.org
28010 Madrid